Introduction to Communication Sciences and Disorders

Introduction to Communication Sciences and Disorders

FIFTH EDITION

Franklin H. Silverman
Lynda Miller

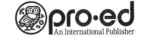
pro·ed
An International Publisher

8700 Shoal Creek Boulevard
Austin, Texas 78757-6897
800/897-3202   Fax 800/397-7633
www.proedinc.com

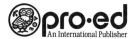

© 2016, 2006 by PRO-ED, Inc.
8700 Shoal Creek Boulevard
Austin, Texas 78757-6897
800/897-3202   Fax 800/397-7633
www.proedinc.com

Library of Congress Cataloging-in-Publication Data

Names: Silverman, Franklin H., 1933– | Miller, Lynda.
Title: Introduction to communication sciences and disorders / Franklin H.
  Silverman, Lynda Miller.
Description: Fifth edition. | Austin, Texas : PRO-ED, Inc., [2016] | Includes
  bibliographical references and index.
Identifiers: LCCN 2015028537| ISBN 9781416410089 ((print)) | ISBN
  9781416410096 ((e-book pdf))
Subjects: LCSH: Communicative disorders.
Classification: LCC RC423 .S5185 2016 | DDC 616.85/5--dc23
LC record available at http://lccn.loc.gov/2015028537

Art Director: Jason Crosier
Designer: Lissa Hattersley
This book is designed in Berkeley and Depot New.

Printed in the United States of America
1 2 3 4 5 6 7 8 9 10   24 23 22 21 20 19 18 17 16 15

acknowledgments

Frank Silverman, who started this project many years ago, and Nancy McKinley, who fostered it after Frank died, were both key figures in the evolution of this book. Without their contributions, I wouldn't have written this latest edition. So, to both, my deepest gratitude in memoriam.

I offer grateful thanks to Dr. Jodelle F. Deem, Associate Professor at the University of Kentucky, for her expertise and guidance, always welcome, and, as usual, precisely on target. Thanks, Jody—your excellent suggestions have greatly enriched the manuscript.

I owe special appreciation to Beth Rowan, Senior Editor at PRO-ED, Inc., whose careful shepherding of this book has resulted in a truly excellent and valuable resource—thank you, Beth.

—*Lynda Miller*

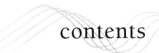

contents

In 2004, Frank Silverman authored the third edition of *Essentials of Speech, Language, and Hearing Disorders*. In his Preface to that edition, Frank said that his primary objective was to "provide users with essential information for understanding 'at a gut level' the symptomatology, phenomenology, and etiology of speech, language, and hearing disorders as impairments, disabilities, and handicaps." When revising the book not long afterward, I retained much of his original objective of providing readers with the essential information they need to understand and help people with communication disorders while at the same time expanding the content to include a description of communication, language development, children's language disorders, and multicultural issues and concerns regarding communication and communication disorders.

This fifth edition includes the information students enrolled in their first course in communication sciences and disorders need to retain an overview, rather than a complete understanding, of the field. As in edition four, I hope this edition stimulates students' interests in particular topics so that they pursue in more depth additional coursework or independent work related to communication sciences and disorders.

Major changes in this edition include the following:

- A less formal writing style that speaks more directly to you, the reader. This less formal style makes the content more readable and easier to grasp for students encountering most of these topics for the first time.
- A reduction from 17 chapters to 14, to reflect my hope that the material included in the book can be covered in one semester.
- Thoroughly updated and reorganized chapters.
- Complete revision of Chapters 11, 12, 13, and 14.
- The addition of sections on assessment for voice and adult neurogenic disorders.
- Updated and expanded sections on diversity and multicultural issues, including several new sections on these two topics.
- A discussion of the impact of the *Diagnostic and Statistical Manual of Mental Disorders–Fifth Edition* on the field of communication sciences and disorders, with an accompanying expansion of information about the communication needs of individuals with autism spectrum disorder.

- A description of how evidence-based practices have emerged as a guiding force for clinicians providing services to clients with communication disorders.
- A new design to make the book more user-friendly and easier to access
- The option of an e-book format.
- Updated graphics to reflect current knowledge and advances in technology since the last edition was published.
- The inclusion of current technologies and methodologies.
- A complete overhaul of references.
- A reorganization into five sections: Introduction to Communication and Communication Disorders (two chapters); Language Development and Disorders (three chapters); Speech Disorders (four chapters); Hearing Disorders (one chapter); and Communication Sciences and Disorders: The Profession (four chapters).
- The boldface terms in the chapters are defined in the glossary.

Throughout this edition, as in the previous one, I use language that reflects the fact that people have disorders, not the other way around. In other words, I refer to people with disorders (e.g., "adult with aphasia," "student with a language disorder") rather than to disorders attached to people (e.g., "the aphasic," "the language-disordered student"). I do this deliberately in order to focus our attention on the human who has a communication disorder rather than on the disorder. Although the field of communication sciences and disorders is based on understanding the science of communication and its disorders, the profession relies on the abilities of speech–language pathologists and audiologists to provide services in a way that is caring, humane, and professional. To do this, I believe, requires that we begin by remembering our human connections.

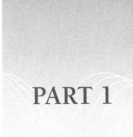

PART 1

Introduction to Communication and Communication Disorders

The two chapters in Part 1 serve as an introduction and orientation to communication, communication disorders, and the field of communication sciences and disorders. In Chapter 1, I describe communication, language, speech, and hearing; how they're related; and how communication is affected by culture.

In Chapter 2, I define in more detail communication, language, speech, and hearing disorders; describe how different cultural groups view these various disorders; and describe how a communication disorder can affect a person's self-image and interpersonal relationships. In the section on multicultural issues and concerns I point out that the United States is becoming ever more diverse, requiring professionals to have considerable knowledge and expertise in providing services to linguistically and culturally diverse populations. I explore the purposes of assessment of communication disorders, the types of assessments used in the field, and the benefits and limitations of assessment. The chapter also includes a discussion of the purposes of intervention, professionals' goals, and the importance of measuring progress throughout the intervention process. The chapter ends with a brief description of the professions included in the field of communication sciences and disorders, typical work roles, and professional organizations.

chapter 1

Communication: How Humans Share Information

Learning Objectives

Define communication and its various modes.

Define language and how it furthers communication.

Define speech and how it is related to communication.

Define hearing and its importance in communication.

Describe how cultural norms and traditions affect communication.

Overview

The professions of communication sciences and disorders are all based on **communication**, **language**, **speech**, and **hearing**. In this chapter, I briefly define each of these topics, explain how they're related, and briefly describe how communication is affected by **culture**.

What Is Communication?

Communication is any exchange of information between people using a common code, or symbol system, that those involved understand. (*Information* is used here to mean ideas, feelings, thoughts, emotions, or facts.) The code or system may involve words, gestures, behaviors, signs, symbols, or sounds. People communicate in order to exchange ideas, feelings, stories, actions, events, and experiences, and they use a variety of modes to communicate: speech, print, sign language, Braille, codes (e.g., Morse codes, semaphore signals), silence, facial expressions, body postures, and gestures. Other examples of communication include art forms such as drama, music, literature, poetry, and dance.

Communication always occurs in some sort of context: an immediate face-to-face conversation, watching a movie, playing a multiplayer online game, participating in an Internet chat room, following someone on Twitter or Facebook, or reading a text written hundreds of years ago. This wide variation of communicative contexts influences such things as

- how close to stand to another person when conversing (this varies by social situation and the relationship between the participants);
- the purpose of the communicative interchange (e.g., engaging in casual conversation, delivering a speech, presenting an argument, giving directions, providing instruction);
- the participants' intent (e.g., to try to change one another's minds, to establish social standing, to form a social or political bond, to preach); and
- the number of participants and their relationships (e.g., family members, social peers, politicians and their constituents, religious figures and their congregants).

Every cultural group communicates according to what Bates (1976), in a well-known book describing the social underpinnings of communication, described as a conversational code of conduct, or an unspoken system that seems to govern communication, summarized in Box 1.1.

Each cultural group interprets these "rules" in its own unique way, which in turn affects what is considered a **communication disorder.** What is considered a disorder in one culture may be considered typical in another culture, and therefore not a disorder at all. (I will discuss this topic at some length in later chapters.) For now, though, consider the following example. A person from a culture in which conversational partners stand closer than 18 inches to each other stands that close to a person from a culture in which the partners stand farther away. Each might then think the other is violating what they perceive as the socially accepted "distance" rule. Along the same lines, someone from a cultural group that typically addresses

---

BOX 1.1   Conversational Code of Conduct (Bates, 1976)

- Cooperate with your conversational partner.
- Tell the truth.
- Offer only information you assume to be new and relevant to your listener.
- Request only information you sincerely want to have.
- Provide your listener with just the right amount of background information so he or she will understand your point.
- Be unambiguous.
- Change your language to fit the current social situation.

elders informally might address an older person from a different culture by his or her first name. The elder might then think the person is violating the socially accepted polite form for addressing an elder.

People communicate not only by following these implicit rules; they also communicate by violating the code, again in ways that vary across different cultural groups. For instance, engaging in a debate violates the dictum "Cooperate with your conversational partner." Saying "Fine" when someone asks how you are and you feel terrible violates the dictum "Tell the truth." So does telling what are called *white lies*—lies considered unimportant and used to be tactful or polite. You'll see in later chapters how, when they are first learning language, children act as if the code is inviolate, and they only gradually develop the ability to use the socially appropriate violations practiced by their cultural group.

Gestural Communication

Facial expressions, and the body postures, poses, and movements people use to impart information, are all considered part of gestural communication. For people who speak English, tilting one's head a certain way, for instance, might be used to convey doubt or humor, especially when combined with raised eyebrows and pursed lips. Romance-language speakers indicate slight differences of meaning through the tilt of their heads and the thrusting of their chins.

One way to think about gestural communication is to examine the list of gestures associated with various parts of the body, listed in Box 1.2. Although cultural groups vary significantly in the meanings they assign to gestures, all groups incorporate the body in communicative interchanges. Combined with vocal inflections, tone of voice, loudness, speech rate, and pitch, gestural communication contributes significantly—approximately 70%—to every communicative interchange.

Although sign languages use gestures, they are not simply gestural—they rely on postures; movements; and orientations of the head, face, arms, shoulders, trunk, arms, and hands. In other words, they *use* gestures, but the gestures are codified into a symbol system just like a spoken language is codified into a symbol system. For this reason, sign languages are considered languages rather than forms of gestural communication.

Oral Communication

Oral communication, also referred to as *spoken language*, is constituted from the speech sounds people combine into the larger units of language we recognize as words and sentences. These speech sounds are ordered in particular ways—differently in each spoken language—so that those speaking any given language can extract particular meanings. For instance, Spanish speakers know that *curandera* means "shaman" (feminine), while for Yup'ik speakers (people living in the village

---

BOX 1.2	Gestures Associated With the Body

Head
- Head tilt
- Chin tilt
- Head shaking
- Head nodding

Face
- Forehead wrinkling
- Eyebrow raising/lowering
- Eyes narrowing/widening
- Nose wrinkling
- Nose wriggling

Mouth
- Lips compressing
- Lips pulled upward at the edges (smile, grin, laugh)
- Lips pursing
- Lips folded inward
- Upper lip raised on one side (sneering)
- Lips pulled downward at the edges
- Lips used to make "raspberry" sound

Chin
- Chin wrinkled
- Chin thrust upward
- Chin pulled inward and down
- Chin wagged side to side
- Chin wagged front to back

Neck
- Neck tensing
- Neck bent to one side (sometimes with raised shoulder)

Shoulders
- Shoulders raised
- Shoulders drooped
- One shoulder raised
- Shoulder(s) moved forward/backward

Trunk
- Chest puffed out
- Chest pulled in
- Trunk turned toward/away from listener
- Trunk bent forward/backward/sideways at waist
- Pelvis tilted forward/backward/sideways

Legs
- Hip cocked
- Knees straight/bent
- Ankles straight/bent

Feet
- If sitting: knees together/apart
- If sitting: legs crossed at knee/ankle on knee
- Foot (feet) still/tapping
- Feet parallel/at an angle to each other
- If sitting: still/tapping/circling
- If sitting: ankles straight/bent

---

of Tuntutuliak, in southwestern Alaska) the word for *shaman* is *angalkut*. In French, *shaman* is *sorcier* or *invocateur*. All three languages include a word that means roughly the same thing, yet the speech sounds used in each are significantly different.

Written Communication

Compared with oral communication, written communication is a recent development, referring to the written or printed symbols used to represent spoken language. The symbol systems used in written communication include the alphabetic system used in English; the **ideographic** system used in Chinese and some other Asian languages; the **syllabary** systems used in the hiragana and katakana syllabic scripts of Japanese; and **pictographic** systems, such as those represented along the Rio Grande in New Mexico and Utah. These written communication systems emerged from spoken language and are used in correspondence with the spoken languages they represent. It is interesting to note that some oral languages have developed written orthographies only recently, as, for instance Afrikaans (a West Germanic language spoken in South Africa and Namibia) and Oromo (an Afro-Asiatic language spoken in Ethiopia and northern Kenya), both of which developed writing systems in the 19th century.

Written communication systems have also been invented to assist people who cannot speak. Some severely communicatively impaired children and adults use such symbols in communication boards. An example of one such system is Blissymbolics (2014), which uses symbols that are both ideographic and pictographic. Both symbol types are illustrated in Figure 1.1.

Codes

Codes are symbol systems based on numbers, letters, symbols, icons, pictures, mathematical formulae, or sounds. The most common codes used today are alphanumeric. Alphanumeric codes combine numbers and letters and are often used as computer, mobile device, and Internet passwords. Computer encryption systems usually use random number strings of varying lengths, longer ones being more difficult to decode. Morse code is an example of a sound-based communication code,

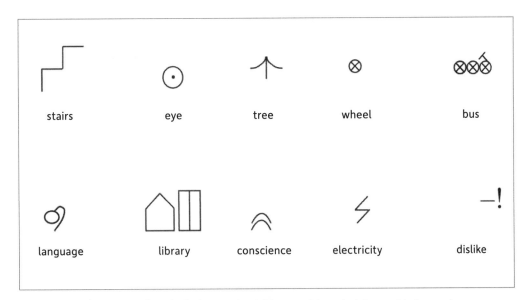

FIGURE 1.1. Examples of symbols that are both ideographic and pictographic from a language called Blissymbolics, which is used on communication boards by some individuals with severe communication impairments. *Note.* From Blissymbolics Communication International (www.blissymbolics.org). Reprinted without changes.

while football referees use a signal system based on body gestures and poses. Bar codes use optical patterns; Braille is a tactile code representing letters and numbers.

Codes often require a key, or a translation between the code and ordinary language, although some codes are accessible only to those who have memorized them or who have access to the technological equipment necessary to decode them. E-mail and instant messaging have produced a steady stream of communication codes in the form of acronyms and emoticons used to represent phrases or feelings. For people new to e-mail or text messaging, breaking the code can be difficult without a key or translation.

What Is Language?

Language is itself a code used for communicating ideas with others. Even though individual languages vary considerably in how they codify ideas, thoughts, events, and experiences, every language is based on an arbitrary set of abstract symbols people use to communicate with each other. These symbols are governed by rules of several types:

- which of all possible sounds humans are capable of producing are actually used;
- how those sounds are ordered and combined;
- what constitutes a word;
- how words are modified to alter meaning;
- how words are strung together into sentences in certain ways to convey specific meanings; and
- how sounds, words, and sentences are modified in differing social contexts.

In the field of communication sciences and disorders, language is usually described in terms of use, form, content, nonverbal language, and figurative language.

In Chapter 3, I will discuss each in more detail as it relates to language development and to disorders manifested by individuals ranging in age from infancy through adulthood.

What Is Speech?

Speech is the production of **phonemes** by the **vocal tract**. The vocal tract is supplied with air from the **respiratory system** and provided with voice by the vocal folds in the **larynx**. The vocal tract, which is illustrated in Figure 1.2, consists of three main cavities (i.e., air-filled passages): the **pharyngeal cavity**, the **oral cavity**, and the **nasal cavity**.

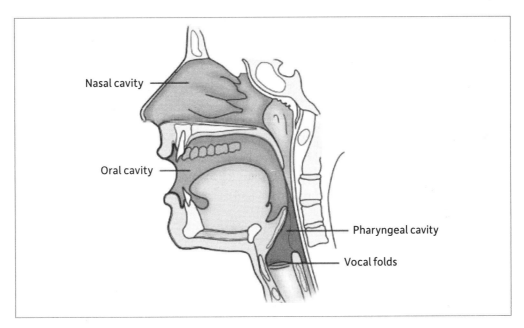

FIGURE 1.2. A section of the head showing the three main cavities (resonators) of the vocal tract.

During speech, air from the lungs passes through the vocal tract and is changed into phonemes. Air from the lungs passes through the larynx and causes the vocal folds to vibrate to produce most speech sounds—all vowel sounds and the majority of consonants—which are referred to as *voiced phonemes*. For the voiceless phonemes, the exhaled air is set into vibration in the oral cavity. During the production of /f/, for example, the air is set into vibration by being forced to exit through the narrow passage between the upper teeth and lower lip.

The configuration (i.e., shape) of the cavities in the vocal tract at a particular moment determines which phoneme will be produced. Each phoneme has a unique configuration. During every second of conversational speech, we are able to perceive between 20 and 50 phonemes per second. This means the configuration of the vocal tract is continually in a state of transformation. Phonemes have been classified in a number of ways, depending on how they are produced. I provide more detail on this classification system in Chapter 8.

When we produce speech, we do so with a moderate amount of what is called **fluency**. Of course, we all hesitate periodically while speaking. We also insert sounds, syllables, words, and even phrases in the course of a conversation. At times, we insert long pauses between words; prolong speech sounds; and stop to correct errors of pronunciation, syntax, and word usage. A certain amount of these pauses, insertions, and hesitations is considered to be a normal part of speaking. Indeed, unless we're listening to trained speakers or actors, we usually notice when someone's speech does not include any of these attributes.

What Is Hearing?

The process of speaking involves the generation of speech sounds; the process of **hearing** involves the perception of sound. Within the context of communication, hearing means perceiving speech sounds. To understand hearing, you need some basic information about how sound is generated and transmitted—that is, the physics of sound. You'll also need to know a few basics about the anatomy and physiology of the ear. The outer, middle, and inner ear are pictured in Figure 1.3. In Chapter 10 you will learn about (1) the physics of sound; (2) intensity; (3) the anatomy and physiology of the hearing mechanism; and (4) the inner ear, **auditory nerve**, and central auditory nervous system.

How Are Communication, Language, Speech, and Hearing Related?

In general, communication takes place through the processes of hearing and speaking, both of which rely on an understanding and command of the rules of the language being used to communicate. Of course, communication also takes place through modes other than speaking and hearing. Children with disabilities may learn to communicate through means other than speaking (e.g., sign language, symbol systems, computer-generated speech), but most children first learn to communi-

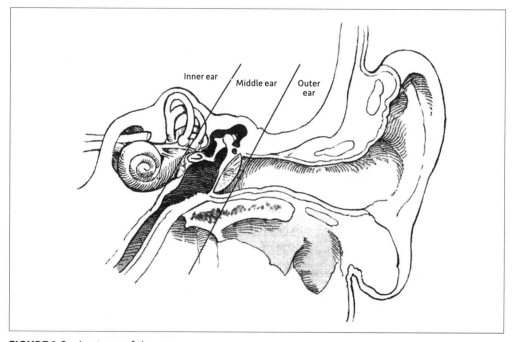

FIGURE 1.3. Anatomy of the ear.

cate through speaking and hearing, and only later in their development are able to communicate through reading and writing.

Culture and Communication

Although communication is a universally shared human process, cultural groups vary significantly in the various rule systems governing how people communicate within each culture, and in how people in each culture view communication. Culture determines how we express (or suppress) emotions, such as happiness, anger, joy, disapproval, and love. For instance, consider how your culture governs the expression of love in public settings. Is it acceptable to hold hands? Hug? Kiss?

Culture governs how we think about and communicate our ideas regarding etiquette, values, norms, rituals, and expectations, to name a few. Try the exercises in Box 1.3 to think about your culture's communication patterns.

BOX 1.3   **Communication in Your Culture**

1. Think about your culture's "rules" regarding personal space, patterns of touch, etiquette and ritual, and the expression of emotions.
   - How close is "too close" when talking to a good friend?
   - Can you touch a stranger on the arm during a conversation?
   - What is the etiquette for how you address your parents' friends (first name, last name)?
   - Does your family have any communication rituals? What are they?
   - How do you express anger or joy in your culture?
2. Think about your culture's ideas about food .
   - Is food viewed as a reward in your culture?
   - Is food viewed as something to enjoy?
   - Is food viewed as simply a necessity?
   - How do people talk about food in your culture?
3. Think about parent–child relationships in your culture.
   - How do children talk to their parents in your culture?
   - How do parents talk to their children?
   - How do nonfamily members speak to other people's children?
   - How do children address adults outside the family?
4. What are some ways of showing respect in your culture?
   - What are the most common polite forms you use? With whom? Under what circumstances?
   - Is it acceptable to show disrespect in your culture? How?
   - Are manners important in your culture? How do they show up?

It is important to remember that every communicative act takes place within a **cultural context**, whether it's enjoying a conversation with a friend, participating in a political rally, listening to a lecture by a world leader, or writing a term paper. Every person exists within at least one cultural context; most of us live in more than one culture. In today's multicultural society, learning to communicate with people from other cultures is becoming more and more commonplace. It is also a prerequisite for becoming a successful clinician. Throughout the remaining chapters, I will revisit the effects of diversity and multicultural factors.

chapter 2

Communication Disorders

Learning Objectives

Understand how communication disorders affect people.

Describe what constitutes a communication disorder.

Explain how a communication disorder can impact personal relationships.

Describe how culture plays a role in the diagnosis of a communication disorder.

Describe the various types of communication disorders.

Describe the primary purposes and types of assessment used with communication disorders.

Explain why it is necessary to track progress during the intervention process.

Define evidence-based practice and explain why it is used to formulate intervention procedures.

Overview

Imagine that when you woke up this morning your tongue was paralyzed and you were completely unable to speak. You could understand **speech** and **language** just as well as ever, and your ability to think and reason was unimpaired. But when you tried to talk, your tongue wouldn't move—it was paralyzed on the floor of your mouth. A physician examined you and concluded that the paralysis was due to damage to the nerves that innervate the tongue musculature and that your condition is unlikely to improve.

Or, imagine instead that you woke up unable to hear even the loudest sound. When your roommate talked to you, you could see his or her lips moving, but you couldn't understand anything because you could no longer hear. Your physician said you'd suffered sudden **hearing** loss, possibly due to two things: a series of upper respiratory infections you'd had over the past several months, or prolonged exposure to loud noise in a music club where you listen to bands. It is possible that your hearing may not ever return to normal because of reduced blood flow to the inner ear.

Consider each scenario. What impact do you think your inability to talk or hear would have on your life? How would these two scenarios affect you differently? Similarly? Would you be able to remain a student with the same major? How would each of these scenarios affect your plans for the future? How would each affect your social life now, including dating? How would it affect how you feel about yourself as a person? Could either motivate you to succeed? For an example, see Temple Grandin's comments in Box 2.1.

If you're like most people, you probably will have a difficult time answering these questions because you take talking and hearing for granted, just as you take for granted your ability to walk and use your hands. This is not particularly surprising because you have been able to do these things for as long as you can remember. Babies begin using their voices to communicate within a few minutes after being born. They communicate feeling uncomfortable by crying, and they cease crying to indicate they are feeling comfortable again. Only those who have had difficulty communicating, either temporarily or permanently, can fully appreciate the impact a **communication disorder** can have on a person.

One of the goals of this chapter is to increase your awareness of the importance of communication in everyday life, and, consequently, the effects a communication disorder can have on one's life. Although the field of communication sciences and disorders is based on scientific facts, professionals who interact with people with

---

BOX 2.1   How Does Visual Thinking Work in the Mind of a Person With Autism?

A Personal Account by Temple Grandin (2009, paras. 2–3)

My mind works similar to an Internet search engine, set to locate photos. All my thoughts are in photo-realistic pictures, which flash up on the 'computer monitor' in my imagination. Words just narrate the picture. When I design livestock facilities, I can test run the equipment in my imagination similar to a virtual reality computer program. I did not know that this was a special skill until I started interviewing other people about how they think. I was surprised to discover . . . [that] the other nonautistic equipment designers could not do full motion test runs of equipment in their minds.

My mind is associative and does not think in a linear manner. If you say the word 'butterfly', the first picture I see is butterflies in my childhood backyard. The next . . . is metal decorative butterflies that people decorate the outside of their houses with and the third . . . is some butterflies I painted on a piece of plywood when I was in graduate school. Then my mind gets off the subject and I see a butterfly cut of chicken that was served at a fancy restaurant approximately 3 days ago. The memories that come up first tend to be either early childhood or something that happened within the last week. A teacher working with a child with autism may not understand the connection when the child suddenly switches from talking about butterflies to talking about chicken. If the teacher thinks about it visually, a butterfly cut of chicken looks like a butterfly.

communication disorders must have tremendous insight into the impact a communication disorder can have. This chapter includes excerpts from people who have communication disorders, in the hope that you can better understand how it feels to live with such a condition.

What Is a Communication Disorder?

In 1993, the **American Speech-Language-Hearing Association (ASHA)** published a definition of communication disorders still in use today. A communication disorder is

> an impairment in the ability to receive, send, process, and comprehend concepts or verbal, nonverbal and graphic symbol systems. A communication disorder may be evident in the processes of hearing, language, and/or speech. A communication disorder may range in severity from mild to profound. It may be developmental or acquired. Individuals may demonstrate one or any combination of communication disorders. A communication disorder may result in a primary disability or it may be secondary to other disabilities. (ASHA, 1993, sec. I.A)

Most professionals in communication sciences and disorders would add two conditions to the ASHA definition:

- The way the person talks or listens must be noticeably different from that of typical peers. If the person is not aware of the difference and most people would not detect it, he or she the person would not likely be looked upon as having a communication disorder. In this situation, the communication difference would not interfere with communication, call adverse attention to the person, or cause the person to be self-conscious or maladjusted.
- The communicative deviation has to be regarded as "abnormal" by at least one person whose judgment the person with the communication disorder respects. This person can be a professional, such as a **speech–language pathologist (SLP)** or **audiologist**, a family member, a friend, or the person him- or herself.

Psychology Today (2014) estimates that 1 in 10 Americans of all ages, races, and genders either has a communication disorder or lives with some type of communication disorder (speech, language, or hearing disorder). Furthermore, "nearly 6 million children under the age of 18 have a speech or language disorder" (para. 2).

Determining What Is "Abnormal"

For a person to be regarded as having a communication disorder, some aspect of his or her speaking or listening behavior must be perceived as deviating from normal.

A necessary first step for deciding whether a particular aspect of communication behavior is abnormal is defining normal limits for it. What is regarded as being normal is almost always a value judgment—an opinion. It depends on the percentage of the population that you are willing to classify as abnormal. Should it be regarded as abnormal, for example, for a 2-and-a-half-year-old child not to be producing the /r/ sound correctly in words?

To view it as abnormal, an SLP would have to be willing to classify more than 75% of 2-and-a-half-year-olds as abnormal. On the other hand, should it be regarded as abnormal for an 8-year-old child not to be doing so? To view it in this way, an SLP would only have to be willing to classify fewer than 5% of 8-year-olds as abnormal. Therefore, two well-qualified SLPs could conceivably evaluate a 5-year-old child and disagree about whether his or her failure to say words containing /r/ correctly is abnormal.

That said, however, in most situations in which a person is thought to have a communication difference that is significant enough to be considered a disorder, the individual will undergo an evaluation conducted by an SLP. During the assessment process, the SLP will administer one or more **standardized tests** (more on this in later sections) that will allow the SLP to compare the individual being tested with his or her peers' scores. The results of the testing will show whether the individual's communication patterns are, in fact, different enough from his or her peers' to be considered a disorder.

Classification of Communication Disorders

Note that the ASHA definition indicates that a communication disorder is present if there are noticeable abnormalities in talking or listening. Because talking and listening are complex and complicated processes, communication disorders are typically described through a classification system based on several factors:

- **Etiology, or the cause of the disorder.** Etiologies include abnormalities in the anatomy or physiology of the individual; neurological conditions; hearing difficulties; cognitive impairments; and environmental factors, including influences on an individual's ability to learn.
- **Onset, or when the disorder first developed or appeared.** A **congenital** onset means that the condition creating the disorder was present at birth and may be because of genetic factors, issues during pregnancy (e.g., maternal use of drugs or alcohol), or difficulties during the birth process. A disorder that appears after birth is referred to as an acquired onset.
- **Receptive, expressive, or receptive–expressive manifestation.** A communication disorder that interferes with the individual's ability to understand speech or language is called a *receptive disorder*. An expressive disorder is one in which the individual has difficulty formulating speech or language or when that individual's speech or language cannot be understood by others.

Individuals with both receptive and expressive difficulties are said to have a receptive–expressive disorder.

- **Severity.** Although the ASHA (1993) definition of a communication disorder indicates that it may range in severity from mild to profound, many clinicians use a 5-point scale to rate severity: borderline, mild, moderate, severe, and profound.

Types of Communication Disorders

Language Disorders

ASHA defines a **language disorder** as

> impaired comprehension and/or use of spoken, written and/or other symbol systems. The disorder may involve (1) the form of language (phonology, morphology, syntax), (2) the content of language (semantics) and/or (3) the function of language in communication (pragmatics) in any combination. (ASHA,1993, sec. I.B)

Note that this definition includes written language as well as spoken language. The Center for Parent Information and Resources defines a language disorder as occurring when a child has problems "expressing needs, ideas, or information, and/or in understanding what others say" (2014a, para. 6). This definition also includes written language.

Paul and Norbury (2012) offered a more robust definition that includes the degree to which the individual's language differs from that of her or his peers. In describing children's language disorders, they stated that a disorder exists if a child has a significant deficit in talking or in understanding, or using appropriately any aspect of language when compared with norm-referenced expectations for typically developing children of comparable developmental age. (I will discuss language disorders in more detail in the chapters in Part 2.)

Speech Disorders

ASHA (1993) defines a **speech disorder** as "an impairment of the articulation of speech sounds, fluency and/or voice" (sec. I.A).

Articulation Disorders

Articulation disorders are characterized by atypical production of speech sounds—specifically, omissions, additions, or distortions—that interferes with the intelligibility of the individual's speech. Articulation disorders occur when children have difficulty with the structures necessary to produce the speech sounds (phonemes) of language, including the jaw, lips, tongue, and soft palate.

Articulation disorders are characterized by consistently making one or more errors in **phoneme** production. These errors can be of several types. One type of error is **sound substitution**. An English-speaking child, for example, might substitute /w/ for /r/ and say "wed wagon" rather than "red wagon." Another error type is sound omission. A child might omit the initial /s/ in a word when it is followed by another consonant and say, for example, "paghetti" instead of "spaghetti." A third type of error is **sound distortion**. A lateralized /s/ (an /s/ production in which the corners of the mouth retract and the air flows between the side teeth rather than the front ones) would be classified as a sound distortion in English because no words in this language contain such a sound. If there were such words, the error would be classified as a sound substitution. Audio Clip 2.1 provides an example of a sound substitution. The individual in this clip substitutes an "r" sound (as in "room") for the "yuh" sound (as in "yellow") in the word "vacuum." (Go to the link http://goo.gl/FTQ3ZK or scan the code.)

Fluency Disorder

Fluent speech is described as smooth, easy, and efficient, with few or no interruptions, hesitations, or interjections. When this **fluency** is interrupted, the resulting **disfluent** speech, sometimes called *stuttering*, can interfere enough with the flow of communication that it is considered a disorder. Specifically, fluency disorders involve "interruptions in the flow of speaking characterized by atypical rate, rhythm, and repetitions in sounds, syllables, words, and phrases" (American Speech-Language-Hearing Association, 1993, sec. I.A.2).

People who stutter often repeat syllables or words (e.g., "W-W-W-Why is the dog running?") or prolong specific speech sounds (e.g., "FFFFFFFind the car keys"). In some individuals, speech is stopped entirely, and they appear to struggle to breathe and to produce sound(s). Audio Clip 2.2 provides an example of stuttering in which the individual repeats a phrase an inserts an interjection. (Go to the link http://goo.gl/R3XHtR or scan the code.)

Voice Disorder

Voice disorders are considered disorders of **phonation**, stemming from a disturbance in the functioning of the **larynx**, particularly the part known as the **vocal folds**. Because voice is the "raw material" from which speech sounds are formed, if you can't produce voice, you can't speak. Other disorders of voice include habitually speaking (1) too loudly or too softly; (2) at a pitch level that is too high or too low; and (3) with a breathy, hoarse, or other type of abnormal voice quality.

Deem and Miller (2000) defined voice disorder as follows: "A voice disorder (**dysphonia**) is said to exist when a person's pitch, loudness, or quality differs from those of [someone of] similar age, sex, cultural background, or geographic location"

(p. 2). Most voice disorders result from some sort of trauma to the larynx, such as vocal abuse, screaming or yelling, using a pitch (frequency) that strains the vocal folds, injury, or burns (Deem & Miller, 2000). Some, however, are caused by congenital or neurogenic factors, including disorders of the central nervous system and vocal tract tumors present at birth.

Some voice disorders arise because of difficulties with air flow through the nose during speech. If too much air flows through the nose, the resulting speech is referred to as hypernasal. **Hypernasality** results in speech that is difficult to understand, and people who have it sound like they are "talking through their nose." **Hyponasality** (i.e., denasality) results if too little air flows through the nose. A person whose nose is "stuffed" as the result of a cold sounds hyponasal.

You can listen to two people with voice disorders on Audio Clips 2.3 and 2.4. In Clip 2.3 you will hear the voice of a woman with an organic voice tremor. The tremor isn't as obvious when she reads aloud as when she sustains a vowel at the end of the recording. (Go to the link http://goo.gl/hxM823 or scan the code.)

In Clip 2.4 you will hear a hoarse voice quality caused by pathology (e.g., a growth) on the vocal folds. I will discuss the various types of speech disorders in more detail in the chapters in Part 3. (Go to the link http://goo.gl/8lusPQ or scan the code.)

Hearing Disorders

ASHA (1993) defines a hearing disorder as

> the result of impaired auditory sensitivity of the physiological auditory system. A hearing disorder may limit the development, comprehension, production, and/or maintenance of speech and/or language. Hearing disorders are classified according to difficulties in detection, recognition, discrimination, comprehension, and perception of auditory information. Individuals with hearing impairment may be described as deaf or hard of hearing. (sec. I.C)

Most individuals who are considered deaf cannot use the auditory channel to receive communicative information, whereas most individuals who are hard of hearing have some ability to do so.

Most hearing disorders are caused by damage to the outer, middle, or inner ear. Damage can be on one or both sides of the head or to some part of the **central auditory nervous system (CANS)**—the parts of the brain that process electrical signals from the ears. The location and extensiveness of damage will determine the amount of difficulty a person will experience in understanding speech. Damage to the ear(s) or CANS can occur either before or after birth.

Hearing loss is classified according to which part of the ear or CANS is affected. When the outer and middle ear are affected, the resulting hearing loss is called a

conductive hearing loss. On the other hand, if the damage affects the inner ear or the CANS, the loss is called a **sensorineural hearing loss**. I will discuss hearing loss in more detail in Part 4.

What Is Significant Enough to Be Considered a Deficit?

Although the various definitions given are useful in describing what constitutes a language, speech, or hearing disorder, clinicians must also consider the significance of any deviation from what is considered typical communication. In most cases, this means the clinician will assess the individual's speech, language, and/or hearing and compare the results with what is known to be typical for that individual's age. Usually, this is accomplished by administering one or more standardized tests, which have been designed and developed so that the questions or prompts, scoring procedures, and conditions for administering are consistent and **reliable** over time and across examiners.

In addition to their consistency, standardized tests reflect the responses of a representative sample of individuals to the same questions or prompts, which allows the clinician to compare the individual's score(s) with those of the standardization sample. Using standardized tests allows clinicians to determine whether the individual's responses on those tests are significantly different from her or his age peers.

Communication Disorders and Interpersonal Relationships

Communication disorders affect interpersonal relationships in several ways, all of which can have profound consequences for the individual with the disorder. One of the most respected authors in the history of the field of communication sciences and disorders, Charles Van Riper, suggested that a communication disorder affects interpersonal relationships in the following three ways (Van Riper & Erickson, 1996).

It Can Interfere With Communication Between Speaker and Listener

People develop and maintain relationships with other people through communicating with each other. If a listener can't figure out what a speaker is saying, that listener may give up, avoid that particular speaker, or exclude that speaker from further conversational attempts. Also, if a speaker cannot remember some of the words needed to communicate messages, cannot control oral musculature sufficiently to form intelligible words, or cannot speak without multiple repetitions, hesitations, blocks, prolongations, or interjections, what the speaker is trying to say can get lost.

It Can Cause a Negative Reaction

Just as there are stereotypes for members of racial and religious groups, there are stereotypes for people who have certain communication disorders. These include stuttering, **lisping**, substituting /w/ for /r/, hearing loss, **dysarthria**, **spasmodic dysphonia**, and **aphasia**. If you expect a person to have certain personality characteristics or to behave in a certain way because he or she has a particular disorder, your expectation can cause you to perceive the person as having these characteristics and exhibiting these behaviors.

What characteristics do listeners ascribe to persons who have communication disorders? The characteristics that people are likely to ascribe to such a person will be determined by the following: (1) the type of disorder, (2) how the person reacts to it, (3) the listeners' previous experiences with persons who have the disorder, and (4) the listeners' cultural background(s).

The type of communication disorder determines to some extent the characteristics that listeners ascribe to a person. A man who has a frontal lisp (who substitutes /θ/ for /s/), for example, is more likely to be viewed as "feminine" than one who speaks with a whistling /s/.

How the person reacts to the disorder influences how listeners will react to it. If listeners sense that the person is embarrassed or ashamed about having the disorder, they are likely to ascribe more negative personality characteristics to the person than they would otherwise (Silverman, Gazzolo, & Peterson, 1990).

A listener's previous experience with persons who have a particular disorder determines, to some extent, the characteristics he or she is likely to ascribe to those who have it. A listener who perceived those he or she met previously who had the disorder as having low intelligence may tend to perceive others who have the same disorder as not being very intelligent.

Finally, cultural background influences the characteristics a listener will ascribe to a child or adult who has a communication disorder (Bleile & Wallach, 1992). For example, an African American preschool-age child who has trouble speaking is likely to have some different characteristics ascribed to him or her by persons in an African American inner-city community than by persons in a white middle-class community. The characteristics ascribed will be determined, in part, by the beliefs in the ascribing person's **culture** about the causes and consequences of disabilities (Smith, 2006). To learn more about the influence of culture on how communication disorders are perceived, see Battle (2012).

Two of the most common traits listeners tend to ascribe to people with communication disorders are relatively low intelligence and immaturity. People who express themselves well are often judged to be more intelligent than those who do not express themselves well. Similarly, people often treat someone with a communication disorder in much the same way they treat a small child, by speaking louder and using short sentences, repeating what they're saying, and using the person's first name in situations in which it is customary to use a title (e.g., Doctor, Ms.) and last name.

It Can Create a Poor Self-Image

Liking yourself is a necessary condition for developing and maintaining enjoyable and beneficial relationships with others. Experiencing negative emotions because of a communication disorder can severely impact a person's ability to form and maintain relationships.

People who have speech, language, or hearing that differs noticeably from their peers often struggle with maintaining a positive self-concept. Having a communication disorder can cause a person to dislike him- or herself, which can result in unhappiness, depression, being overly sensitive, frustration, suicidal thoughts or actions, embarrassment, pessimism, emotional instability, defensiveness, introversion, being frightened, or feeling tense.

A person who has a communication disorder may attempt to maintain a positive self-image by frequently employing one or both of the following strategies: (1) avoiding situations in which he or she would be expected to communicate or (2) participating in those situations but reducing speaking to an absolute minimum. Either strategy can reduce the number of times the person becomes embarrassed as a consequence of communicating abnormally, but they can seriously impair interpersonal relationships. In fact, using them may contribute more to the person being impaired than the communication disorder itself. Some of the responsibilities of SLPs and audiologists include encouraging people with communication disorders to communicate, teaching them ways to better communicate, and supporting their communication efforts.

A communication disorder's impact on a person's self-image is, in part, a function of how others react to the person in his or her culture (Ndung'u & Kinyua, 2009). Persons from different cultures may react differently to a child who has a particular communication disorder. To learn more about how a person's culture can affect a communication disorder's impact on his or her self-image, see Battle (2012).

Multicultural Issues and Considerations

People from different cultural groups may communicate differently from each other and hold different beliefs about what constitutes appropriate and, therefore, disordered, communication. But what is culture, exactly? Most people think culture consists of the characteristics of a particular group of people who speak the same language and who share similar social habits, musical taste, religion, and arts. People in a given cultural group share attitudes, values, goals, and practices over a period of time, passing them along to succeeding generations.

Stockman, Boult, and Robinson (2004) wrote that

> culture can be viewed broadly as the socially constructed and learned ways of believing and behaving that identify groups of people. Verbal and nonverbal

communication behaviors readily identify cultural groups. By attaching the prefix *multi-* to the word *culture*, we can refer to more than one socially constructed and learned way of believing and behaving. (p. 6)

These authors suggest that the term *multicultural* applies to everyone because everyone belongs to a multicultural group. Specifically, they say that people in every culture have "multiple and complex identities" (p. 6) that are created by their membership in various sorts of groups, including race, ethnicity, gender, social class, religious preference, geographical region, sexual orientation, and linguistic community.

For more than 30 years, ASHA has been engaged in guiding SLPs and audiologists in developing culturally sensitive practices (ASHA, 1985). In addition, ASHA has developed a wide range of resources for faculty offering coursework in communication sciences and disorders, professionals offering clinical services, and students (ASHA, 2014p).

One of ASHA's major contributions has been to identify that just as each client has a culture, so, too, does every clinician (ASHA, 2014r). Consequently, as clinicians, we have a responsibility to appropriately modify the services we provide to clients from cultures other than our own. We also have a responsibility to recognize that culture is not necessarily immediately apparent from how a person looks because "culture is not limited to race or ethnicity. Multiculturalism includes issues dealing with race, ethnicity gender, gender identification, age, sexual orientation, and ability. It is important to realize that a person may identify with more than one culture" (ASHA, 2014r, para. 4).

Differentiating between what constitutes a communication disorder and what is merely a cultural variation in communication style or custom requires knowing how different cultural groups communicate, what is considered "normal" in each cultural group, and what is considered "disordered." For instance, in virtually all cultures, severe language disruptions following a stroke constitute a language disorder, but dialectal variations in grammatical constructions do not. Similarly, in almost all cultures, a child who does not speak by age 3 would be at least evaluated for a language disorder, but a teenager with a hoarse voice might be sent for an evaluation in some cultures but not others.

People living in cultures that are heavily dependent on print (i.e., reading and writing) view difficulties in learning to read or write as communication disorders, while people from cultures that rely more heavily on oral language may not. Similarly, people from cultures in which oral language is prized may view people who cannot tell complex, entertaining, and lengthy stories to be communicatively impaired, while those from cultures in which storytelling is not particularly valued may not.

A related issue concerns cultural perceptions of hearing loss and the use of sign languages. Most people with normal hearing view profound hearing loss and the inability to speak as a communication disorder, while most people with hearing impairment who use a sign language to communicate do not. Rather, people who sign argue that theirs is a culture separate from the hearing culture and thus should be considered a cultural entity separate from any conceptualization of disorder imposed by the hearing community. One way to think about cultural groups is to examine the demographic characteristics of the United States.

Demographic Profile of the United States

As of July 28, 2014, the total population of the United States was 318,463,000 (U.S. Census Bureau, 2014). According to the 2010 U.S. census, 63.7% of the population is non-Hispanic white, 16.4% is Hispanic or Latino, 12.6% is African American, 4.8% is Asian American, and 0.9% is Native American or Alaska Native; and 20.2% is age 14 or younger (U.S. Census Bureau, 2010).

The Annie E. Casey Foundation (2014) reported that the total number of children under age 18 is 74.2 million, of which ethnic children comprised 46%. Of particular interest to our field, two ethnic groups of children grew substantially between 2000 and 2010—the number of Hispanic children grew by 4.8 million (39%), and the number of Asian and Pacific Islander children grew by almost 800,000 (31%).

According to the American Community Survey, more than 60 million individuals in the United States speak a language other than English at home (Ryan, 2011). Of those, 62% speak Spanish or Spanish Creole, 4.8% speak Chinese, 4.6% speak Tagalog, 2.3% speak Vietnamese, 1.6% speak Arabic, and 1.5% speak African languages (Ryan, 2011). In all, the survey found that 39 major languages are reportedly used as the primary language spoken at home (Ryan, 2011).

These findings make clear that, as professionals in the communication disorders field, we must attend to the widening circles of diversity that make up our society to ensure that our clients can participate fully. Becoming familiar with multicultural issues and concerns affords us the opportunity to develop the necessary sensitivities and tools.

The Basics of Assessment and Intervention

Two approaches to assessment and intervention are used in communication sciences and disorders: medical and developmental. The medical approach is used for conditions arising from a specific and known cause—a particular disease, injury, or condition—that has resulted in a communication disorder. Labeling the approach "medical" does not imply that the focus is strictly on medical aspects; rather, it means that the process of gathering data and diagnosing the disorder follows that used in the field of medicine, which is to identify and label the disorder and specify its cause. In the medical approach, management of the disorder arises directly from this identification, labeling, and specification of cause.

The developmental approach, on the other hand, focuses not on diagnosis but on deciding whether there is a significant problem in communication relative to what is known about normal development. Issues of cause are not of primary concern; rather, attention is given to describing the client's communication and determining what should happen next developmentally. Even when a potential cause can be identified or a developmental condition categorized, the focus remains on the developmental sequence of communication rather than on "treating" or managing the underlying cause.

Within the field of communication sciences and disorders, the medical approach is most often utilized when assessing and diagnosing voice disorders, dysarthria and **dysphagia**, hearing loss, adult neurogenic disorders, and fluency. The developmental approach is most often used when assessing children's language development and consequent disorders; intervention is designed to facilitate and enhance language development. A combination of medical and developmental approaches is used to assess children's articulation and phonological disorders. Because these two approaches differ in their basic goals, the process of assessment for each is somewhat different. I will discuss assessment in more detail in Chapter 13.

Purpose of Assessment

Assessment in the medical approach focuses on three goals: (1) identifying the underlying cause of the disorder and its severity, (2) diagnosing the disorder, and (3) arranging for treatment.

Assessment in the developmental approach focuses on (1) screening to find out whether there is a problem; (2) establishing the client's **baseline** function; (3) establishing goals for intervention, consisting of appropriate targets and procedures; and (4) measuring change across time in intervention to determine whether intervention goals have been met and when to dismiss the client from intervention.

Types of Assessments

Professionals in communication sciences and disorders use several types of assessments. They range from informal conversations and interviews with family members, to standardized tests that are administered in quite specific ways, to measurements taken with sophisticated instrumentation, such as an **audiometer**. There are five primary types of assessments used when evaluating communication systems.

Standardized Assessments

Standardized assessments, known as norm-referenced tests, are based on the data collected from a large number of people in statistical groupings based on chronological age. These groups are the norms against which an individual client's scores are compared (Polloway, Miller, & Smith, 2012). Standardized tests are called standardized for two reasons: (1) they are administered, scored, and interpreted in a standard (i.e., specifically described) manner and (2) because they are based on a set of norms (i.e., standards) collected from a representative population to which the client is then compared.

Nonstandardized Assessments

Nonstandardized assessments include criterion-referenced procedures, developmental scales, and dynamic assessment. Criterion-referenced procedures are methods that compare the client's performance to a performance standard (e.g., Which components of a story does the child include when telling a story?). Developmental scales provide what is known about a particular aspect of communication development. The clinician then compares the client's current developmental progress against the scale. Dynamic assessment is a method in which the clinician assesses the client's ability to learn a new skill or ability with graduated levels of support.

Interviews With Families and Caregivers

Families and caregivers represent a rich source of information about a client, more so when the client is unable to communicate fluently. The clinician can design an appropriate interview with family or caregivers, depending on the communication disorder exhibited by the client. For instance, when interviewing a family member of a child with a language disorder, the clinician will focus on the child's developmental history (including any medical and health issues or concerns), understanding and use of language, and hearing acuity. When interviewing a family member of a client who has suffered a stroke, the clinician will want to obtain information about the client's health prior to the stroke; communicative ability and habits before the stroke; special interests or hobbies; personality characteristics; motivation level; current language ability; hearing acuity; and any medical or health problems beyond those associated with the stroke.

Observation of the Client in Familiar Environment

Although clinicians cannot always observe their clients at home, in school, or at work, the ideal scenario would be to make at least one visit to a place with which the client is familiar. Outside the clinic setting, the clinician will almost always be able to discover aspects of the client's communication abilities that were not apparent inside the clinic, hospital, health-care facility, or rehabilitation center. Children, especially, are more noticeably comfortable in their own surroundings, and observing their play and routines offers invaluable information that can be utilized in both the assessment and intervention processes. Visiting a client with a voice disorder may reveal aspects of everyday life that impinge directly on the client's ability to progress during the management phase. Similarly, making a home visit to a client who has had a stroke and is back in a familiar environment may yield important clues about how to design subsequent intervention sessions that focus more directly on communication that will be functionally useful to the client in this setting.

Use of Calibrated Instrumentation

Audiologists rely to a large extent on calibrated instruments to measure various aspects of hearing acuity and function. To measure hearing acuity, they make use of audiometers of varying degrees of technological complexity. Assessing middle-ear function is done with an instrument called a **tympanometer**. Central auditory function—how the hearing system functions once sound is translated from physical energy to neural energy in the inner ear—is measured with a variety of instruments, including electrodes and audiometers. All of these instruments are **calibrated**.

Speech–language pathologists often use calibrated instruments when assessing voice function, particularly when evaluating respiratory and laryngeal function. Noninvasive instruments used include the spirometer (which measures respiratory volume) and strain gauges, magnetometers, and plethysmographs (which all measure respiratory movement). Invasive instruments, which are usually used by an **otolaryngologist** rather than an SLP, are used to assess vocal fold condition and function and include the endoscope and the stroboscope. The endoscope is a fiber-optic tube, often with a video camera attached (which makes it a videoendoscope or videoscope), that is inserted into the nose or mouth to view the vocal folds. The stroboscope is a flashing light that is used to view the vocal folds during movement. (Topical anesthesia is required for both.) Speech–language pathologists working with clients with dysphagia often use a videofluoroscope. This instrument combines video and x-ray to provide a dynamic record of swallowing.

Benefits and Limitations of Assessment

The chief benefit of the assessment process is that it offers a way to collect information regarding a client's communication abilities, organize the resulting data, and generate relevant and meaningful goals for intervention. Without the assessment phase, developing intervention goals becomes virtually impossible. In addition, the assessment period allows the clinician to develop a relationship of trust with the client, who will then more likely participate fully in the intervention process knowing the clinician is trustworthy and has his or her best interests at heart.

The assessment process also carries a serious limitation—it can only show limited "peeks" at the client's communication system. Assessment occurs at certain periods, in certain places, and for a limited period of time. In other words, by its very nature assessment cannot be ongoing, nor can it be totally thorough. For this reason, clinicians strive to use assessment procedures and instruments that will yield representative samples of the client's communication abilities and not just snippets that may or may not be representative. Using **valid**, reliable, and efficient assessment methods and procedures in combination with an always-growing ability to make accurate clinical judgments, the clinician aims at gathering the most representative information possible during the assessment process. However, clinicians know that the collected information is always just a sample and not a complete picture of the client's communication abilities.

Management and Intervention

Managing communication disorders involves designing therapeutic intervention based on the outcomes of the assessment process I described in the previous sections of this chapter. In this section I describe the purposes of intervention, the types of goals utilized in designing intervention, and how to measure progress.

Purpose of Intervention

The intervention process is guided by the results of assessing and evaluating the communication disorder. The primary purpose of intervention is to assist in improving (a) the client's communication abilities as much as possible, given the nature and severity of the disorder; (b) the client's desire and ability to make changes; and (c) the resources necessary for making changes.

Types of Intervention Goals

Several types of goals are used in management and intervention. Generally, clinicians set both **long-term and short-term goals** (the latter are often called **objectives**). A long-term goal usually specifies the communication abilities and skills that will result from a course of management or intervention. For a client with an articulation disorder in which he substitutes /w/ for /r/, for instance, the long-term goal would be that he successfully produce /r/ in all positions in words 100% of the time. The clinician may want to establish a series of short-term objectives written for shorter time periods. For example, one of the first short-term objectives might be for the client to make a close approximation of an /r/ sound once every five tries. A later short-term goal might be for him to correctly produce an /r/ sound at the end of the words *clear*, *fire*, and *bear* 50% of the time he produces the words.

Clinicians working with students in school settings are sometimes required to write goals known as benchmarks, performance standards, or objectives. Benchmarks and performance standards are usually linked to abilities considered essential to school success and codified by each state in a set of learning standards to which all schools must adhere. For instance, a benchmark for a child in early elementary school might be to "restate and carry out a variety of oral instructions." The clinician would then write a series of steps the client would need to carry out in order to reach that particular benchmark.

Measuring Progress

For intervention to be considered successful, the client must demonstrate measurable change directly related to the intervention process. To demonstrate the change, and to determine whether the intervention goals or methods need to be modified, the clinician collects data periodically and compares it with the information and data collected during the initial assessment. In this way, the clinician demonstrates **efficacy** of intervention.

Collecting data can range from use of a simple tally sheet to the administration of a standardized test. However, standardized testing is used more often at the beginning and end of the intervention process. Monitoring ongoing intervention progress usually involves designing some sort of data collection system that summarizes client progress. Table 2.1 shows an example of a data collection sheet designed for the client described earlier, who substitutes /w/ for /r/.

Evidence-Based Practices

Closely related to the concept of efficacy of intervention is **evidence-based practice**, a concept originally borrowed from the field of medicine but now used in many health-care professions and services. The idea of evidence-based practice (EBP) is to provide the best possible intervention for each client through utilizing a combination of evidence from scientific studies, clinical experience and judgment, and the unique needs of each client. More specifically, ASHA describes EBP as "the integration of (a) clinical expertise/expert opinion, (b) external scientific evidence, and (c) client/patient/caregiver perspectives to provide high-quality services reflecting the interests, values, needs, and choices of the individuals we serve" (American Speech-Language-Hearing Association, 2014j, para. 1).

ASHA proposed that clinicians follow a four-step process in employing EBP (2014j, para. 1).

1. Frame the clinical question through an analysis of the specific communication disorder presented by your client; a comparison of possible intervention approaches to determine which offers the best outcome; and the formulation of the desired outcome for this client.
2. Find the evidence you need to plan intervention through an analysis of existing practices that are considered highly efficacious; a systematic review of scientific evidence related to a particular clinical question; an

TABLE 2.1 Data Collection Form (/w/ for /r/ substitution)

	Sessions				
Initial /r/—Word imitation	**1**	**2**	**3**	**4**	**5**
Correct production					
Incorrect production					
Total attempts					
% correct					

analysis of individual studies that relate to the clinical question you are posing for a particular client.

3. Assess the evidence through determining its relevance to the specific clinical question you are asking about your client and through considering who wrote and published the evidence you're analyzing. Of particular concern is whether the clinical practice being described in any of the literature is actually evidence-based rather than opinion or consensus among a group of "experts."

4. Make the clinical decision, which involves combining your clinical experience and expertise with the evidence you've gathered to determine which intervention approach would best serve your client.

At this point you may be thinking that the concept of EBP and the steps ASHA proposes for following EBP are rather abstract. As you learn more about the profession and begin developing your clinical skills, you can keep up to date on the latest evidence regarding best practices on ASHA's Evidence-Based Systematic Reviews webpage (2014d). The reviews are conducted annually and include information regarding the various types of disorders you are most likely to encounter in your clinical work.

PART 2

Language Development and Disorders

The three chapters in this part of the book are devoted to language development and language disorders. Chapter 3 is an overview of typical child and adolescent language development. This chapter is important because understanding language disorders depends on a thorough understanding of how language develops.

In Chapter 4, I describe language disorders within the context of the components of language form, content, use, narrative language, and figurative language. You will learn about the language characteristics of children with specific etiologies and conditions, such as autism, language-learning disability, hearing loss, and others. I have also included a section on differentiating between a language disorder and a language difference, emphasizing again the importance of taking a multicultural perspective in order to assess language disorders and to design appropriate intervention programs for children exhibiting the various characteristics of language disorders.

In Chapter 5, I focus on language disorders in adults arising from conditions, diseases, and traumatic events. I begin with a brief discussion of the causes of brain damage and then move to a description of aphasia, how it is classified, and its symptomatology. I also describe right-hemisphere deficits that result from trauma and those that are associated with dementia and Alzheimer's disease. In the assessment and management sections I focus on how to reduce the severity of the deficit and augment the client's remaining communication abilities.

chapter 3

Preschool, Child, and Adolescent/Young Adult Language Development

Learning Objectives

Identify the types of students with language disorders served by speech–language pathologists in school settings.

Describe the five building blocks of language: use, form, content, nonverbal language, and figurative language.

Summarize language development from infancy through young adulthood.

Describe metalinguistic development and its impact on academic achievement and social acceptance.

Describe the relationship between oral language development and the development of writing.

Describe factors contributing to students' literacy development.

Overview

To understand **language disorders** you will need a thorough understanding of how **language** develops. Knowledge of language development is the cornerstone for the decisions **speech–language pathologists (SLPs)** make regarding whether a client exhibits a language disorder or uses language that is merely different from that of his or her age peers, perhaps because of cultural background. To help you better understand language disorders and their effects, I first describe the building blocks of language: use, form, content, nonverbal language, and figurative language. Then I present an overview of how language develops from infancy through young adulthood. Following this, I describe the relationship between oral and written language and how children make the shift from being primarily oral, which is relatively concrete and literal, to being able to communicate using written forms, which include more abstract and nonliteral concepts and processes (i.e., the development of literacy). In the last section, I discuss the importance of literacy for academic success.

Language Use, Form, Content, Nonverbal Language, and Figurative Language

Language Use

Language use, also called **pragmatics**, refers to how people use language to negotiate socially in a variety of situations and with a wide range of other people, some of whom are familiar and some not (Polloway, Miller, & Smith, 2012). To do this, people follow—and violate—the set of implicit rules I described in Chapter 1 as a conversational code of conduct. Individuals who have difficulty figuring out what these rules are or how to follow and violate them may be referred to as having a language use problem, a pragmatic language disorder, or a social language disorder (these terms are used interchangeably).

How people use language varies according to numerous factors, including the following:

- *The relative ages of the conversational partner(s).* We use different language when we talk to babies, familiars, and elders.
- *The power dynamic between conversational partners.* We usually use less formal language when the power relationship with a conversational partner is roughly equal, while we use more formal language if we perceive that our conversational partner has more social power. The person in the more powerful position can choose whether to use formal or informal language.
- *The gender of the conversational partners.* In most **cultures**, both men and women change how they use language depending on whether they're conversing with someone of the same or different gender.
- *The degree of respect we wish to convey.* Again, the specific ways in which people change their language to convey (or not convey) respect vary by culture, but, in every culture, people make adjustments for this purpose. Interestingly, in some situations, using less formal language indicates a higher degree of respect, while other contexts call for using more formal language. For instance, fans addressing a well-liked athlete often use informal forms of address to show their respect, while these same people would most likely use much more formal language to address a member of the clergy in their faith.
- *The degree to which we know our conversational partners.* When speaking to someone we don't know, most of us use less slang, fewer idiomatic expressions, and more careful diction than when speaking to someone we know. When speaking to a stranger, we use vocabulary we assume the stranger will know, while when speaking with friends, we often use terms known only to our circle of friends.

Try the mind experiments in Box 3.1 to learn more about how you use language differently for different purposes.

Another aspect of language use is **discourse**, which Polloway et al. (2012) defined as a linguistic unit larger than a sentence: a conversation, a story, a speech. People use many discourse types (e.g., conversational, narrative, classroom, argumentative–persuasive), each of which consists of its own set of rules and conventions.

Narrative Discourse

Narrative discourse is the discourse people use to tell and understand stories. Cultural groups vary in the degree of importance placed on telling stories, but in many cultures, children are included in the oral traditions of storytelling. In most cultures, children grow up hearing and telling stories, first in their families and later in their peer groups.

When they enter school, children are expected to know the basic elements of story structure, and as they begin learning to read, to apply that knowledge to what they are reading. In most classrooms, children are also expected to be able to begin writing primitive stories as soon as they can write.

BOX 3.1   **Pragmatics Mind Experiments**

In your mind . . .

1. Think about how you would ask your best friend if you can borrow some money until next month.
2. Think about how you would ask your parents if you can borrow some money until next month.
3. Imagine you are going to the credit union or the bank where you have a checking account. Think about how you would ask a loan officer to borrow some money until next month.

How did you change what you said and how you said it in each instance? Did you explain more in any of the situations? Was your language more or less formal? Did you use a different tone of voice? Different vocabulary? Did you use any softeners or qualifiers? When?

In your mind . . .

1. Tell your little brother or sister you are angry at him or her for ruining your favorite CD.
2. Tell your father or mother you are angry at him or her for giving away your favorite pair of jeans.
3. Tell your boss you are unhappy that the promotion you wanted was given to someone else.

Did you change your language in each situation? How? How did you change your vocabulary? Did you change your tone of voice? The length of your sentences? The formality of the language you used? Did you use any softeners or qualifiers? When?

Classroom Discourse

Classroom discourse is the language education professionals use to teach in the classroom. Polloway et al. (2012) listed six characteristics of classroom discourse:

- The teacher talks the most and limits the amount and frequency of student talking.
- The teacher determines the topic(s) to be discussed.
- The teacher regulates how students talk (e.g., direct response to a question, brief personal comments, short explanatory summaries).
- The students' language is evaluated continuously by the teacher.
- The context for the language used is often situated outside the classroom, as compared with conversational discourse, which is situated in the here and now.
- Students are often required to use **metalinguistic skills** to talk about language or parts of language. For instance, students might be asked to list several words that all sound alike (e.g., *to, too, two*), or to list different words that mean the same thing (*couch, sofa*).

Expository Discourse

Expository discourse refers to nonnarrative discourses, such as those used in textbooks, magazine articles, news editorials, advertisements, and political speeches. Expository discourse is also used orally, as in lectures or presentations. In most classrooms, children begin encountering expository discourse by third grade, when they make the switch from learning to read to reading to learn. According to Polloway et al. (2012), the three most common types of expository discourse are descriptive, explanatory, and argumentative–persuasive.

Language Form

Three basic categories are usually used to describe language form: **phonology**, **morphology**, and **syntax**.

Phonology

Phonology consists of the set of rules governing how the sounds in a given language are pronounced, which sounds are actually used, and how they can be combined. Different languages use different sets of rules for phonology (e.g., in Spanish, *millón* is pronounced "mee YONE," while in English, *million* is pronounced "MILL yun"). In English the *l* is pronounced as /ɛl/ ("ell"), and in Spanish it is pronounced as /jə/ ("yuh").

The smallest linguistic units to carry meaning are **phonemes**, the pronounceable sounds in a language. This means that in any given language, some sounds carry meaning and some do not.

Morphology

Morphology governs how phonemes can be combined into larger units (e.g., syllables and words) to convey meaning (Polloway et al., 2012). Morphological rules govern language aspects such as tense markers (e.g., present tense: "He *drives* me to school" and past tense: "He *drove* me to school"), plurals (more than one: "The *trees* were shaking in the wind"), and possessives (e.g., "That's *my* car in the garage"; "Where's *your* sandwich?").

Morphemes are the smallest grammatical units that carry meaning (phonemes can *change* meaning, but, individually, they don't carry meaning). An example of a morpheme is the word *cat*, which is considered a **free morpheme** because it can stand alone. Another example of a morpheme is the plural marker -*s*, which, when added to *cat*, results in *cats*. The -*s* plural marker is known as a **bound morpheme** because it cannot stand alone; it must attach to either a free morpheme (as in *cats*) or another bound morpheme that is already attached to a free morpheme. An example of a bound morpheme attaching to another bound morpheme that is already attached to a free morpheme is -*s* in the following: *calculate+tion+s* (*calculations*).

Each language has its own set of morphemic rules for marking meanings, such as

- plural (-*s*, as in *dogs*),
- possessive (-*'s*, as in "the girl's dress"),
- verb tenses (-*s*, as in "He walks every day"; -*ed*, as in "He walked there yesterday"; -*ing*, as in "He is walking there now"), and
- **negation** (*un-*, as in "undesirable"; *dis-*, as in "disinterested"; *im-*, as in "impossible").

Syntax

Syntax governs how phrases and sentences must be built in order to convey meaning. For example, in English, the following sentence makes no sense because it doesn't follow the rules of syntax: "Boy the followed dog white brown and the." English syntax requires that the sentence be ordered like this: "The white and brown dog followed the boy" in order to be understood.

Syntax allows you to create an infinite number of different sentences using the same basic rules. In other words, syntax is **generative** rather than regurgitative—you utter unique sentences rather than imitate others with whom you are conversing.

Among other things, syntax explains

- word order;
- when to use active or passive voice;
- how to make declaratives, imperatives, or interrogatives;
- how to form negatives;
- how to make conditional statements; and
- how to combine sentences into compound or complex sentences.

Some languages, such as English, rely on word order (i.e., syntax) to convey meanings, while other languages, such as German, rely on adding markers to words (i.e., morphology).

Language Content

The most common way professionals refer to language content is in terms of **semantics** (Polloway et al., 2012), or the meaning level of language. Semantics provides a way to describe how people understand ideas, feelings, events, relationships, processes, and things (Polloway et al., 2012). The primary component of semantic ability is **vocabulary**, although semantics also addresses the relations between specific words, such as homonyms (words that sound the same but have different meanings, such as *pare–pear–pair*), synonyms (words that have similar or identical meanings, such as *couch–sofa*), and antonyms (words that are considered to have opposite meanings, such as *top–bottom, big–little, sweet–sour, antonym–synonym*).

Semantics involves the relationship of words to the things (objects, experiences, ideas, processes, events) they refer to, called **referents.** It is important to note that these relationships between words and their referents are **arbitrary.** What this means is that there is no *necessary* relationship between the sounds and words used to refer to something and the thing itself. For example, there is no inherent reason a chair is called a chair or an idea is called an idea. Another important concept is that the relationships between words and the things they represent are **symbolic.** This means that words are symbols that represent things, ideas, or concepts. Words are not the things they represent; they are symbols of those things.

The arbitrariness of the symbols used in language allows for tremendous power in representing the ideas, feelings, thoughts, events, actions, experiences, possibilities, and wishes we want to communicate. Consider, for a moment, the word *apple* and the object to which it refers. There is nothing inherent in the actual apple that implies anything about which sounds are used to represent it, the order of those sounds, how they are pronounced, or how they look when written on the page. In short, the apple you see in your mind's eye is totally unrelated to the word *apple* except that it has become customary to call it by that name. There is nothing inherent in an apple to suggest that it be called an apple; hence, *apple* is an arbitrary symbol used to represent the object we're describing.

Semantic development in children is often discussed in terms of vocabulary. In young children, their oral vocabulary reveals the semantic knowledge they are acquiring. As they begin reading, their vocabulary is usually measured through tests of reading vocabulary, and as they begin writing, their written vocabulary is used to assess their semantic knowledge.

Nonverbal Language and Paralinguistic Signals

When people converse with each other, they use not just vocalizations but also a variety of nonverbal signals, such as head and body postures, hand gestures, facial expressions, eye contact, and physical distance (known as **proxemics**). These non-verbal signals convey a significant amount of the meaning in any conversation. For instance, you probably know people who use their hands and arms to gesture while they talk, or you may know someone whose eye contact is different from most other people's. I'll talk more about this in later sections on how **communication disorders** affect people's lives.

Communication also involves using **paralinguistic signals**, which include stress, intonation, rate of delivery of **speech**, and hesitations and interjections. These paralinguistic signals also convey a considerable amount of the meaning in any given conversation. For instance, think how rising or falling intonation completely changes the tone, and, therefore, the intended meaning, of the following sentence: "Are you kidding me?" (rising intonation), compared with "Are you kidding me!" (falling intonation). In the former, you might conclude that the speaker is sincerely asking a question, whereas in the second sentence you would probably conclude that the speaker is expressing anger, frustration, or displeasure, depending on the context.

Figurative Language

Language exists along a continuum from the concrete and literal on one end, to the abstract and figurative on the other end. On the concrete, literal level, words and phrases have only one primary meaning, while on the figurative level, words, phrases, sentences, essays, and books may convey meaning on two or more levels. For example, the sentence "The dog followed the girl" conveys a direct, literal message that means exactly what it says. On the other hand, the idiom "The chickens have come home to roost" does not mean exactly what it says. Instead, according to the *Free Dictionary* (2014), the meaning is that someone must face the consequences of her or his actions. All idioms, parables, fables, parodies, and the like are examples of **figurative language**, or language that says one thing but means another.

Think about this sentence: "Flying planes can be dangerous." On one level it means that flying planes can be dangerous to the people flying them, while on another it means that planes flying through the air can be dangerous. Or consider the **idiom** "It's raining cats and dogs." On the literal level, it means cats and dogs are falling from the sky, but on the figurative level, it means it's raining hard. To illustrate the idea of multiple levels of language, Box 3.2 shows examples of double meanings.

Language Development From Infancy Through Young Adulthood

Children develop an awareness of the arbitrariness of language gradually. When they are first developing language, they do not understand that language has multiple levels; their ability to understand the different levels of language develops over time.

BOX 3.2   **Examples of Double Meanings**

1. Read the following sentence and describe the two levels of meaning.

   Visiting relatives can be a nuisance.

2. Read the following sentence and describe its literal and figurative meanings.

   He's been under the weather for a few days.

3. Read the following words and imagine how you would use each to refer to something.

   hare–hair

   pare–pear–pair

   there–their–they're

   two–to–too

   Mary–merry–marry

Children typically learn language in the social context of a family, although different cultures hold different views about how and when to talk to children, and some children grow up in different settings (e.g., foster homes, hospitals, group homes). Most children learn to speak well-formed sentences in spite of hearing the fragments and ill-formed scraps of conversations that are typical of normal communication. For this reason, most language researchers believe that children are born hardwired to learn language, although they differ on the specifics of what constitutes the hardwiring. At the least, children must be in the presence of people using language in order to develop their own language system, whether it is oral or signed. At best, children engage in social interactions with people they trust and who attend to their emerging language skills with delight and pride.

Children who do not grow up hearing (or seeing, in the case of sign language) language will have a more difficult time learning anything beyond simple vocabulary words. In other words, there seems to be an optimal period for developing the capacity to understand and use language fluently; the child who has not learned any language system before puberty will most likely demonstrate deficits in one or more language forms.

Although first spoken words do not appear in most children's communication before 9 to 12 months of age, children are actively engaged in learning important communication skills beginning in infancy.

For many years, very little was known about language development beyond the preschool years. Gradually, the professionals who studied language development contributed more and more information about what happens in the language development of school-age children and adolescents. Today, one of the best-known descriptions of language development is a five-stage model first described in landmark work by Roger Brown (1973) and later expanded by Rhea Paul (2007):

1. The prelinguistic period: communication up to the emergence of the first words.
2. Emerging language: from first words to the first combination of words.
3. Developing language: from two-word utterances through the basic structures of language.
4. The language of learning: language used to learn to read and write.
5. Adolescent language development: abstract language used to read and write the various forms of expository discourse.

The Prelinguistic Period

Very quickly after birth, infants begin attending to the primary adults around them. They are highly dependent on caring adults who will talk to them and respond to them as if they are communicating, which in a short time they actually are. The earliest communicative behaviors infants show is to look at their primary caregiver, usually a mother or a father, and slow down the movements of their arms and legs while the adult talks.

This talk is called "**parentese**" regardless of who is speaking—a mother or father or grandparent. Parentese, which adults use to talk to infants for the first 6 months or so, emphasizes the interaction rather than any particular meaning. The adult uses only a few words at a time, usually words of endearment, and varies pitch, loudness, speed or rate of speech, the rhythm of what she is saying, and her intonation patterns (e.g., rising intonation for questions, falling intonations for declarations). If you talk to a baby, you will notice that you use a higher pitch, you use singsong intonation ranging from very high to very low, and you increase the emphasis you place on certain words. For instance, if you are talking to a baby, you might say something like this: "*What* a happy baby you are. *Such* a happy baby. *So* happy." All the while you are probably smiling, pausing between each utterance, and maybe even putting one of your fingers out so the baby can grasp it with her hand.

While you are talking, the baby is watching your face, maybe smiling, and she is slowing down her movements a bit. When you stop, she is likely to look away and then back to your face, jiggle her arms and legs, smile and perhaps vocalize. Then, when you start speaking again, she will bring her gaze back to your face, and she will slow down her movements again. In this way, you and the baby begin taking turns "talking."

Parentese focuses on things the infant can see, feel, and hear. When you were talking to the baby, you were probably looking directly in the infant's eyes and smiling throughout the "conversation." If the infant vocalized, you responded as if the baby were saying something and has taken a conversational turn.

Adults continue using parentese until their babies reach approximately 6 months of age, after which the adults change their communication patterns to include the use of more informational language (Penman, Cross, Milgrom-Friedman, & Meares, 1983).

One of the most important prelinguistic developments during infancy is the infant's emerging skill in engaging in joint attending and joint referencing (Bruner,

1975). Both are necessary foundations for the acquisition of language. Joint attending is when the infant and adult both look at the same thing, first each other (mutual attending) and then at objects or one of the baby's limbs, for example. Joint referencing emerges out of joint attending. As the baby develops, the adult tells the baby what things are called, naming them as they jointly attend to them. Gradually, the baby begins gesturing toward what the adult is talking about, to which the parent responds with enthusiasm. Soon, both adult and baby point to things to indicate joint reference. The baby develops the ability to refer to things through this process of jointly referring with an adult. As first words emerge, they replace pointing.

As babies and infants get to know one another, parents quickly develop the ability to judge from the quality of their infant's crying whether he or she is hungry, needs to be changed, is frightened, or wants to be held, and soon after that, at around 6 months of age, the baby begins producing consonant–vowel (CV) syllables called **babbling**, which seems to consist of experimenting with sounds, although no real words are produced. When babies begin babbling, their conversations with their parents change (Polloway et al., 2012). They begin to imitate their parents and eventually to initiate conversations with them. During this period, babies develop considerable skill at communicating nonverbally to get what they want. As their mobility and motor abilities increase, they become adept at combining pointing, body gestures, and vocalizations to get adults to respond. They communicate their desires for more juice, a cookie, a visit to a grandparent's, or a hug. As most parents know well, babies in this period develop clear abilities to communicate interrogatives (i.e., questions) and negation.

Toward the end of the prelinguistic period of development, children begin expressing different **communicative intentions**

1. to seek attention or conversational interaction;
2. to request something;
3. to protest or reject something;
4. to respond to or acknowledge something; and
5. to inform their conversational partner of something.

They express these intentions through a combination of babbling, intonation patterns, and body and facial gestures.

As mentioned, another development at the end of this period is that children begin to express both negation and **interrogative forms**. Negation usually takes the form of a clear "No!" while their interrogative forms utilize rising intonation, as in "Go?" or "Eat?"

Emerging Language Period

Language Use/Pragmatics

Children in the emerging language stage communicate verbally with greater and greater frequency as they develop, engaging in conversations that increasingly take into consideration what the listener already knows or needs to know. Children become better able to ask for information in order to learn about the world, let the listener know that his or her message was received, and respond appropriately to someone's request for information (Polloway et al., 2012).

At the beginning of the emerging language stage, adults have to do most of the conversational work because children assume everyone else knows exactly what they know, what they are thinking, and what they mean in their communication. Even though children become better able to understand that others do not know what they know (and to adjust their communication accordingly), they still have difficulty providing enough information for listeners who do not know them well.

Turn taking, a crucial aspect of successful communication, has its foundation in the earliest give-and-take "conversations" mothers and fathers have with their babies. Joint attending and joint referencing provide early opportunities for babies to learn the rudiments of turn taking, and by the time they reach 18 months of age, most demonstrate basic turn-taking rules in their conversations (Bloom, Rocissano, & Hood, 1976). However, their turn-taking abilities continue to develop well into the elementary school years.

During the emerging language period, the frequency of children's attempts at communicating more than double between 18 and 24 months (Paul, 2007). During these attempts, verbal communication becomes more frequent than nonverbal, which allows us to observe what Polloway et al. (2012) call "an increased sophistication in their communicative intentions and their abilities to take the listener into consideration during conversation" (p. 22). Children's communicative intentions expand so that, in addition to those they used during the prelinguistic period, they can now use communication to

- name something (e.g., "door," "car," "cup");
- comment, for instance, by noticing an attribute of something ("big"), possession ("mine"), location ("here");
- request something that is not physically present (e.g., "car" to indicate a toy in another room); and
- protest or reject with words in addition to "no" (e.g., "ick," "bad").

Another major development during the emerging language period is that children's awareness of the social-interactive requirements of conversations increases. For instance, they become able to acknowledge to a conversational partner that they understood what their partner has just said by nodding or repeating all or part of what was said. Also, by the end of the emerging language period, most children are able to respond appropriately to questions and provide information a conversational partner requests, and can clarify what they're talking about.

Children begin producing two-word phrases around 18 months of age, which marks a leap in the ability to communicate about relationships rather than being limited to referring to one thing at a time.

Content/Semantics

The emerging language period begins when children start using one-word utterances and ends when they begin using two-word phrases. For most children, their first words name important people, objects, or processes, for example, "Mama," "Dada," "da" (for "dog"), and "ee" (for "eat"). At first, their vocabulary is relatively limited; they use one word to refer to several objects or processes, for instance, saying "da" whenever they see any animal with four legs. Gradually, however, their vocabulary increases. Around 12 months of age, they can understand 20 different words, but by the time they reach 24 months, their vocabulary has increased to approximately 200 words (Gillam & Bedore, 2000).

Syntax

Syntax in the emerging language stage remains relatively simple. Children's earliest syntactic structures are single words, accompanied by gestures, facial expressions, and intonation. At the end of this stage, they begin using two-word combinations, which are limited in the syntactic structure they can incorporate.

The most typical kinds of syntactic constructions children demonstrate in their two-word phrases include the following:

- Agent + Action (*Car go*)
- Agent + Location (*Cup table*)
- Action + Location (*Go home*)
- Agent + Object (*Girl dress*)

During the emerging language stage, interrogatives and negations expand into two-word phrases. Negation is typically expressed by saying "No" and naming whatever is to be negated (e.g., "No coat," meaning, "I don't want to put my coat on!"). Questions are usually indicated through rising intonation, as in, "Go Nanny's?" meaning, "Can we go to grandmother's?"

Phonology

Children's phonological abilities develop well into elementary school age, and children in the emerging language stage exhibit wide variations in their phonological systems. Perhaps the most notable is that most children choose phonological forms that are obviously not adult forms, but they use them consistently so that their conversational partners recognize their meaning. For instance, when I was small, I was unable to say my name and called myself "Leelaw," which my family understood to mean "Lynda." Similarly, unable to say "Granddad," I called my grandfather "Lanlad" long enough that everyone in my family adopted it as his nickname.

Although children's phonological abilities change considerably during the emerging language stage, the phonemes they are able to use consistently vary tremendously among them. Gillam and Bedore (2000) report that the first set of phonemes acquired by most children by age 3 is /m, b, n, w, d, p, h/. During this stage, children's word choices are somewhat dependent on the phonemes they can produce readily.

During this stage, children tend to simplify adult phonological forms, a process known as **phonological processes**. Gillam and Bedore (2000) found that the most common of these phonological processes in children between 2 and 3 years of age are

- deleting unaccented syllables (e.g., "Saturday" becomes /ˈsædeɪ/ "Saa-day");
- deleting final consonants (e.g., "dog" becomes /dɑ/ "Da"); and
- velar fronting, or the substituting of frontal sounds such as /t/ and /d/ (which are velar stops) for back stops /k/ and /g/, as in /tʌp/ "tup" for /kʌp/ "cup."

Developing Language Period

The developing language stage in typically developing children begins at around 27 months and extends until about 46 months. During this period, children's language develops rapidly, elaborating on structures and competencies acquired during the emerging language stage. By the time children are around 4 years of age, they have acquired most of the basic structures of language, which they will refine and fine-tune as they enter the educational process and begin using their language abilities to learn in school.

Pragmatics

During the developing language stage, children become much better at engaging in conversations, which means that their adult conversational partners have to do less work to keep the conversation going. By the end of this stage of development, children can take turns conversing over several turns, and they interrupt less. They also understand when their listener doesn't know what they're talking about and can make adjustments and provide more information. Their initial attempts at revising or repairing something for a listener may not actually result in a clarification the listener can use, but children become more adept at clarification toward the end of the period.

Early in this stage, children's ability to take turns during conversations remains relatively basic, and they can stay on the same topic for only one or two conversational turns (Polloway et al., 2012). They do not hesitate to interrupt their conversational partners and conclude that any falling intonation indicates the end of an utterance and, therefore, an opportunity to begin speaking. Later in this stage, children become able to wait longer before they begin speaking, but if they hear a relatively long pause, they will initiate their turn to speak (Polloway et al., 2012).

Throughout this developmental period, children make significant gains in their ability to provide clarification if a conversational partner doesn't understand something they have said—a process known as **conversational repair**. Their repairs become considerably more relevant as they gain an understanding of what their conversational partners already know and what they don't know—known as **presuppositions**, which affects what and how much the child must say in order to be understood.

One of the most interesting aspects of children's pragmatics during this stage is their increasing ability to make indirect, as opposed to direct, requests. At the end of the emerging language stage, most children who want something say, for instance, "I want more milk." During the developing language stage, children learn to soften their requests by becoming less direct, saying, for example, "I need more milk" or "I want more juice, please." These less direct requests are correlated with what are considered polite forms, the indirect language that social groups have developed for saying what one wants, thinks, believes, or desires. Without the ability to use polite forms, children may be regarded as rude, unintelligent, arrogant, or disrespectful.

While children's conversational discourse abilities show significant changes during this stage of development, they also begin learning about another form of discourse, narrative discourse, the language of stories. Stories and storytelling exist in all cultures and begin appearing in children's communication in the developing language stage. By the end of this period, children begin telling stories with fictional elements, and they begin retelling their own experiences using a narrative format. The earliest stories children tell usually take the form of a **basic episode**, which consists of an initiating event (some problem that begins the action), followed by an attempt by a character to solve the problem, and a consequence, or resolution of the problem. The ability to engage in narrative thinking and expression becomes especially important when children enter school and are expected to understand stories and produce stories of their own.

Syntax and Morphology

Syntax. One of the most dramatic developments during the developing language stage is children's syntax. At the beginning of the period, children's syntax is defined primarily by two-word phrases. By the end of the period, their language includes sentences with adjectives, prepositional phrases, and subordinate clauses. These more complicated sentences include inverted word forms for interrogatives ("Is she eating?"); tag questions ("You're the mama now, OK?"); conjoined clauses, usually with *and*; and embedded relative clauses ("That's the bike he rode"; Hulit & Howard, 2006).

Once children begin embedding clauses, they are able to express more complicated relationships than they were able to express using only added modifiers (e.g., adjectives, such as "big," "scary," "blue"). One type of embedding that appears during this developmental stage is the use of **prepositional phrases**, such as "in the box," "over the bridge," "on the desk," "in front of the car."

Morphology. Children in the developing language stage begin using morphological markers to refine word meanings, adding -s to *dog*, for example, to indicate more than one, or adding -*ing* to *eat*, to indicate present tense. As children learn the rules for morphological markers, they tend to overgeneralize them to those tricky irregular words, saying things like "eated," "drived," and "mouses." First they learn the rules; later they learn the exceptions, a process that lasts well into elementary school.

The earliest morphemes children acquire during this stage are the plural marker *-s* to mark more than one ("The kid<u>s</u> are playing"), the possessive marker *-s* to indicate possession ("The teacher'<u>s</u> desk"), and the progressive *-ing* to indicate ongoing action ("The cat is purr<u>ing</u>"; Gillam & Bedore, 2000). Soon after these markers appear in a child's speech, two additional markers emerge: the third-person singular verb morpheme *-s* ("The man sit<u>s</u>") and the past-tense marker *ed* ("The kids walk<u>ed</u> to school"). In the last part of this stage, children begin using the **copula** ("Daddy <u>is</u> hungry") and the "to be" verb forms ("The cat <u>is</u> purring").

Learning the exceptions to morphemic rules (e.g., irregular past tense, as in "ate" and "drove"; irregular plurals, e.g., "mice," "children," "sheep") takes time. Although most children manage to learn some of the exceptions during the developing language stage, many continue learning them well into the next developmental stage.

Figurative Language

When children first enter the developing language stage, most of them understand only that language exists on one level—the literal. They use language in a relatively direct and efficient manner, and what they say is exactly what they mean. As their abilities emerge, however, they discover that words and phrases can be separated from the things they represent and thus come to mean something else entirely. For instance, they discover that different things in the world can have the same name (e.g., several people with the name "José" or "Mary"), that one thing can have several names (e.g., "table," "buffet," "counter"), that several things can have names that sound the same (e.g., "pair," "pear," "pare"), and that some words have more than one meaning (e.g., "sweet," "warm," "bad").

During the developing language stage, children become increasingly aware of the metaphoric aspect of language. Among the first **metaphors** they understand and use are idioms. Idioms are sayings that on the figurative level mean something entirely different from what the actual words imply. For instance, *straight from the horse's mouth* means *from a dependable source* in some areas of the English-speaking world, but the *dependable source* is nowhere implicit or explicit in any of the words: *straight*, *horse's*, or *mouth*. Children in the developing language period learn, first, that there are such things as idioms (though they may not have any idea what these funny sayings are called) and, later, what some of them are. In fact, children may learn an idiom as a literal phrase, not knowing, for example, that *hang* in *hang out* has any meaning separate from the entire phrase.

Children's verbal humor begins to appear during the developmental language stage, although they do not become fully adept until they are between 8 and 10 years old. Among the first humorous forms to appear are knock-knock jokes and riddles, both of which first appear as unfunny routines in which the child learns the general format and only later develops the ability to juggle the demands of the format and the content. Box 3.3 provides examples of children's developing abilities with

---

BOX 3.3   Examples of Children Retelling a Joke

4-year-old Sue Ann's knock-knock joke:

> Sue Ann: Knock, knock.
>   Mom: Who's there?
> Sue Ann: Sue Ann! [laughs with glee]

4-year-old Brian and 5-year-old Sid are told the following riddle on Halloween:

> Adult: Why didn't the skeleton cross the road?
> Both boys: Why?
> Adult: Because he didn't have the guts. [Both boys laugh knowingly.]

Here's how each boy retold the riddle to his parents:

> Brian: Why didn't the skeleton cross the road?
> Parents: Why not?
> Brian: Because he fell down [laughs].
>   Sid: Why didn't the skeleton cross the road?
> Parents: Why?
>   Sid: He, he . . . [rubs his stomach] . . . he was afraid.

In this example, Brian clearly understood and could use the riddle format, and he may even have understood the double meaning of "guts." However, he was unable to tell the riddle using the double-meaning word. Sid, by rubbing his stomach, showed that he understood that "guts" can refer to stomach, and saying "he was afraid" indicates he knows that "guts" also refers to fear. He is developmentally closer to being able to manipulate both the riddle format and the double-meaning content.

---

knock-knock jokes and riddles. Table 3.1 summarizes the primary characteristics of language development at this stage.

The Language of Learning Period

Between the time most children enter the formal schooling process in kindergarten or first grade and leave for middle school or junior high, their language continues to develop at a rapid pace. Their language expands and becomes more complicated and precise as they shift from learning language to using their language to learn in the classroom. Their burgeoning language skills shift from oral language to reading, writing, figurative language, and narrative and expository discourse. During this stage of development, children are expected to make what Westby (1991) called the *oral-to-literate shift,* making the transition from using language primarily as a means to regulate social interactions and communicate in face-to-face conversations to using language as a vehicle for regulating thought, constructing abstract ideas, communicating over time and distance, and reflecting. Making this oral-to-literate

TABLE 3.1. Primary Characteristics of Developing Language

	Emerging language stage: Birth–26 months	Developing language stage: 27–46 months
Syntax and morphology	• Expands from first word to 2-word combinations • Expands use of declaratives, interrogatives, imperatives, and negatives into 2-word utterances	• Begins using morphological markers to indicate grammatical meanings (e.g., using -s to indicate plurality) • Learns most of the syntactic structures
Phonology	• Does not yet use adult forms but is consistent in the forms used	• Develops almost all the phonemes in language; fine-tuning still to come
Semantics	• Expands vocabulary knowledge and use significantly: uses approximately 20 words at the beginning of this stage to over 200 at the end	• Expands vocabulary comprehension and use significantly: uses approximately 200 words at the beginning of the stage to more than 1,800 at the end; understands somewhere between 3,000 and 4,000 words at the end
Pragmatics	• Uses few (if any) indirect speech acts • Has little ability to take the listener's perspective • Has limited ability to respond appropriately to requests for clarification • Becomes increasingly adept at turn taking in conversations	• Extends turn taking over several turns during a conversation • Requires listeners to do less work to keep the conversation going • Begins using indirect speech acts (e.g., polite forms and softeners)
Figurative language	• Does not understand figurative language forms	• Begins using nonliteral language forms such as idioms and colloquialisms • Begins to use verbal humor
Discourse	• Does not yet combine words into larger units to tell stories or explain/describe things	• Begins using basic story-telling abilities (although most children in this stage cannot tell a complete story)

shift depends on the oral language abilities children develop earlier in pragmatics, semantics, syntax, morphology, phonology, figurative language, and writing.

Pragmatics

Conversational competence. Children's conversational competence during the school-age years increases significantly. They become more proficient at taking turns during conversations with several other people, they learn how to interrupt appropriately, and they learn how to signal their readiness for taking and yielding turns. Their ability to clarify when their listeners don't understand also improves enough that they can use their listener's request for clarification as a guide for exactly how to repair (i.e., clarify) their previous sentences.

Indirect requests become much more frequent when children enter school, largely as a function of their discerning that they have a much better chance at getting what they want if they utilize less direct (i.e., polite) forms. After around age 8, most children have developed enough facility with indirect requests to know which ones to use with each listener.

Learning polite forms is tied to a child's development in understanding that language exists on several levels (described in an earlier section on metalinguistic ability), and that what one says is not always exactly what one means. For instance, in many cultures, people greet each other by saying some version of "Hi, how are you?" The response is usually "Fine" or "Doing well," even though that may or may not be true. Consider your own behavior when you're greeting a casual acquaintance (we often suspend polite forms with close friends). How often have you wanted to say, "I feel horrid!" even as you respond in the appropriate, socially sanctioned way? Another example of people saying one thing and meaning another is when an adult will ask a child a question but what he or she really intends is to give a direction. For instance, the adult might say to the child, "Do you want to look at this book?" when what he really means is, "Look at this book." Children in this stage begin to understand these subtle social language skills.

Narrative development. As I noted earlier, when children enter school, the stories they tell are not yet true narratives because, although they contain a basic episode, their stories do not yet include what is considered a complete story episode that includes the main character's feelings or intentions regarding what is happening in the story; the main character's plan about what to do and why; and a reaction or ending that shows the character's reaction to the consequence of the story (Miller, Gillam, & Peña, 2001). However, around the age of 7, most children begin including plots, usually undeveloped at first, and then, later, after about age 8, their narratives begin to resemble adult stories.

Expository discourse. Unlike narrative discourse, expository discourse has as its main objective explaining or describing something or presenting an argument intended to persuade the listener or reader of something. The language used in expository discourse is usually **decontextualized**, that is, removed from the here and now, and the internal structure of expository language is very different from the structure of most narratives. Table 3.2 shows the basic structure of common types of expository discourse.

The "Metas." During the school-age years, children develop not only metalinguistic skills, but also a set of **metapragmatic and metacognitive abilities**.

As I mentioned in an earlier section, when children enter elementary school, many academic tasks require that they reflect on and talk about language (metalinguistic ability), how language is used (metapragmatic ability), and how they themselves think and reason (metacognitive ability).

TABLE 3.2. Classroom Discourse Types and Characteristics

Classroom discourse: Lecture & giving directions	Classroom narratives: Story-based	Expository: Explanation & description	Argumentative/Persuasive
• Teacher chooses topic • Teacher takes most of the turns • Teacher determines: □ whether student talks □ when student talks □ how long student talks □ when student should relinquish a turn □ if student's response is correct • Follow IRE format: □ Teacher Initiates the topic □ Student Responds □ Teacher Evaluates student's response • Language often decontextualized • Requires metalinguistic skill	• Follows a story grammar • Contains setting, characters, and episodes • Predictable language and form • Highly contextualized language • Sequence = plot driven • Information familiar to student	• Decontextualized language: □ states facts □ states hypotheses □ asks questions □ draws conclusions □ interprets □ classifies □ synthesizes □ summarizes □ hierarchic organization • Paragraph format: □ topic sentence stating main idea □ clincher sentence summarizing main idea • Abstract cause–effect • Enumerative • Comparison–contrast • Sequence = logical • Information new to student • Requires metalinguistic skills	• Takes others' perspectives & viewpoints • Puts forward a fact or statement as proof or evidence • Expresses disagreement • Uses a set of statements so that one follows logically as a conclusion from the others: □ a statement of fact □ a set of supports for the fact OR □ a set of supports for a fact □ a statement of fact derived from the supports □ a statement of belief □ a set of reasons the belief is "true" OR □ a set of reasons a belief is "true" □ a statement of belief • Requires skill with the "metas"

Note. Adapted from *Language Instruction for Students With Disabilities* (4th ed.), by E. A. Polloway, L. Miller, and T. E. C. Smith, 2012, Denver, CO: Love. Copyright 2012 by Love. Adapted with permission.

A large number of prereading activities present metalinguistic challenges, especially to children who may be struggling with language learning in the first place. Polloway et al. (2012) listed six sets of reading and prereading activities that require metalinguistic ability:

1. defining words
2. identifying **homonyms**, **synonyms**, and **antonyms**
3. recognizing **homophones** and subsequent semantic ambiguity
4. identifying syntactic and morphological elements in sentences
5. diagramming sentences
6. and matching sounds to letters. (p. 47)

When children consciously think or talk about the behaviors and choices they make regarding how they are using language, they are demonstrating metapragmatic ability. Their metapragmatic abilities grow as they become able to attend to their listeners' perspectives and prior knowledge (and consequent conversational needs), engage in different types of conversations (e.g., explanations, descriptions, reports, disagreements, arguments, persuasion, benign teasing), and engage successfully in classroom discourse. They are reflecting on and talking about their use of language, which is more abstract than merely using language without reflection.

Beginning around third grade, students shift from learning to read to reading to learn. At the same time, they are asked to develop metacognitive skills, or the ability to reflect on and assess how they think and learn. One aspect of metacognitive skill is students' ability to recognize when they do not understand or have questions about what they are learning. Before the age of 8, children usually know when they do not understand something, but they have not yet developed a strategy for remedying their lack of understanding. After age 8, most children know they can ask for something to be repeated; can look for clues in the context of what is being said or what they are reading; reason logically about the sequence of events to figure out what comes next; or see if the teacher has provided the information in another form (e.g., on a laptop or tablet; Polloway et al., 2012).

Another aspect of metacognitive skill is the ability to organize oneself for learning, which involves the following:

1. Knowing strategies for learning and when to employ each one according to the contextual demands of the learning environment (e.g., "What is required for me to learn in this situation? Do I have everything I need? Have I had trouble before with this kind of task? If so, what can I do differently this time?").
2. Taking the steps necessary to analyze the results of a given learning strategy (e.g., "Did this approach to the learning task work? Did I learn what I need to learn? Do I need to try a different approach? Should I double-check my results?").

3. Recognizing when one needs to ask for help (e.g., "I've used all the approaches I know, but I still don't understand. Who is available and likely to help? Which questions do I need to ask to get help that is relevant and to the point?").

Semantic Development

Vocabulary development, which showed a significant increase during the developing language stage, continues during the school-age years. Most children during this period are exposed to increasing amounts of print, and their vocabulary development reflects their interactions with print. Children during this period learn to use words they already know in new ways, to differentiate among words with similar meanings, to select among many words the one that is best suited for their purpose, and to use the same word to mean different things in different contexts (Polloway et al., 2012).

Vocabulary development at this age includes homonyms, antonyms, and synonyms (which also require metalinguistic abilities, as I described in an earlier section). Much of this ability stems from their developing competency in reading as they encounter words used in ways that do not occur in oral language usage.

Two important semantic developments during this period are learning to classify words and learning the English pronoun system. Children first begin classifying words during the developing language stage into categories such as "animals," "runny things," "people I know," and "things I have experienced." At the end of that stage and into the beginning of the language-for-learning development period, children begin elaborating their categories to include, for instance, "wild animals," "animals likely to be at a zoo," "pets," and "extinct animals." These elaborations form hierarchical subcategories, which continue to develop into and through adulthood. Box 3.4 contains an exercise that lets you explore how you think about and categorize words.

The pronoun system is one of the few holdovers from Old English (i.e., Anglo-Saxon) still in general use in English. Old English, like many other Romance and Teutonic languages, used a declension system to differentiate gender (masculine, feminine, neutral), person (first, second, third), position in the sentence (nominative, possessive, objective, or reflexive), and singular and plural. Table 3.3 shows the modern English pronoun system, on which children in the developing language stage begin to elaborate. Children vary widely in their pronoun usage, some becoming consistent in their use of pronouns referring to self and not so consistent with pronouns referring to others. Other children will demonstrate just the opposite, or they will develop consistency using first- and second-person pronouns but not third-person. By the end of the developing language stage, typically developing children have mastered most of the pronouns, though not all, and their pronoun systems will generally reflect their unique approaches to figuring things out.

BOX 3.4 **Categorizing Words**

1. List as many categories as you can to describe how you classify animals. Don't think about it before you start; just write down the categories that come to mind. Here are the categories I listed without any planning:

wild	free	beautiful	ugly
domesticated	nonmammals	slow	slimy
four-legged	insects	striped	whiskered
feline	arachnids	multicolored	spotted
canine	two-legged	smart	speedy
equine	slithery	mammals	vertebrates
feathered	graceful	reptilian	invertebrates

Notice that my list is simply an associative list rather than a hierarchically arranged system. Do your categories fit into a hierarchical system? What would be the main categories?

2. Now think about how you categorize words themselves. List as many categories of words as you can without any planning. Here are the categories I thought of without any planning:

nouns	verbs	pronouns	adverbs
adjectives	prepositions	gerunds	participles
articles	proper nouns	locatives	interrogatives
imperatives	indicatives	negatives	names
modifiers	antecedents	conjunctions	predicates
antonyms	synonyms	homonyms	contractions
interjections	collectives	abbreviations	portmanteaus

You can tell from my list that I've probably studied language and know the names of some types of words you've never heard of! Not to worry—look at your list and think how you could arrange the types of words into a hierarchical system. What would be the main categories?

Syntax

Because children have learned most of the syntactic structures of English in the developing language stage, their syntactic development once they enter school consists primarily of expanding on the forms they have already learned. In addition, they gradually acquire most of the more difficult forms. Polloway et al. (2012) described several syntactic processes typical of children in the school-age language learning period.

TABLE 3.3. English Pronouns

		Singular			Plural		
		1st	**2nd**	**3rd**	**1st**	**2nd**	**3rd**
Subjective	Female	she	you			you	
	Male	he	you			you	
	Neutral	I*		it, one	we*		they
Possessive	Female	her, hers	your, yours			your	
	Male	his	your, yours				your
	Neutral	my, mine*		its, one's	our*		their, theirs
Objective	Female	her	you			you	
	Male	him	you				you
	Neutral	me*		it, one	us*		them
Reflexive	Female	herself	yourself			yourselves	
	Male	himself	yourself			yourselves	
	Neutral	myself*		itself, oneself	themselves*		themselves

*Self-referring pronouns are assumed to carry the gender of the person using them.

1. *Expanding noun and verb phrases.* Children in this stage expand their noun and verb phrases through the addition of more adjectives and adverbs and through incorporating more prepositional phrases (e.g., "We went *into the mall* yesterday") and subordinate clauses (e.g. "We went to the store *that has the cool shoes*"). During this stage children also fine-tune their usage of irregular plural and tense markers (e.g., *deer, mice, cattle, sheep; ate, drove, swam*), and they include articles appropriately (e.g., "*The* big dog barked at me" when the listener knows which dog is being referred to; "*A* big dog barked at me" when the listener does *not* know the specific dog). Box 3.5 tells the story of two 12-year-olds who experienced a "eureka" moment about verb-tense markers, one example of the fine-tuning that continues throughout childhood and into adolescence.

2. *Decoding passive sentences.* Passive sentence constructions present special difficulties because the order of the words is opposite the order of the events being described, a cognitive mismatch that children at the beginning of this stage are unable to decipher. During this stage, children first figure out how to understand and use *nonreversible passives*, which are sentences in which the meaning can be expressed only one way. For example, "The mouse was eaten by the cat" is nonreversible since it is extremely unlikely that a mouse could eat a cat, which would be the case if the sentence was "The cat was eaten by the mouse." Later in this period of development, children understand and use *reversible passives*, sentences

---

BOX 3.5 **Dennis Figures Out "Have Tooken"**

I began my professional career as a junior high school English teacher in Westminster, Colorado, where I taught seventh- and eighth-grade English language arts and English literature. Dennis, a bright seventh-grade student, had learned Spanish and English simultaneously in a family of migrant workers. He was adept at both languages and used a vernacular speech style in both.

At the end of Dennis's sixth-grade school year, his family had moved into the area on a more permanent basis because his father had gotten a year-round job. When Dennis entered seventh grade, he discovered that he liked to read, an activity he hadn't had much opportunity to explore outside school.

I noticed that in his oral speech, Dennis (and several other students) would say things like "I've *tooken* the book to the library" or "My mom and dad have *tooken* the car to the garage." When we began studying past participles in English class, I had the students practice writing sentences using "have taken" to see if Dennis would figure out that the "standard" past participle of "take" was "have taken."

For a period of several weeks, none of the students remarked on "have taken" or "have tooken," and they continued using "have tooken" in their oral language. Then, one day when the students were reading during free time, Dennis came up to where I was sitting and excitedly pointed to a sentence in the book he was reading. "Miss Miller, guess what I just learned!" Thinking he'd read about an interesting event or idea, I asked him what it was. "You can't say 'have tooken'! This guy keeps saying stuff like, 'I've taken the kids to the store,' and 'He's taken the book to school.' Nobody says 'tooken'!"

When I asked him what had caught his attention about "have tooken," he said he didn't know and that it had just started to sound funny to him. When the students were sharing their new learning after their free period, Dennis excitedly shared his new knowledge with his classmates. Mark, another student whose language included "have tooken," was taken aback because he, too, suddenly realized he had been using a form that didn't coincide with the standard English usage. Both boys continued to point out examples of "have tooken" when they heard them, although not all their classmates were entirely happy having their language usage scrutinized.

The story illustrates how the finer points of language usage continue developing well into late childhood and adolescence, particularly for children who are bilingual.

---

in which the meaning can be expressed with either of two word orders. For instance, because either "The girl was chased by the dog" or "The dog was chased by the girl" is possible, the word order doesn't help children in their attempts to decode the sentence.

3. *Embedding.* Embedded phrases can encode a variety of complicated relationships. One of the first syntactic strategies children learn is to use word order as a primary cue for understanding sentences. To interpret a sentence, children assume that the order of words reflects the order of the events or relationships being described. Hence, they understand a

sentence such as "The girl who won the election is my sister" as meaning something like "The girl won the election. That girl is my sister." Later in this stage of development, children begin to understand that some sentences cannot be relied on to provide clues to their meaning through word order alone. Children come to realize that a sentence such as "The girl the dog bit ran away" means that the girl ran home, not the dog.

4. *Conjoining.* Children at the beginning of the school-age language stage are able to manipulate straightforward conjoined sentences, most typically those with *and.* During this period, they develop proficiency with the other conjunctions as well. First, they develop the ability to express cause–effect conjunctions, such as "We came inside *because* it was raining." Next, they begin using conjunctions that express a contrastive relationship, such as "It was raining, *but* we didn't get wet." Later, as their cognitive understanding develops, they are able to use constructions using conditional conjunctions, such as "*If* I do all my chores, I can go to the movie."

Sentences that do not express things in a logical order are more difficult for children to grasp; thus, they develop in children's language later in this period. For instance, putting the effect in front of the cause, as in, "He was late *because* he missed the bus," does not follow the "logical" order of the cause, missing the bus, followed by the effect, being late. Facility with sentences that are "illogical" develops at the end of this stage, at around 10 or 11 years of age.

Morphology

Like syntax, morphology during the school-age language stage becomes a process of learning aspects of English morphology that elaborate on linguistic relationships to further extend their meaning. One example is learning how to produce *gerunds,* which are verbs turned into nouns by adding *-ing* (e.g., *build–building*). Another example of a morphological elaboration that occurs in the school-age language stage is learning to add *-er* to a verb in order to identify the person as the one engaged in the action of the verb (e.g., *paint–painter*). At the beginning of this period, children typically add the *-er* ending to every verb to produce this *agentive* effect (e.g., *type–typer,* or *draw–drawer*). By the end of this stage, children have learned which of these forms are correct in usage and which are not. A third example of a morphological elaboration occurring in this stage of development is forming adverbs by adding *-ly* to adjectives (e.g., *slow–slowly*). By the end of the stage, children have figured out the special cases in which adding *-ly* does not work, as in *fast.*

Phonology and Phonological Awareness

Early in the language of learning development period, children's use of phonology is fine-tuned. Typically developing students can produce all phonemes correctly by approximately age 7. Once children enter school, **phonological awareness** skills become necessary in order to begin learning **phonics**, which includes

- identifying rhyming words,
- counting syllables in words,
- segmenting words into syllables and sounds, and
- matching speech sounds to letters (i.e., **graphophonemic awareness**).

Most children acquire these phonological awareness skills by age 8, although some children require more time and may experience difficulty learning to read and write because both depend on these metalinguistic abilities.

Figurative Language

Figurative language, which emerges in the developing language stage, becomes more frequent—as well as more fluent—in children's language during the language of learning period. Children's interactions with print through both reading and writing provide encounters with various forms of figurative language and afford opportunities for them to develop facility with figurative language they might not develop if they don't read.

Children's ability to manipulate idioms increases considerably during this period, especially after age 7 or 8, when their abilities to understand the multiple levels of language seem to spurt. They begin understanding that idiomatic expressions are best understood not literally, but in a more abstract (i.e., figurative) manner. Where earlier a child might envision cats and dogs pouring down from the sky when someone said, "It's raining cats and dogs," now he or she understands that the phrase offers a humorous way to depict a particularly hard storm.

During this period, children encounter metaphors and **similes**, and develop an understanding that each is a particular way of comparing two ideas, events, people, feelings, or experiences. A metaphor implies a comparison between two dissimilar things (e.g., "She's a sunbeam," meaning she's cheerful), while a simile is an explicit comparison (e.g., "She's like a sunbeam"). Children also become more adept with **proverbs**, **adages**, and **maxims** such as "A penny saved is a penny earned" or "Don't bite the hand that feeds you."

Children's humor continues to develop during this stage (and long after) as they become more proficient with juggling different levels of meaning to produce punchlines. By age 9 or so, children have developed the ability to utilize multiple meanings of words in order to tell jokes that are actually funny, as in this riddle: "Why do leopards have a hard time hiding?" "Because they're always spotted."

Writing

Writing during the school-age years develops almost directly from children's oral language skills and from their emerging reading abilities (Polloway et al., 2012). When children first begin writing, their writing ability is considerably less well developed than their oral language abilities, but, as their reading becomes more fluent, their writing usually follows. Therefore, children who experience difficulties learning to read will likely experience similar difficulties in their writing.

Most writing in elementary school is done in response to teacher assignments or emerges from a particular child's enthusiasm for writing. Sometime around fourth grade, children are expected to use their writing abilities to write for people other than themselves and their teachers. For instance, students may be asked to write to further a cause in their community, solicit information from a local business, or thank a visitor for coming to their classroom.

Children from homes in which writing and print are available and used as part of everyday life often arrive at school with the ability to write their own names and a few additional words, usually the names of others in their household. These children usually possess what is called *graphophonemic awareness*, the ability to associate letters of the alphabet with speech sounds. They know that print is speech written down and often play with "writing" squiggles, lines, and shapes along a line that suggests the linearity of print. As children explore and experiment with writing, they gradually gain mastery over their writing and begin trying new forms, such as poems, letters, or short essays.

While in the lower elementary grades children's writing is usually story based, in the upper elementary grades, they start writing basic expository discourse (i.e., book reports, short descriptive or explanatory passages, and brief arguments in favor of or against a cause or program). As their reading skills continue to develop, their writing ability increases in complexity as well. The writing of children who read fluently in the upper elementary grades is typically more sophisticated than their oral language. Table 3.4 summarizes the primary characteristics of school-age language development.

Adolescent Language Development

Larson and McKinley (2003) have described adolescence as unfolding across three stages, each of which can be characterized according to the developmental tasks and stages that are unique to adolescence. Table 3.5 shows their characterizations for the early, middle, and late stages of adolescence.

Language development during adolescence marks the transition from childhood to adulthood. The forms, contexts, and styles of language used by adolescents accompany a reduced reliance on family and the increasing importance of friends, music, popular culture, mobile devices, movies, and the Internet. According to Paul (2007), typically developing adolescents extend the language competencies they have already learned for use in

- peer social interactions, which are often intensive;
- literate contexts, such as debate, presentations, and written discourse; and
- critical thinking.

TABLE 3.4. Primary Characteristics of the Language of Learning Stage of Development: 4–11 Years

Syntax and morphology	• Expands syntactic structures already in use • Learns the most difficult syntactic forms, including passives, conjoining, and embedded phrases • Uses the most complex and least frequent morphological markers, such as gerunds, agent *-er*, and adjectives
Phonology and phonological awareness	• Becomes able to use all phonemes appropriately • Develops phonological awareness skills, such as rhyming, syllableness, and matching speech sounds to letters
Semantics	• Continues expansion of vocabulary, which is now influenced by rapidly improving reading skills • Elaborates classification of words • Masters most of the English pronouns
Pragmatics	• Becomes proficient in turn taking • Understands subtle social language rules • Interrupts appropriately • Develops metapragmatic ability • Uses conversational repair strategies • Follows classroom pragmatics • Uses indirect requests
Figurative language	• Develops the ability to use more sophisticated figurative language forms (e.g., metaphors, similes, proverbs, adages, maxims) • Becomes more proficient with different levels of meaning used in humor
Discourse	• Makes the oral-to-literate shift, from being primarily oral to being able to understand and use written language • Becomes aware of audience (both oral and written) and develops the ability to speak or write from that perspective • Becomes able to tell complete stories • Develops the ability to understand and use various forms of expository discourse, though this continues to develop throughout adolescence and young adulthood
Writing	• Uses writing skills that reflect the development of reading skills (i.e., the better the student reads, the better he or she will write) • Becomes able to write complete stories, poems, letters

Because language development after the childhood years is not as immediately obvious as the development that occurs during the preschool and elementary school years, it is easy to think that not much development is actually taking place. However, those who study language development in older children and adolescents have shown that two crucial aspects of language development occur during this period: (1) the development of meta-awareness about one's own thinking, speaking, listening, and writing and (2) the development of skills in written language. Adolescent development is characterized by growth in their metalinguistic, metacognitive, and

TABLE 3.5. Development of the Cognitive Patterns of Typical Adolescence

Early (10–13 years females; 12–14 males)	Middle (13–16 years)	Late (16–20 years)
• Concrete operational thought: present more real than future; concrete more real than abstract • Egocentrism • Personal fable • Imaginary audience	• Emerging formal operations: abstraction, hypotheses, and thinking about future; personal interests and identity emerge	• Formal operations: thinking about the future, things as they should be, and options; consequences can be considered

Note. Adapted from *Communication Solutions for Older Students* (p. 36), by V. L. Larson and N. L. McKinley, 2003, Austin, TX: PRO-ED. Copyright 2003 by PRO-ED, Inc. Adapted with permission.

metapragmatic abilities. The metalinguistic skills adolescents need include being able to analyze, reorganize, synthesize, and talk about both oral and printed language. Writing puts a particularly heavy demand on adolescents' metalinguistic skills because it cannot be done effectively without reflecting on and manipulating various aspects of language and language levels. Adolescents must develop metacognitive skills in order to understand and comprehend information; organize information and materials; reflect on their own learning processes and skills; and monitor themselves as they progress through the curriculum. To develop facility with written discourse, for instance, adolescents need to develop competence in outlining logical hierarchies; devising numerical schemes to illustrate ordinate and subordinate relationships; and construct diagrams to represent how information or ideas are related.

Larson and McKinley's (2003) summary of the contrasts, general trends, and specific trends between early and later language learning, shown in Table 3.6, describes some of the most salient characteristics of language development during this stage. The specific aspects of language development during adolescence are described in the following sections.

Pragmatics

Though some parents would disagree, I find that most adolescents are fluent conversational partners. That is, they usually understand what they need to say so listeners will understand what is being said; they know how to take turns appropriately during the conversation; they know how to repair a conversational breakdown; they can interrupt appropriately in various social contexts; and they know how to ask for clarification if they don't understand something that is being said. Of course, one of the characteristics of adolescents is that they don't always see the need to demonstrate their knowledge of appropriate pragmatic language use, especially with their parents.

TABLE 3.6. Contrasts, General Trends, and Specific Trends Between Early and Later Language Learning

	Young children	Adolescents
Contrasts	• The major goal is to acquire spoken language. • The primary source of language stimulation is spoken communication. • They learn language in nondirected, informal settings. • Language development does not require metalinguistic competency. • They are literal in their interpretations of language. • Their language and reasoning are concrete. • They do not always take others' perspectives when communicating.	• The major language goal is to acquire written communication skills. • The most significant sources of language stimulation are spoken *and* written communication. • They learn many aspects of language through formal instruction. • Metalinguistic competency is required, especially as they learn to read and write. • They demonstrate increasing ability to appreciate figurative meanings. • They are learning language and acquiring reasoning processes that are abstract. • They are aware of listeners' and readers' needs and can adjust their spoken and written messages accordingly.
General trends	• Developmental language milestones are relatively universal across children. • Language is acquired rapidly, and the changes that occur from year to year are highly visible. • Written language is not critical for communication. • First indications appear of meta-awareness (ability to think about one's own thinking, listening, and speaking performance).	• Language, thinking, and communication development is highly individual. • Changes in language knowledge are more subtle and individual. • Written language is as critical as oral communication after about fourth grade. Written communication may influence oral communication and vice versa during the preadolescent years and beyond. • Increased development of meta-awareness and the ability to revise communication performance based on evaluative feedback occur.
Specific trends	• Lexicon (word development) increases based on what the child hears. • Syntactic structure is greatly affected by the context in which the utterances occur (e.g., home, school). • Focus is on learning to read. • They can think about and operate on tangible objects and events. • Figurative language begins to emerge. • Ability to comprehend linguistic ambiguity is limited. • They are able to tell simple stories.	• Lexicon, especially word usage, improves greatly, in part as a result of reading vocabulary. Quantitatively, upon graduating from high school, the average adolescent has learned the meaning of at least 80,000 different words. • Qualitatively, old words take on new and subtle meanings, and it becomes easier to organize and reflect on the content of the word meanings. • Syntactic structure becomes more formal, complex, and complete with exposure to and experience with different discourse genres (e.g., narrative, expository).

TABLE 3.6 (*continued*)

	Young children	Adolescents
Specific trends (*continued*)		• Focus shifts from learning to read to reading to learn. • Thinking becomes more abstract. They are able to think about and operate on ideas. • Figurative language increases to include metaphors, similes, idioms, and proverbs. • They are able to understand and use linguistic ambiguity (e.g., isolated sentences, humor, advertisements). • At 7 to 11 years of age, they are producing stories with multiple, embedded narrative structures. • Between 13 and 15 years of age, they are capable of analyzing stories. • From 16 through adulthood, they are capable of more sophisticated analysis (i.e., can generalize about story meaning, formulate abstract statements about the message or theme of the story, and focus on their reaction to the story).

Note. Adapted from *Communication Solutions for Older Students: Assessment and Intervention Strategies* (pp. 53–54), by V. L. Larson and N. L. McKinley, 2003, Austin, TX: PRO-ED. Copyright 2003 by PRO-ED, Inc. Adapted with permission.

Metapragmatic ability is needed to engage in virtually all literate discourse because one must know the purpose of each type of writing, who the audience is and what they already know, which discourse genre best matches the purpose and the audience, and how to build sentences for the particular discourse genre and audience (Polloway et al., 2012).

Figurative Language and Slang

Adolescents develop considerable fluency with figurative language of various sorts. Much of adolescent humor depends on multiple meanings and levels of language, especially idioms. Adolescent slang requires a sophisticated metalinguistic ability and plays a major role in how adolescents are perceived and accepted by their peers. Polloway et al. (2012) described slang as the punctuation of teenage language. The ability to use the slang characteristic of one's peer group may be the single most important language development to occur during adolescence. Being unable to figure out how slang works and how to use it can have severe social consequences for teenagers.

Discourse

Adolescents also develop considerable expertise with the multiple types of discourse they encounter in school, both through different teaching styles manifested by multiple teachers and through the diverse expository texts they are required to read and comprehend. After children leave elementary school, they are expected to be relatively fluent with more extensive forms of expository and narrative discourse in both oral and written form.

Semantics

Vocabulary development during adolescence reflects the ever-increasing importance of the literate language forms used in writing. Paul and Norbury (2012) described adolescent vocabulary development in the following categories:

- Advanced adverbial conjuncts (e.g., *moreover, similarly, consequently, nonetheless*)
- Adverbs of likelihood (e.g., *possibly, probably, definitely, likely*) and adverbs of magnitude (e.g., *considerably, significantly, greatly*)
- Terms related to specific curriculum content (e.g., *photon, obtuse, quadrangle, axis*)
- Specific verb types, such as presuppositional (e.g., *regret*), metalinguistic (e.g., *predict, infer*), and metacognitive (e.g., *hypothesize, conclude*)
- Multiple-meaning words (e.g., *sore, pitch*)
- Multiple-function words (e.g., *soft opening, soft water, soft blanket*)

Adolescents also come to understand how words are related through the following:

- Derivation (e.g., *music–musician; phonetics–phonetician*)
- Meaning (e.g., antonyms such as *pleased–disappointed*; synonyms such as *mesa–butte*; sound such as *pear–pare–pair*)

Syntax and Writing

Adolescents typically produce longer, more complicated sentences than they used in the previous stage of development, and they become adept at using specific sentence structures for each type of discourse (e.g., descriptive, explanatory, argumentative). Their sentences contain more interrogatives, negatives, and verb tense markers than younger children's, and they use more literate forms in their writing (e.g., embedded phrases or subordinate clauses). Adolescent writing begins to reflect a knowledge of the intended audience, how much information the reader already has (or does not have) regarding the topic, and an organizational framework appropriate for each type of writing. Table 3.7 summarizes the primary characteristics of adolescent language development.

TABLE 3.7. Primary Characteristics of Adolescent Language Development: Ages 12–19

Syntax and writing	• Produces longer, more complicated sentences • Uses specific sentence structures for each type of discourse • Uses more literate forms in writing • Begins to reflect a knowledge of the intended audience in writing
Semantics	• Vocabulary development reflects literate language forms used in writing • Comes to understand how words are related through derivation and meaning
Pragmatics	• Becomes fluent conversational partner • Increases metalinguistic, metapragmatic, and metacognitive ability
Figurative language	• Bases humor on multiple-meaning words • Use of slang plays a major role in peer perception
Discourse	• Develops expertise with multiple types of discourse types in school and with peers • Becomes relatively fluent with more extensive forms of argumentative and persuasive discourse

Young Adult Language Development (Ages 20+)

Language development continues throughout adulthood; however, language development in adulthood has not been studied as thoroughly as language development at younger ages. According to Owens (2008), although language continues to grow in all areas during adulthood, the most prevalent changes occur in the semantic and pragmatic areas. Semantic development continues throughout adulthood as people continue to add new words to their lexicons. Young adults enrolled in higher education typically add significantly to their lexicons as they take courses replete with terms specific to particular fields of study. Their reading assignments also introduce them to words they would not encounter in oral language. Young adults continue to expand their abilities to understand relationships among words, particularly if they study foreign languages, many of which have contributed substantially to the English vocabulary.

A recent examination of persuasive writing in children, adolescents, and adults found that the syntactic, semantic, and pragmatic language used improved steadily from childhood to adulthood (Nippold, Ward-Lonergan, & Fanning, 2005). The changes included

> gradual increases in essay length; mean length of utterance; relative clause production; and the use of literate words, including adverbial conjuncts (e.g., *typically, however, finally*), abstract nouns (e.g., *longevity, respect, kindness*), and metalinguistic and metacognitive verbs (e.g., *reflect, argue, disagree*). (p. 125)

Pragmatic development in young adults reflects their continuing cognitive growth, especially their ability to take the perspective of others and to communicate on an abstract level about topics with many dimensions and perspectives (Owens, 2001). As young adults gain competency in understanding other people's viewpoints, they gain greater control of language structure in their efforts to take their audience into account.

Because they use language in a variety of different situations and contexts, adults typically use more than one style of speech, or register (Owens, 2008). The language they use when conversing with their family and close friends is different from the language they use when talking with people at their work or when speaking at a town meeting. In addition, adults learn a specific set of terms related to their job, their politics, or their identity, which includes ethnic, racial, or sexual orientation minorities (Owens, 2008). In addition, workplace environments use different styles of language; young adults may find themselves using a variety of language styles within one workplace, as, for instance, in talking on the phone, writing reports, sending e-mail or text messages, talking to superiors or subordinates, and presenting information to colleagues.

Communicating on an abstract level about topics with different dimensions and perspectives requires the young adult to use language that can describe coordinated, multiattributional descriptions of objects, events, and ideas (Owens, 2001). This sort of language use is a distinct change from the more personal, one-dimensional descriptions used by younger children and adolescents. I mentioned earlier that young adults' lives take place in more than one communication context, including those requiring the use of more formal, literate language. Young adults frequently find themselves in situations in which they must make a bridge between one topic and another in order to change the subject of conversation, which necessitates using a sentence or two to segue from one topic to another, perhaps unrelated, topic. Young adults also become more adept with what are called **conjuncts** ("She was sick. *Therefore,* she couldn't go swimming") and **disjuncts** ("*In my opinion*, the movie was awful" **or** "*Luckily*, we were able to duck inside a store when the rain started"). The primary characteristics of young adult language development are shown in Table 3.8.

Oral Language and the Bridge to Written Language

In previous sections I referred to the oral-to-literate shift children undergo as they make the transition from primarily using oral language to using print language for learning and communication. Although social, cognitive, and motor skills are involved in moving from orality to literacy, language development remains the most important and necessary component of the shift.

Several factors contribute to children becoming literate. Among the earliest influences is the literacy level of the child's family. Children from families in which

TABLE 3.8. Primary Characteristics of Young Adolescent Language Development: Ages 20+

Syntax and writing	• Develops skills in tandem with educational achievement • Increases essay length • Increases mean length of utterance • Produces relative clauses
Semantics	• Uses literate words • Continues to add new words to lexicon • Adds terms specific to a field of study in higher education
Pragmatics	• Takes the perspective of people whose experiences are not shared • Takes greater command of language structures to speak and write for a particular audience • Uses more formal language • Uses the discourse style of various groups • Learns the pragmatics of the work setting • Segues from one topic to another

literate language is a part of everyday life arrive at school with many of the preliteracy skills necessary for making the shift into literate language. For instance, these children already know the following:

- Print generally represents speech (though what print represents changes as children become more adept at using written symbol systems).
- Words have smaller components (syllables, phonemes).
- You can talk about language and about talking (metalinguistic and metapragmatic ability).
- Letters correspond to sounds (graphophonemic awareness).
- Stories involve a problem, characters who try to solve the problem, and a solution to the problem; a specific setting or settings; conflicts between and among characters; plot twists and reversals; and characters talking to each other, among others.
- English print is read left to right, and book pages turn from right to left (of course, this varies across cultures).
- Pencils, pens, markers, and crayons can be used to write; mobile devices and computers can be used to write using a keyboard (real or virtual).
- Signs (e.g., road signs, billboards, advertisements) contain messages, sometimes ironic or with double meanings.

A second factor contributing to children's emerging literacy is their own language ability. Children whose language development is atypical may experience difficulty acquiring the literacy skills necessary for school success, particularly if they have a **language disorder** associated with cognitive disabilities, severe **hearing** loss, behavior disorders, or moderate to severe **autism.** Even children with mild or moderate language disorders not associated with other disabilities may struggle to acquire the literacy skills they need.

A third factor affecting literacy development is **bilingualism.** Recent research with bilingual (Spanish–English) children in kindergarten and first grade by Uccelli and Paez (2007) showed a strong association between these children's oral vocabularies (in both languages) and their storytelling abilities (again, in both languages). These authors found that children in kindergarten with higher scores on an English vocabulary test used a greater number of distinct words in their English story narrative, and those who scored high on story structure in their Spanish narratives had higher-quality English narrative scores in first grade than children whose scores were lower on these three measures. In addition, the authors found that kindergarten Spanish vocabulary scores were highly correlated with children's first-grade Spanish narrative scores.

In interpreting Uccelli and Paez's results, Fusaro (2010) pointed out the "supportive relationship between early storytelling skills in Spanish and later storytelling proficiency in English" (para. 11). Although the Uccelli and Paez study included a relatively small number of children, the results seem to indicate that children's early experiences in telling stories in their native language carry over to the development of what Fusaro calls "the same structural and organizational skills in English" (para. 11). Regarding the children's vocabulary skills, however, the results indicate that if bilingual children's vocabulary skills are not well developed in the language in which they're learning to read (e.g., English), they will most likely have difficulty acquiring the literacy skills necessary for success in reading and writing (Fusaro, 2010).

As I pointed out in Chapter 2, more than 60 million individuals in the United States speak a language other than English at home (Ryan, 2011). Among those individuals, 62% speak Spanish or Spanish Creole, which means that a large number of children entering school each year speak Spanish as their first language, and the majority of research studies done on bilingualism focus on Spanish–English speakers. In a typical school district in the United States, 37% of students are from racial minorities, and up to 12% of the total population in the schools is either bilingual or becoming bilingual (learning English as a second language; Peña, Summers, & Resendiz, 2007). Literacy development for these children differs from that of children who are monolingual English speakers, which carries implications for how we assess language disorders and how we structure intervention programs for those with true language disorders. In the sections on Assessment and Intervention in Chapter 4, I will address these implications in more detail.

The Importance of Literacy for Academic Success

As children progress in school through the early elementary grades, literacy and academic success become more entwined. By the time children exit elementary school, they are expected to use their language abilities to understand and produce a variety of literate language forms, both oral and print. These language abilities include

- applying phonological awareness skills (e.g., segmenting words into smaller units, synthesizing sounds and syllables into words);
- using an extensive vocabulary;
- defining words;
- applying metalinguistic, metapragmatic, and metacognitive skills;
- understanding and producing compound, complex, and compound-complex sentences;
- understanding and using advanced morphological markers (e.g., exceptions to general rules and markers for infrequent grammatical constructions);
- understanding who they are writing for (their audience) and their purpose in speaking or writing (e.g., to persuade their audience of something; to explain how something works; to tell a funny story); and
- using appropriate organizational and stylistic conventions for each discourse genre.

Most children develop the skills listed above by becoming fluent readers so that, by the time they reach adolescence, reading and writing are reciprocal processes (Polloway et al., 2012). The more experience children have with reading, the more they know about writing. And, conversely, the more experience they have with writing, the more they learn about reading. Of course, strong oral language abilities are required for both reading and writing. Consequently, children with poorly developed oral language abilities will most likely have difficulties reading and developing skills in writing.

chapter 4

Preschool, Child, and Adolescent/Young Adult Language Disorders

Learning Objectives

Describe language disorders of form, content, use, nonverbal language, and figurative language.

Describe the language characteristics of children and adolescents with language disorders of various etiologies, including autism spectrum disorder (ASD), specific language impairment (SLI), attention-deficit/hyperactivity disorder (ADHD), intellectual disability, traumatic brain injury (TBI), and abuse and neglect.

Differentiate between language disorder and language difference, specifically in relation to multicultural populations.

Describe the various types of assessments used by SLPs.

Explain the purposes of intervention for language disorders.

Explain the principles involved in designing language assessment and intervention for multicultural populations.

Describe the primary types of language intervention used with children and adolescents, including augmentative and alternative communication (AAC).

Overview

The National Institute on Deafness and Other Communication Disorders (NIDCD; 2010a) reported that between 6 and 8 million people in the United States have a specific **language** impairment (SLI). Of these, approximately 6% are children in preschool and early elementary school. The NIDCD reports that children whose parents have less than a high school education are three times as likely to have an SLI as children whose parents are college graduates (NIDCD, 2010b). Furthermore, children identified in kindergarten with an SLI have a much greater likelihood of having a reading disability in second and fourth grade when compared with their typically developing peers (NIDCD, 2010b).

Children with other, related disorders, such as cognitive disabilities and learning disabilities, may have language disorders related to their primary disorders. Some SLIs can occur after a period of normal development because of infection, tumor, stroke, epilepsy, or brain injury. Other language disorders may result from developmental conditions such as brain damage, chromosomal anomalies, **hearing loss**, or motor functioning disorders. **Speech–language pathologists (SLPs)** provide language services to all these populations of children and adolescents.

The majority of SLPs providing services to children with language disorders work in school settings. Figure 4.1 shows the types of students served by SLPs in schools. As this shows, SLPs in school settings spend considerable time providing services to children and adolescents with language disorders related to various conditions. It is estimated that between 2% and 19% of preschool children have some sort of language impairment (Nelson, Nygren, Walker, & Panoscha, 2006).

The main symptom of a childhood or adolescent **language disorder** is the lack of ability to understand or formulate language as well as other children the same age. A child or adolescent with a language disorder may have difficulty with any or all areas of language—pragmatics, semantics, syntax, morphology, phonology, nonverbal language, or figurative language. With older children, adolescents, or young adults who have a language disorder, the deficit may be relatively subtle. For instance, they may have poorer comprehension of humor or figurative language than peers, or they may have difficulty writing.

It is important for you to have read Chapter 3 carefully in order for the material in this chapter to make sense. The information on language development will help you understand the discussions of how language disorders are described, identified, and remediated.

Disorders of Language Use, Form, and Content

Children and adolescents can exhibit language disorders in use, form, content, nonverbal language, or figurative language. Disorders of **language use** appear as difficulties adjusting language form and content to match varying social settings and conditions (i.e., **pragmatics**). Disorders in language form include difficulties with **phonology** (i.e., speech sound system), **syntax** (i.e., use of grammatical structures), or **morphology** (i.e., use of markers). Disorders in **language content** typically appear as problems with vocabulary development, word meaning, (i.e., **semantics**), and word retrieval.

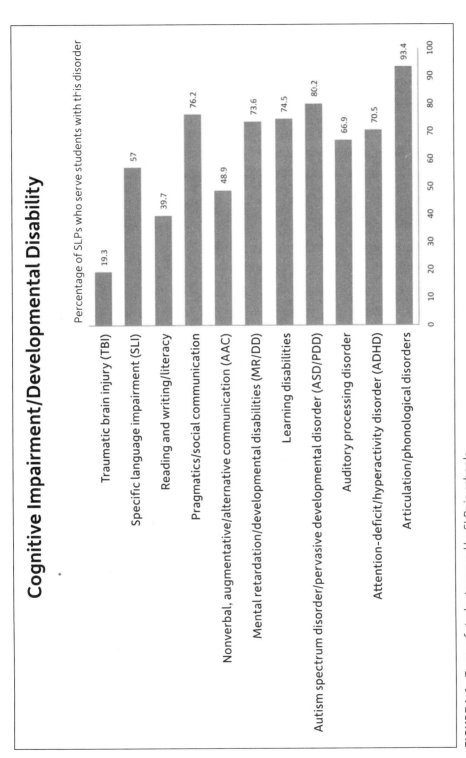

Cognitive Impairment/Developmental Disability

Percentage of SLPs who serve students with this disorder

Traumatic brain injury (TBI) — 19.3
Specific language impairment (SLI) — 57
Reading and writing/literacy — 39.7
Pragmatics/social communication — 76.2
Nonverbal, augmentative/alternative communication (AAC) — 48.9
Mental retardation/developmental disabilities (MR/DD) — 73.6
Learning disabilities — 74.5
Autism spectrum disorder/pervasive developmental disorder (ASD/PDD) — 80.2
Auditory processing disorder — 66.9
Attention-deficit/hyperactivity disorder (ADHD) — 70.5
Articulation/phonological disorders — 93.4

FIGURE 4.1. Types of students served by SLPs in schools.

Note. Adapted from *ASHA 2012 Schools Survey: SLP Caseload Characteristics* (p. 7), by American Speech-Language-Hearing Association. Available from http://www.asha.org/uploadedFiles/Schools-2012-Caseload.pdf

Disorders of Language Use

Children and adolescents who struggle with language use are described as having a **pragmatics disorder**. These students often are unable to participate effectively in conversations because they are unable to take the perspective of their listeners, they may not know how to take turns appropriately, and they may be unable to provide clarification if a listener asks for it. These students also have difficulty participating in the various discourses they encounter in school because they are unable to shift the form and content of their language to fit individual settings and contexts. In 2012, the American Speech-Language-Hearing Association (ASHA) reported that 83% of SLPs in schools provided services to students with pragmatic disorders (ASHA, 2012).

Students with pragmatic language disorders often experience difficulty with figurative language and **metapragmatics**. As a result they struggle with humor, idioms, slang, using language to learn, and reflecting on their own language use and learning strategies. They may ask questions in class that seem irrelevant or disrespectful, interrupt at inopportune times, and use non sequiturs. Because of their difficulty with metalinguistic processes, students with pragmatic language disorders continue to use direct rather than indirect language, which often results in others thinking them impolite or rude. In addition, they have difficulty discerning the difference between facts, opinions, arguments, and hypotheses.

Disorders of Language Form

ASHA describes a **phonological disorder** as "impaired comprehension of the sound system of a language and the rules that govern the sound combinations" (ASHA Ad Hoc Committee on Service Delivery in the Schools, 1993). The committee indicated that compared with their age peers, children with phonological disorders have difficulty producing the speech sounds of their language and that for 80%, the disorder is severe enough to require treatment by a speech–language pathologist.

Many (50%–70%) children who are identified as having a phonological disorder at a young age experience subsequent difficulties with reading, writing, spelling, and mathematics (ASHA Ad Hoc Committee on Service Delivery in the Schools, 1993). In a 2012 survey, just under 93% of school-based SLPs indicated that they provided services to children with phonological or articulation disorders (ASHA, 2014j).

Children and adolescents with **syntactic** and **morphological disorders** may demonstrate reduced ability to understand or produce longer or more complex sentences. They frequently use short, simple syntactic structures. Their syntax and morphology is slow to develop and often remains at a relatively unelaborated level. They rely on the most common morphological markers and may have difficulty learning exceptions to morphological or syntactic rules. In addition, children with syntactic and morphological disorders produce a limited variety of syntactic structures, their sentences may exhibit persistent errors, and they have difficulty using connectives (e.g., *because, but*) and words indicating relationships, such as *moreover* and *therefore*.

Disorders of Language Content

Children and adolescents who experience difficulty with language content are usually identified as having **semantic disorders**. They may have problems with word retrieval in conversational speech, which can result in various disfluencies (e.g., repeating, starting over, revising). In addition, they may have difficulty defining words and may not be able to elaborate on word meanings beyond simple, basic statements. Another characteristic of the language of children and adolescents with semantic disorders is difficulty in using specific referents that actually name what they are referring to. Instead, they use words such as *stuff, thing, this, that,* or nonverbal cues to indicate what they are referring to.

Students with semantic disorders also have difficulty understanding word relationships, such as derivatives (e.g., *science–scientist),* antonyms (e.g., *graceful– clumsy),* synonyms (e.g., *couch–sofa),* and sound (e.g., *two–to–too).* They may be unable to form adverbs (e.g., *happily, slowly, gracefully)* or use adverbial conjunctives (e.g., *therefore, nonetheless).*

Language Disorders With Specific Etiologies

Language disorders arise from a variety of etiologies or conditions, such as

- specific language impairment (SLI), also called *language-learning disabilities* (LLD);
- genetic factors that result in cognitive or sensory impairments; and
- physical–social–environmental factors, including neglect or abuse, drug exposure in utero, malnourishment, and disease.

Language-Learning Disabilities

The terms *language-learning disabilities* (LLDs) and *specific language impairments* (SLIs) are often used interchangeably. However, some SLPs use *SLI* to refer to children prior to their entering elementary school and *LLD* to refer to children once they have entered elementary school. The relationship between language and learning disabilities, although not linear, certainly seems to suggest that early language problems often reappear in the school years as a learning disability sometimes called **dyslexia.** The National Center for Learning Disabilities (2014) described dyslexia as a language processing disorder.

ASHA (2014o) explains that language-based learning disabilities interfere with reading, writing, and spelling, while dyslexia refers to learning disabilities with reading only. The term *LLD* is used in this book because it highlights the importance of language for learning and the relationship between language disorders and learning disabilities. However, because states use their own terms to define disorders related to language and learning disabilities, you may encounter different terminology in your own state.

Children are identified as having an LLD when their difficulties are specific to language and not secondary to some other disability. The cause of LLD is not known, nor do these children exhibit associated conditions such as cognitive disabilities, neurological impairment, or sensorimotor problems.

Children with LLD frequently begin talking later than their peers, acquire words relatively slowly, and have **word-finding** (i.e., word-retrieval) **problems.** Although children with LLD have delayed language skills, their language development usually follows the same sequence as that of their typically developing peers in spite of their difficulties with specific components of language.

Many children with LLD have problems with articulation and phonology. These children are often difficult to understand (i.e., their speech is relatively **unintelligible**), and their phonological development proceeds at a considerably slower rate than their typically developing peers'. Children with LLD commonly have problems with phonological awareness. They often struggle to learn the alphabet and to understand the relationship between print and speech. They have difficulty sequencing the sounds in a word, particularly if the word is more than one syllable in length.

Children with LLD often have difficulty with syntax and morphology. Their utterances are frequently short and simple, retaining essential meaning but omitting smaller grammatical units, such as *the, a,* and *an*. Their syntax is usually simple and contains few compound, complex, or compound–complex sentences. In addition, they may have difficulty comprehending directions, questions, or complex sentences. Children with LLD may show errors in singular and plural forms of words (e.g., "That a cats" for "That is a cat"), possessives (e.g., "There is the dog bed" for "There is the dog's bed"), the present progressive -*ing* (e.g., "Dog eat" for "The dog is eating"), third-person singular noun form (e.g., "He go outside" for "He goes outside"), *is* verb forms (e.g., "Dog eating" for "The dog is eating"), past-tense markers (e.g., "He walk" for "He walked"), and pronoun forms (e.g., "Him is at the movie" for "He is at the movie").

The pragmatic abilities of children with LLD are often affected. Some children with LLD are relatively passive conversationalists, expressing and responding little to their conversational partners. Others may be expressive yet unresponsive to their partners. These children experience difficulties with turn taking, introducing and maintaining topics appropriately, interrupting appropriately, maintaining coherence throughout a story or explanation, and repairing conversations that have suffered a breakdown. They seem relatively unable to take the perspective of their listeners and have little concept of varying audiences.

Children with LLD often do not understand how stories are constructed and organized, nor can they tell stories using the usual story structures that include a problem, a character attempting to solve the problem, and a resolution of the problem. They also find expository discourse difficult to comprehend and may not be able to see the organizational frameworks of the various types of expository discourse (e.g., descriptive, explanatory, cause–effect, compare–contrast, argumentative persuasive).

Cognitive–Sensory Impairments

Cognitive disability is also called *intellectual disability* and in the past was referred to as *mental retardation*. A cognitive disability is characterized by significantly below average intelligence and limitations in daily life functions. More specifically, intellectual disability results in an individual's having limitations in mental functioning, communicating, taking care of him- or herself, and social interactions (Center for Parent Information and Resources, 2014a, para. 3). Cognitive disabilities, which are the most common developmental disability (National Center on Birth Defects and Developmental Disabilities, 2005), may arise any time before age 18. Approximately 1 in 6 (approximately 15%) children in the United States has a cognitive disability (Centers for Disease Control and Prevention, 2014).

Because they can arise from a wide range of conditions, cognitive disabilities affect a diverse group of individuals. They can be caused by injury, disease, or brain abnormality. The most common known causes are fetal alcohol syndrome, Down syndrome and fragile X syndrome (both caused by genetic and chromosomal factors), and conditions such as toxoplasmosis (caused by a specific infection during pregnancy; National Center on Birth Defects, 2005). Some cognitive disabilities are mild, while others are severe. The more severe the disability, the greater the consequences to communication and language development.

The language development of individuals with mild cognitive disabilities usually follows the same sequence as seen in typically developing children, albeit at a slower pace. Thus, their language abilities often resemble those of younger children. However, if the disability is severe, the individual may exhibit language that is **idiosyncratic** and unlike younger children's.

Children with even a mild cognitive disability may show difficulties with all aspects of language form, content, and use. Their articulation and phonological skills are often delayed, making it difficult to understand their speech. Their semantic abilities are compromised by their relatively small receptive and expressive vocabularies and difficulties in understanding relationships between words. Their syntax is more typical of younger children; that is, they understand and use short, simple utterances and have difficulties comprehending and expressing longer, more complex syntactic structures.

The morphological abilities of children with cognitive disabilities are often more compromised than their syntactic abilities, primarily because of the abstract nature of morphological markers (Roseberry-McKibbin & Hegde, 2010). Last, their pragmatic abilities suffer. They have difficulty understanding the nature of less direct language forms, understanding the nature of turn taking, taking others' perspectives, and organizing and telling a story.

Autism Spectrum Disorder (including Asperger's Syndrome)

Several conditions with associated **communication disorders** are classified by the American Psychiatric Association (APA) in the *Diagnostic and Statistical Manual of Mental Disorders, Fifth Edition* (DSM-5; APA, 2013). Among them are autism spectrum disorder (ASD). In previous editions of the DSM, ASD and Asperger's syndrome (and several other related conditions) were treated as separate conditions. However, in the DSM-5, Asperger's syndrome has been incorporated into the diagnostic criteria for ASD.

ASD is defined by ASHA as

> a neurodevelopmental disorder characterized by deficits in social communication and social interaction and the presence of restricted, repetitive behaviors. Social communication deficits include impairments in aspects of joint attention and social reciprocity, as well as challenges in the use of verbal and nonverbal communicative behaviors for social interaction. Restricted, repetitive behaviors, interests, or activities are manifested by stereotyped, repetitive speech, motor movement, or use of objects; inflexible adherence to routines; restricted interests; and hyper- or hypo-sensitivity to sensory input. (ASHA, 2014g, para. 1)

Children with ASD often have difficulty with various aspects of communicating, such as understanding what others are talking about, how to talk to other people, and with reading or writing. In addition, individuals with ASD often do not understand gestures such as pointing or showing something to another person or engaging in conversations through using turn taking and knowing what their listeners already know.

Social Communication Disorder

Social communication (pragmatic) disorder is a new category in the DSM-5 and applies to individuals who have difficulties with a variety of social-interactive behaviors, including making eye contact, understanding and using facial expressions and body language, using vocal tone and inflection, using polite forms, and understanding their own and others' emotions.

The DSM-5 (APA, 2013) states that this disorder is characterized by

> a primary difficulty with pragmatics, or the social use of language and communication, as manifested in deficits in understanding and following social rules of verbal and nonverbal communication in naturalistic contexts, chang-

ing language according to the needs of the listener of situation, and following rules for conversation and storytelling. The deficits in social communication result in functional limitations in effective communication, social participation, development of social relationships, academic achievement, or occupational performance. (p. 48)

Specific Language Impairment

Specific language impairment (SLI) is the diagnosis given to children whose difficulties with language cannot be explained by deficits in oral structure, hearing loss, intellectual/cognitive impairment, or deficits in perceptual abilities. The NIDCD (2015) stated that approximately 8% of kindergarten children have SLI. Children with SLI often begin talking later than their typically developing peers, and when they do begin to talk, they may be very difficult to understand.

It is not surprising that if it is not caught and treated early in a child's life, SLI can have a profound effect on academic achievement. Ervin (2001) reported that 50% to 70% of children with SLI also have reading disabilities. Children whose language comprehension is also affected tend to have greater difficulty with acquiring literacy skills (Simkin & Conti-Ramsden, 2006).

The Merrill Advanced Studies Center (2014) at the University of Kansas offers a list of the top 10 things you should know about children with SLI:

1. SLI is called by many different names and is very common.
2. Children who are late to begin talking may very well have a disability.
3. Children with SLI do not have low IQs or poor hearing.
4. SLI is a language disorder—most children with SLI do not have a speech disorder.
5. Children with SLI typically have difficulty with the intricacies of verb forms (e.g., plural markers, forms of the copula, past-tense markers).
6. Children with SLI will likely have difficulties with reading and learning.
7. It is possible to diagnose SLI with great accuracy.
8. There seems to be a genetic factor (or factors) associated with SLI.
9. Because children with SLI have difficulty forming language easily, they miss opportunities to explore their world through language, thus limiting their exposure to language.
10. Intervention for SLI can begin as soon as the first signs appear, generally by age 3.

Attention-Deficit/Hyperactivity Disorder

According to the Centers for Disease Control and Prevention (2014), attention-deficit/hyperactivity disorder (ADHD) is a chronic **neurodevelopmental** disorder and is one of the most common disorders of childhood. Inattention, hyperactivity, and impulsivity are the primary characteristics.

Inattention seems to stem from difficulty concentrating; sensory stimuli and one's own thoughts impede focusing and attending. Consequently, students with ADHD appear as if they are not listening. Inattention seems to vary according to the interest of the person affected. This means that an individual may be able to attend to and concentrate on some activities for extended periods but be unable to plan, organize, or complete other tasks of less interest. In addition, students with ADHD may not be able to monitor their own behavior in some situations and contexts.

Hyperactivity and impulsivity often appear together, although they are somewhat different. Hyperactivity means difficulty sitting still—fidgeting, squirming, moving about, tapping pencils, wiggling, and touching things. Students with hyperactivity often switch quickly from task to task without completing any of them. Students exhibiting impulsivity appear to have problems thinking before they act. For instance, these students may barge into a game, interrupt speakers, or hit someone when they are frustrated.

Students with ADHD often have difficulties with various aspects of communication, language, and speech. Pragmatic language is often affected because of the impulsivity, hyperactivity, and inattention associated with ADHD. Students with ADHD frequently have problems modifying their language to fit specific settings and conversational partners, which often appears to others as being rude or impolite. Students with ADHD frequently barge into conversations without knowing the topic, without acknowledging that someone else (e.g., a teacher) is speaking, and without any apparent knowledge of likely consequences. In addition, these students do not seem to consider their listener's background and knowledge, resulting in statements that cannot be understood by their listeners. Pragmatic language in students with ADHD is also affected by their relative inability to switch from the informal language of home and the playground to the more formal and literate forms required for participation throughout school. These students may talk to authority figures using the same casual language they use with their friends, again resulting in being thought rude or disrespectful.

Discourse in students with ADHD is often disorganized. They frequently have difficulties telling stories because they cannot put together all the necessary components and because they cannot sustain attention throughout the entire story. In addition, they may experience considerable difficulty following what is being said in stories and in other discourse forms, particularly those with relatively abstract organizational schemes, such as argumentative–persuasive, explanatory, compare–contrast, and descriptive.

Hearing Impairments

Normal hearing is essential to acquiring spoken language, but individuals without normal hearing may learn other communication systems, such as a sign language (e.g., American Sign Language, or ASL); augmentative and alternative communication, or AAC; and communication boards or communication books. Hearing loss that occurs before a child begins acquiring language is called **prelingual deafness**, while hearing loss that occurs after the language acquisition process has begun is called **postlingual deafness**. In general, the more severe the hearing loss, the more likely it is that it will affect language development. In addition, children whose hearing loss occurs before they begin developing language are more likely to experience difficulty with language acquisition than those whose hearing loss occurs after they have begun learning language.

There are exceptions, however. Children with prelingual deafness whose families are fluent in sign usually experience little difficulty acquiring the rule systems governing sign language, and many are able to develop proficiency in written English as they learn to read, thus becoming bilingual. In addition, some individuals with relatively severe hearing loss use language well, while others with the same onset and degree of loss struggle to acquire language.

When prelingually deaf children are exposed only or primarily to oral language, they frequently exhibit specific characteristics, including

- limited oral communication;
- reduced understanding of oral communication;
- difficulties with pragmatic language, especially providing background information and maintaining topic;
- reduced understanding and use of compound and complex syntactic structures;
- difficulties using various morphemes such as tense markers, possessives, present progressive -*ing*, conjunctions, articles, prepositions, and indefinite pronouns (Roseberry-McKibbin & Hegde, 2010);
- low reading comprehension; and
- poor writing skills.

Traumatic Brain Injury

Traumatic brain injury (TBI) can result whenever an individual sustains any injury to the head, including concussions. ASHA (2014w) identifies two types of TBI: **penetrating injuries** and **closed head injuries**. Penetrating injuries affect those areas of the brain along the pathway the object travels once inside, with symptoms varying according to the parts of the brain affected.

According to ASHA (2014w), two types of damage result from closed head injuries: primary brain damage and secondary brain damage. Primary brain damage is what occurs at the time of the impact and can include skull fracture, damage to nerves, tearing of brain lobes or blood vessels, hematomas (blood clots), and contusions (bruises). Secondary brain damage occurs after the trauma and unfolds over time. Secondary brain damage includes any or all of the following (ASHA, 2014w):

- edema
- pressure inside the skull

- seizures
- infection inside the skull and/or brain
- fever
- abnormal blood pressure
- low sodium level
- anemia
- abnormal carbon dioxide
- changes in cardiac function
- changes in lung function
- changes in nutritional needs

The communication problems that occur after TBI range widely and depend on both the severity of the injury and its location and extent. Among the communication difficulties experienced by people with TBI are oral and written word finding, understanding speech or writing, spelling, reading, and writing. The most affected area of communication for individuals who have had a TBI is social communication. Most have trouble with turn taking, staying on topic, following the pace of ordinary conversation, modulating their voice appropriately for the conversational context, and differentiating between the literal and metaphoric levels of language (thus having difficulty discerning humor, idiom, sarcasm, or irony).

In addition, people who have had a TBI may have problems forming speech sounds and combining them into words, difficulties speaking loudly enough to be heard in oral conversation, or difficulties chewing and swallowing.

Poverty, Abuse, and Neglect

Many children who grow up in families with low income and limited access to health care develop excellent language skills. However, among families in which educational and literacy levels are low, children's language development suffers. Language development is adversely affected by inadequate oral stimulation from adults; few (if any) opportunities to engage in the preliteracy activities that are known to enhance language development (e.g., being read aloud to, seeing print used as an integral part of everyday life, hearing adults talk about language); little exposure to enriching activities that stimulate language development (e.g., going to a children's museum, an art fair, or a zoo); and limited access to toys and books that stimulate language development (Roseberry-McKibbin & Hegde, 2000).

However, one of the biggest causes of dysfunction in children's acquisition of communication skills is living in an impoverished family with poor maternal health, poor nutrition, lack of social supports, teenage parents with less than a high school education, parental difficulty accessing pediatric care, parental substance abuse, and inadequate nutrition (Welc, 2010). Sullivan and Knutson (2000) reported that physical, sexual, or emotional abuse affects 35% of children with speech–language delays.

Abuse and neglect in young children have a dramatic impact because the brain is growing rapidly and is particularly sensitive to environmental input (Lee & Hoaken, 2007). Abuse and neglect can have profound effects on the biochemical and structural changes in the brain, which can result in generalized language deficits, difficulty using language to articulate one's needs and wants, difficulty conveying abstraction, and difficulty maintaining cohesive narrative discourse (Westby, 2007). Rogers-Adkinson and Stuart (2007) found that children who have been abused and neglected showed problems in both receptive and expressive language and pragmatic language (especially interpreting peers' body language and nonverbal cues) and understanding the figurative language used in sarcasm and indirect commands.

Cultural Considerations

In Chapter 2, I discussed the increasingly diverse population of the United States and the importance of culturally sensitive practices when providing services to people with communication disorders. A corollary involves differentiating a true language disorder from a language difference. A language *disorder* is a disruption in an individual's ability to understand or express the conventional symbols of his or her native language in use, form, or content. A language *difference*, on the other hand, refers to dialectal or cultural uses of a language that may differ from the conventions used by a linguistic majority.

Because of the diversity of the U.S. population, many speakers' use of English differs from what is called **Standard English**, or the national norm in the United States. In fact, just as language itself is constantly changing, so too is the national norm, transforming in response to the many and varied cultural groups who speak English or are in the process of learning to speak it. What this means for professionals delivering services for people with communication disorders is that sometimes what looks like a language disorder is not, in fact, a disorder but a language difference that does not need intervention.

Bilingual children who are learning English as a second language, or who speak a dialect other than Standard American English, frequently exhibit language characteristics that might be mistaken for a language disorder unless careful consideration is given to each child's situation. Children learning two languages, whether simultaneously or sequentially, often demonstrate growth bursts in one language while development in the other language plateaus. These growth bursts can continue throughout the course of acquiring the languages, seesawing between the two. If viewed in isolation, the child's development in the plateauing language compared to the one showing a growth burst may appear to be delayed or even disordered in comparison.

In addition, children learning two languages, especially in the early stages, often engage in what is called **code switching**. Code switching, while it may call attention to itself, is not considered a communication disorder because it is a normal progression in the acquisition of a second language. The child's overall language system includes both languages, and if this overall language system contains the forms, content, and usages that are customary and appropriate in the child's environment and **culture**, then a communication disorder is not present.

Dialects

People in different geographic regions of the United States speak different dialects of English. In addition, racial and ethnic groups in various regions of the United States often speak different dialects. Owens (2008) provided the example of Southern American English, which varies according to race in most southern states but is complicated by the Cajun–Creole American English used by both African Americans and whites in Louisiana.

According to Owens (2008), African American English (AAE), Spanish-influenced (Latino English), and Asian English are the three major racial and ethnic dialects in the United States. Within these dialects, there is considerable variation related to country of origin (e.g., Puerto Rico, Mexico, Spain; Vietnam, Indonesia, or Thailand), geographic region in the United States (e.g., West Coast Spanish-influenced English or Texas Spanish-influenced English), and socioeconomic characteristics (e.g., "upper class" dialects and "lower class" dialects).

Each dialect uses its own unique semantics and syntax. Texans, for instance, are recognized by their use of "y'all" (you all) and "fixin' to" (preparing). New Englanders agree by saying "Ayup," get a drink from a "bubbla" (drinking fountain), and eat a "grindah" (sub sandwich or hoagie) for lunch. Dialects also follow their own syntactical rules. African American English (AAE), for example, repeats the noun subject with a pronoun (e.g., "My father, he work there") and uses the same form for singular and plural nouns (e.g., *one girl, five girl*). Dialectical differences such as these are examples of language differences, not disorders.

Cultural Views of Communication

People from different cultures view communication in different ways, often using different means to accomplish the same end, such as having a request met. For instance, people who live in cultures oriented toward the individual tend to use direct language that can easily be understood outside the immediate context of the conversation, which is called *low-context* language (e.g., if someone writes, "I bought a shirt yesterday," you understand all the referents without having to be present in the immediate context). In these cultures, being too indirect can be seen as a sign of weakness or a lack of self-assuredness, or as a sign of a feminine way of communicating. On the other hand, people from cultures oriented more toward the collective, or larger social group, tend to use language that is more indirect and tied to the immediate context. Language with these characteristics is called *high-context* because it is not as easily understood outside the context of the immediate conversation (e.g., "I bought one, too" isn't immediately understandable unless you are present to know what *one* refers to). In these cultures, people use language to promote group cohesion, and being too direct can be seen as bringing too much attention to the individual.

Different cultures also have different ideas about how status and connection influence communication. Tannen (1992) reported that in some Asian cultures, such as Japanese, Chinese, and Javanese, people in close relationship (e.g., parents and their children) tend to communicate in a more hierarchical manner, while those in less close relationship (e.g., business associates) tend to communicate in a more egalitarian way. In contrast, people in Western European cultures who are in close relationship communicate in a more egalitarian manner, while those in less close relationship communicate in a more hierarchical manner.

Cultural variations also exist regarding appropriate distance between conversational partners. Edward T. Hall (1966), an anthropologist who studied spatial relationships in communication, found that in the United States, people who are engaged in conversation stand between 4 to 7 inches apart—just close enough to touch. In many countries, the expected social distance is roughly half that. In Arab countries, for example, friends are expected to stand close enough to smell each other's breath because "to deny the smell of your breath to a friend is considered an insult in most Arab cultures" (Gudykunst, 1998, p. 101).

Other cultural variations in communication include the following:

- In Japan, a collective culture, people are viewed as more truthful the less they speak (i.e., silence is seen as directly connected with truthfulness). In individualistic cultures (e.g., American), silences are seen as awkward and in need of filling.
- In Arab cultures, the use of assertion and exaggeration is the norm, while in Western and most Asian cultures, these characteristics are often viewed as offensive.
- French and Italian cultures use a more animated style of communicating, using a far wider range of intonation, volume, and body gestures than people in many other cultures.
- In many cultures, not making eye contact is a nonverbal sign of respect for someone in authority rather than the dishonesty or avoidance associated with it in other cultures.

It would be impossible for any individual SLP to know all the characteristics of the languages and dialects spoken by schoolchildren today. However, SLPs can become attuned to multicultural issues and develop a set of resources for making certain that children receive appropriate assessments and intervention when warranted. ASHA recommends that SLPs develop an understanding of the myriad ways in which cultural differences impact the delivery of services to individuals from different cultural groups. The ASHA website (2014t) offers several tools for checking your cultural competence, including an interactive web-based evaluation instrument.

Assessment and Intervention

Managing language disorders usually occurs in three phases: (1) assessment, (2) intervention and ongoing data collection, and (3) reassessment. The assessment process determines what the intervention will be and how it will be provided, although other factors, such as where intervention will take place (e.g., school or clinic), also contribute to the design of intervention. For instance, language intervention in a clinic may not include classroom collaboration between the SLP and the child's teacher, while school-based intervention may take place entirely in the child's classroom, necessitating ongoing collaboration.

A number of factors affect how language disorders are managed, including

- the age of the person with a language disorder—child, adolescent, or adult;
- the cause, or etiology, of the disorder, if known;
- the developmental level of the client's language;
- the severity of the disorder;
- the age at which the disorder was first identified or diagnosed and what has been done to remedy it since;
- the family's and client's attitudes toward the disorder and the processes of assessment and intervention;
- the setting in which the assessment and intervention will take place (e.g., school, clinic, hospital);
- whether English is the native language of the client;
- if the client speaks a dialect of English; and
- if the client is unable to speak and is a candidate for augmentative and alternative communication.

Purposes of Assessment

The primary purpose of language assessment for individuals of any age is to discover which language skills the individual already does or does not possess in order to design the most appropriate intervention, if warranted. Assessment in young children and preschoolers focuses on their level of language development so that intervention can help them move to the next developmental stage.

For school-age children, however, the purpose of assessment is heavily influenced by the interaction between the individual's language skills and the demands of classroom instruction. The assessment process determines whether an individual's language abilities are well-enough developed to make the shift from orality to literacy, and if they are sufficient for the individual to succeed academically (Polloway et al., 2012). Polloway, Patton, Serna, and Bailey (2013) suggested that for elementary students, language assessment is used to determine "how (and how well) children use language to

- participate successfully in the classroom;
- talk about language and its parts;

- understand and tell stories;
- learn to read, write, and spell; and
- comprehend the various types of expository text" (p. 89).

For adolescents, the purpose of language assessment is somewhat different, both because their language abilities have typically developed considerable more breadth and complexity and because they are expected to use language appropriately in a wide variety of spoken and written contexts. Polloway et al. (2013) indicated that there are three main purposes guiding language assessment in adolescents, which are to discover

- how adept they are with the social discourse used by their peers;
- how they interact with literate language forms, including the various discourse genres characteristic of the secondary grades; and
- the extent of their metalinguistic, metacognitive, and metapragmatic abilities and how successful they are in exercising them appropriately for learning. (p. 89)

Types of Assessment

SLPs use a variety of assessment types:

- standardized assessment
- developmental scales
- criterion-referenced procedures
- observations or interviews
- dynamic assessment

Standardized Assessments

Standardized assessments are used to determine how individuals compare with their age peers on some aspect of language. Standardized instruments consist of a set of items that have been administered to a large group of other individuals constituting a representative sample of the U.S. census. The responses from these individuals are collected into statistical groupings based on age, called the **norms**, against which children who are suspected of having a language disorder are then compared.

SLPs often choose to use standardized tests because, among other benefits, they offer clear administration and scoring criteria; they are valid (they measure what they say they measure); and they are reliable (they measure the same thing no matter who administers them) (Paul & Norbury, 2012). Although the results of standardized testing give the clinician information about how an individual's language development compares with that of her or his same-age peers, the results are limited because they reflect how children use language only in a testing situation and not in any other context. Furthermore, for an individual whose native language is not English, a test standardized in English may seriously underestimate her or his language abilities.

Paul and Norbury (2012) emphasized that once standardized test results show that an individual's language abilities differ from those of a normal population, the clinician's job is to then use other assessment procedures "to establish baseline function, to identify goals for intervention, and to measure progress in an intervention program" (p. 44). In the next sections I describe some of those other procedures.

Developmental Scales

Developmental scales offer clinicians a way to look more thoroughly at specific areas of an individual's language abilities, such as sound and speech discrimination, grammatical structures, speech sound production, number of disfluencies in a given sample of speech, and inventory of vocabulary words.

Criterion-Referenced Procedures

Criterion-referenced procedures are used to determine whether the child can attain a certain level of performance on a specific language target, such as prepositions or pronouns. Criterion-referenced procedures range from highly formal, question-and-answer formats, in which the clinician asks the child direct questions; to role-play or games, in which the clinician attempts to elicit particular structures, content, or functions; to informal, naturalistic formats, in which the clinician records a spontaneous sample of the child's conversation, and then transcribes and analyzes the sample to see which structures, content, or functions appear or do not appear in the sample. Criterion-referenced procedures are an effective way to track an individual's progress throughout intervention.

Case History, Observations, or Interviews

Usually, when seeing a new client, the clinician's first step is to take a case history in order to learn how the individual's speech, language, and communication have been developing. Specifically, the clinician will ask questions regarding

- how the individual uses language and engages in conversations (pragmatic language);
- the individual's ability to manage language content—specifically, oral vocabulary in young children; oral and reading vocabulary in primary-grade children; and oral, reading, and written vocabulary in upper-primary-grade and older children; and
- the individual's ability to understand and use the various formal aspects of language expected for her or his age—specifically, tense markers, plural markers, age-appropriate sentence type and structure, temporal and spatial terms, pronouns, and prepositions.

Clinicians often observe an individual in several contexts (e.g., classroom, playground, a one-to-one setting) in order to describe the individual's language within or across contexts. Usually the clinician is focusing on particular aspects of the individual's language structure, content, or function, such as verb forms, vocabulary, or story elements. Most observational tools are designed by clinicians as checklists or rating forms that can be used to track an individual's specific language forms, content, or structures across time or contexts.

When assessing the communication and language abilities of infants, toddlers, and preschoolers, clinicians often interview the child's parent(s) in order to determine the child's developmental level. Because interviewing requires skill and sensitivity, you should not attempt interviewing clients or parents without considerable practice. Paul and Norbury (2012) emphasized that the clinician must

- understand and respect the cultural group to which the family belongs,
- convey to the family the purpose of the interview, and
- ask nonleading and nonjudgmental questions.

Dynamic Assessment

Miller, Gillam, and Peña (2001) described dynamic assessment as a test–teach–retest approach in which the clinician, using an informal method such as a checklist, obtains a baseline measure of a particular language structure, content, or usage—the test phase. Next, the clinician presents the client with one or two teaching sessions based on what the clinician learned during the testing phase. In the teaching phase, the clinician's goals are to help the client understand the goal of the lesson(s), why that particular aspect of language is important and how it's related to what she or he already knows, and ways to remember to use it outside the context of the lessons (Miller et al., 2001).

The retest phase involves the clinician testing the individual again on the same aspect of language in order to determine whether there has been any change from the first testing phase and, if so, which strategies worked best.

Purposes of Intervention

Olswang and Bain (1991) believed there are three purposes for language intervention with students: (1) changing or eliminating the problem causing the disorder, (2) changing the language disorder itself, and (3) teaching compensatory strategies. Changing or eliminating the problem causing a language disorder is difficult or impossible, in most cases, because the underlying cause is either unknown or unchangeable. Changing the language disorder involves teaching the client specific language components, which is the approach that the majority of SLPs use. Teaching compensatory strategies is also used, although it may require the client to use metalinguistic, metacognitive, or metapragmatic abilities, which makes it a more suitable approach for upper elementary students, adolescents, and young adults.

Of course, deciding which option to choose depends on the nature and severity of the language disorder, the age of the individual, previous successes or failures, the individual's support system (family, teachers, peers), and the individual's communication needs in everyday life. For instance, while young children may not always know exactly why they are receiving intervention, adolescents must not only know the purpose but also be full partners in planning their goals and objectives (Larson & McKinley, 2003).

Types of Intervention

All language intervention is not alike. As you might imagine, the type of intervention selected for any particular client with a language disorder will be affected by the same factors that influence the choice of purpose for the intervention, including age, severity of the disorder, degree of support from family, previous intervention successes or failures, and the individual's specific communication needs in everyday life. Intervention can be family based, individual or group based, classroom based, intervention with adolescents, and augmentative and alternative communication.

Family-Based Intervention Programs

Often, young children and clients with severe language disorders receive intervention through a family-based program. In family-based intervention, the SLP works directly with the family members closest to the child, teaching them how to interact with the child (or adolescent or young adult, in the case of a severe disorder) to promote the child's acquisition of specific communication and language skills. For children just learning to use words, for example, the SLP demonstrates to family members how to draw the child's attention to an object, name the object, offer it to the child, and play with the child and the object, all the while emphasizing the name of the object throughout the interaction.

The SLP provides the family with a list of the words to emphasize in their interactions with the child and specific behaviors to look for in the child to indicate comprehension of the words on the list. The SLP also teaches the family members how to generally interact with the child in such a way as to facilitate language development, both comprehension and expression, perhaps through reading aloud to the child, singing songs, or reciting rhymes.

Family-based intervention for an older child who has suffered a TBI might involve providing family members with a list of language behaviors characteristic of the particular injury suffered by the child, along with information on how to respond to emotional outbursts and frustration. Immediately following the TBI, the SLP may function more as a resource for parents rather than providing face-to-face intervention for the child. As the child regains brain function, the SLP may take a more direct role in the intervention process.

Individual and Group Therapy

Clients in hospital and clinical settings receive intervention in individual sessions, group sessions, or both. Students in schools also receive language intervention individually or in small groups; they can also receive intervention in their classrooms.

Whether to provide intervention in individual or group sessions is not determined only by the type of intervention needed to address the disorder but sometimes also by the SLP's scheduling constraints. Some children benefit greatly from interacting with their peers throughout the intervention process, while others respond much more favorably when they receive one-to-one intervention. The primary factor in deciding whether to see individuals alone or in groups is determining which would be most beneficial to each client.

Classroom-Based Intervention

SLPs who work in schools increasingly provide language intervention in classrooms, working with classroom teachers to design and deliver the intervention. In a 2008 ASHA convention presentation, Kent Brorson reported that 63.93% of the SLPs surveyed in five states indicated they provided language intervention services within the regular education classroom for students ranging in age from prekindergarten through high school. Brorson's survey indicated that while most of those SLPs (53%) felt that teachers are willing to be involved with them in coteaching models, 28.79% did not (Brorson, 2008). In addition, he found that more than 30% of the SLPs he surveyed do not provide language intervention in the classroom because of uncooperative teachers.

Some SLPs design an intervention plan and consult with the classroom teacher about how it can most effectively be implemented by the teacher. Other times, the SLP and the teacher collaborate in the design of intervention and then coteach the plan in the classroom. In this situation, the SLP and the teacher jointly plan the intervention and then take turns teaching the plan, acting as the lead teacher and teaching consultant during the lesson, or using flexible groupings to each work with a group of students. In these situations, the language targets are embedded in the lesson and taught to all students. A third situation involves the SLP coming into the classroom to teach a small group of students with language disorders using a plan designed by the SLP. Although students without language disorders may be part of the group, the primary focus of the intervention is on specific language skills and processes.

Intervention With Adolescents

Because of their developmental needs, language intervention with adolescents requires a somewhat different approach from that used with younger children. Larson and McKinley (2003) described some general guidelines to use with adolescents at three different stages. For preteens and youth in early adolescence, they advocate developing the language students will need in order to be successful academically and to be accepted by their peers. For students in middle adolescence, language goals include seeing academic growth, interacting successfully with peers, and beginning to think about vocational considerations. For students in late adolescence, language goals shift away from the academic to focus more on the language students will need for vocational success and for establishing and maintaining one-to-one personal relationships.

Larson and McKinley (2003) emphasized that one of the SLP's most important roles is to help adolescents take responsibility for their communication disorder and the behaviors necessary to change it. They offer these specific suggestions for SLPs:

- Take time to sit down with the student to listen and to talk.
- Ask the student questions about his or her communication and organization problems.
- Suggest ways the student could address his or her communication and organization problems.
- Stick to what the student wants to talk about.
- Assist the student in knowing his or her legal rights and becoming a self-advocate.

In addition to their suggestions regarding how SLPs can best support adolescents in learning to take responsibility for their communication disorder and how to manage it, Larson and McKinley (2003) offered a list of things SLPs should avoid when communicating with an adolescent:

- Jumping to conclusions before the student finishes talking
- Ignoring the topic the student raises
- Hurrying the student
- Avoiding talking with the student about her or his concerns
- Showing a flat affect
- Ignoring the student as he or she is talking (e.g., working on something else)

Language intervention with adolescents requires that clinicians be flexible, be willing to counsel when necessary, listen attentively and thoroughly, and offer guidance grounded in their professional knowledge and experience.

Augmentative and Alternative Communication

ASHA (2014e) describes augmentative and alternative communication (AAC) as referring to any form of communication other than speech that is used by an individual to articulate thoughts, needs, wants, observations, and feelings. AAC systems are used by individuals with little or no verbal ability to supplement (augment) existing speech or to replace speech that is either nonexistent or nonfunctional. Most AAC systems involve picture and symbol communication boards and electronic devices, such as iPads, specially programmed computers, and iPhones. However, some individuals use paper and pencil, communication books, speech-generating devices, or written output systems.

The most commonly used AAC system for individuals with little or no verbal ability is the Picture Exchange Communication System (PECS), which is used to help the individual build a vocabulary and consistently express desires, observations, and feelings through the use of pictures. When the clinician begins using the PECS system with an individual, he or she teaches the individual to exchange a picture for an object (e.g., a picture of a ball for an actual ball). Gradually, the clinician introduces both symbols and pictures so that the individual can use both to form sentences. Clinicians can also use the PECS system to reinforce verbal communication.

However, as I will discuss in Chapter 5, AAC technology is evolving at a rapid pace. Mobile devices are being used more frequently because they offer multiple functions within one device, and almost anyone can develop apps (software applications) that specifically target communication in various settings. For individuals with autism, for instance, Light and McNaughton (2010) reported that Hewlett Packard launched the Hacking Autism website (http://www.hackingautism.org/) where anyone can post their ideas for apps that would benefit individuals with autism. In response, software programmers develop apps of touch-enabled technologies that are then offered free of charge.

Reassessment

For a variety of reasons, intervention always includes reassessment (reevaluation) to assess client progress, make decisions about continuing therapy or changing intervention strategies, or provide **documentation** to outside parties, such as insurance companies or employers. In Chapter 13, I provide details about these various aspects of reevaluation.

chapter 5

Adult Language Disorders

Learning Objectives

Describe the neurology of aphasia.

Identify the primary causes of brain injury and resulting aphasia.

Identify the primary types of aphasia and their language characteristics.

Describe the most common nonlanguage characteristics of people with aphasia.

Describe right-hemisphere deficits and language characteristics.

Describe dementia and associated language characteristics.

Discuss the primary types of intervention used with aphasia, right-hemisphere deficits, and dementia.

Describe the factors the SLP must take into account when providing services to a bilingual (or multilingual) client with aphasia.

Overview

Adults, like children, can be impaired in their ability to comprehend or use **language**. Most adults who have such impairments were able to comprehend and use language normally when they were younger but lost their language abilities because of damage to their brain, usually somewhere in the **left cerebral hemisphere** (see Figure 5.1).

Although a range of neurological disorders can result in adult language disorders, in this chapter I will focus on **aphasia**, **right-hemisphere deficits**, **dementia**, and **traumatic brain injury (TBI)**.

According to Engelter et al. (2006), 15% of individuals under age 65 have aphasia, while 43% of individuals 85 and older have aphasia. People who have aphasia have lost some ability to understand or formulate language because of damage to the brain—specifically, to the **cerebral cortex**. Language abilities that may be impaired

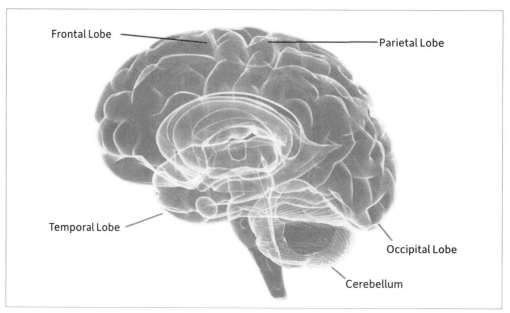

Frontal Lobe

Parietal Lobe

Temporal Lobe

Occipital Lobe

Cerebellum

FIGURE 5.1. Left cerebral hemisphere.

include understanding and expressing **speech**, speaking, reading, writing, calculating (e.g., doing simple addition, subtraction, multiplication, and division), and communicating appropriately across varying social contexts. Although it is possible for only one or two of these language abilities to be impaired, in most cases all are impaired to some extent. The degree of impairment, however, varies across abilities and between people. One person who has aphasia, for example, may be more impaired in the ability to speak than in the ability to understand speech, while the opposite may be true for another person. Part of these differences depends on the exact nature and extent of the damage to the brain.

Furthermore, the degree of impairment of a particular language ability can range from minimal to profound. Impairment of the ability to comprehend speech, for example, can range from an inability to understand highly abstract words to not being able to understand any words. Fortunately, the impairment is more likely to be mild or moderate than it is to be profound. If the degree of impairment in all language abilities is profound, the person is referred to as having **global aphasia.**

Neurology of Aphasia

The brain sits at the top of the **central nervous system (CNS)** and is thus able to communicate with the rest of the body through the various nerves constituting the CNS. The right and left hemispheres of the brain are connected by a structure called the **corpus callosum**, which facilitates neural communication (motor, sensory, and cognitive information) between the two hemispheres. In most people, language functions are processed in the left hemisphere, while nonlinguistic and paralinguistic information is processed in the right hemisphere. For this reason, damage to the left hemisphere produces more severe and long-lasting language disturbances than does comparable damage to the right hemisphere.

As you can see in Figure 5.1, each hemisphere of the cerebral cortex is divided into four lobes: **frontal, temporal, parietal,** and **occipital.** Just as the two hemispheres of the cerebral cortex are important for mediating different functions, so too are the lobes and specific locations within each lobe. This specialization of the nerve cells in the cerebral cortex is referred to as cerebral **localization of function.** Recent investigations into localization indicate that the cortex is organized in a hierarchy of three types of areas:

- primary sensory areas at the bottom of the cortex,
- sensory association areas in the middle, and
- higher-order association areas at the top.

Sensory information first comes in contact with the cerebral cortex at its own specialized area (e.g., from the ears, eyes, tongue). Then, each different type of sensory information sends its signals through the sensory association areas to the part of the cortex that processes higher-order associations. For example, sound enters the ear, where it is transduced into electrical signals. These electrical signals are picked up by the auditory pathway, which sends them to the primary auditory cortex at the top edge of the temporal lobe.

The **cerebellum**, which was seen until recently as dedicated to regulating and coordinating motor functions, also plays a role in language processing. In particular, Murdoch (2010) reported that the cerebellum, in particular the right cerebellar hemisphere, is involved in the modulation of a wide range of language functions, such as "verbal fluency, word retrieval, syntax, reading, writing and metalinguistic abilities" (p. 866).

The cerebral cortex that covers both hemispheres mediates all motor, sensory, and "intellectual" (including language) functions. The disturbances that result from damage to specific nerve cells are determined by the functions those nerve cells mediate. Aphasic-type language disturbances can result from lesions at specific sites (i.e., to specific nerve cells) in all the lobes of the left hemisphere of the cerebral cortex: the occipital, temporal, parietal, and frontal. Impairment of the ability to read is caused by lesions in the occipital lobe. Impairment of the ability to understand speech is caused by lesions in the temporal lobe. An impairment in the parietal lobe results in the inability to repeat. And an impairment of the abilities to formulate speech and to write is caused by lesions in the frontal lobe. It is important to note, though, that no one knows *exactly* where speech and language actually occur in the brain because both are so complex and are handled by several different areas. I'll go into more detail about this in the section on types of aphasia.

Conditions that damage nerve cells that are important for mediating language functions usually also damage cells that are important for mediating other functions. Damage to the cerebral cortex is rarely limited to a small group of cells. As a result, people with aphasia are also likely to have certain other impairments, usually resulting from damage to nerve cells that lie in close proximity to the damaged cells that produce aphasia.

One of the most common of these impairments is a **right hemiplegia**. Nerve cells within the left hemisphere of the cerebral cortex control muscle contractions on the right side of the body. When the lesion that produces aphasia is on the left side of the cerebral cortex, the hemiplegia that results will be on the right side of the body. I'll describe some other impairments that people with aphasia may exhibit in a later section in this chapter.

Aphasic impairments often decrease in severity during the first 6 months posttrauma, a phenomenon known as *spontaneous recovery*. When there is trauma to the brain, some brain cells are destroyed while others are only damaged. At least some of the damaged cells are likely to begin functioning again during the first 6 months posttrauma. However, cells that have not begun functioning after 6 months are highly unlikely to change. Consequently, the prognosis for improving a client's ability to comprehend speech, formulate speech, converse, read, or write a year or more posttrauma is usually poor. Note, though, that this is not the same as saying that the prognosis for a client learning to communicate better is not very good. It often is possible to improve a client's ability to communicate through the use of what are known as augmentative and alternative communication (AAC) strategies, which I'll discuss in a later section of this chapter. An excellent way to learn more about the neurology of language is to read *Conversations With Neil's Brain: The Neural Nature of Thought & Language* (Calvin & Ojemann, 1994), which is available online.

Causes of Brain Damage and Resulting Aphasia

Aphasia, which literally means "without language," is caused by damage to specific areas of the brain that are responsible for language processes. The leading cause of aphasia is stroke, which causes approximately 80,000 new cases of aphasia per year in the United States (National Stroke Association, 2014a). Currently, the National Stroke Association estimates that there are approximately 1 million Americans who have aphasia. Other causes of aphasia include

- tumors,
- traumatic brain injury (TBI),
- brain surgery,
- brain infection, and
- dementia (discussed in a separate section in this chapter).

Three conditions can stop the flow of blood through a cerebral artery and thereby cause a stroke. In the first—which results in what is known as a **thrombotic stroke**—a blood clot forms in a cerebral artery and blocks blood flow. In the second—which results in what is known as a **thromboembolic stroke**—a clot forms in an artery outside the brain, a piece (i.e., **embolus**) breaks off, and the embolus is carried to a cerebral artery and blocks it. Note that the only difference between these two is where the clot originated. Both are collectively called **ischemic strokes**. The third condition that can cause a stroke differs from the first two in that it does not result in a blockage. Instead, a cerebral artery bursts and **hemorrhages**. Because there is now an opening in the artery, blood no longer flows through it to the areas of the brain it nourishes. Also, the blood that is released through the opening rips into the brain tissue, causing intense inflammation and swelling. Such strokes are called **hemorrhagic strokes**.

Another cause of aphasia is **neoplasms**, or **tumors**. Some are malignant (i.e., cancerous) and some are benign (i.e., noncancerous). Both types can impede the functioning of adjacent tissue by pressing against it or by obstructing blood circulation to it. In addition, malignant tumors can impair tissue function by invading and destroying it. Aphasia can also result from TBIs. TBI is the most common cause of brain damage in children and young adults. As with strokes and tumors, the site and the amount of damage will determine the severity of the language or other disorders. Brain surgery and brain infections can also result in aphasia, though sometimes surgery to remove a brain tumor that is affecting language function can improve the aphasia. ASHA's (2014b) website describes aphasia in considerable detail.

Language Characteristics of Aphasia

Although the language of individuals with aphasia varies according to which general area of the brain has been damaged, some of the language processes that are commonly affected are

- the ability to name objects, pictures, events, experiences;
- language fluency;
- conversational speech;
- expository speech;
- auditory comprehension;
- the ability to form speech sounds;
- the ability to repeat what has just been said;
- reading; and
- writing.

As you can see, aphasia affects language comprehension and language expression in both oral and written language. Some individuals with aphasia may have few of these symptoms while others may have all or almost all of them. Severity also varies considerably, with some individuals exhibiting minor symptoms that are hardly noticeable and others exhibiting more obvious and disabling symptoms. My point is that individuals with aphasia each present a unique and complex set of symptoms that must be thoroughly assessed in order to provide intervention that is tailored specifically to each client's unique pattern of speech and language needs. Box 5.1 lists several websites that offer detailed information about aphasia.

Classification of Aphasia

Aphasia is generally classified as **fluent** or **nonfluent aphasia**, based on the ease or effort required to produce speech. More specifically, aphasia is classified by type.

Wernicke's Aphasia–Fluent

Wernicke's aphasia (also called *receptive aphasia*) is a disturbance in the ability to comprehend speech. It usually is caused by a lesion on the part of the temporal lobe known as the **first temporal convolution**. This location is also referred to as *Wernicke's area*. Carl Wernicke, a 19th-century German neurologist, is thought to be the first to attribute receptive aphasia to a lesion in this area.

BOX 5.1 **Informative Aphasia Websites**

American Academy of Neurology
http://patients.aan.com/resources/neurologynow/?event=home.showArticle&id=ovid.com:/bib/ovftdb/01222928-201107030-00016

American Speech-Language-Hearing Association
http://www.asha.org/PRPSpecificTopic.aspx?folderid=8589934663&section=Overview

Mayo Clinic
http://www.mayoclinic.org/diseases-conditions/aphasia/basics/definition/con-20027061

National Aphasia Association
http://www.aphasia.org

National Institute of Neurological Disorders and Stroke
http://www.ninds.nih.gov/disorders/aphasia/aphasia.htm

National Stroke Association
http://www.stroke.org/site/PageServer?pagename=aphasia

WebMD
http://www.webmd.com/brain/aphasia-causes-symptoms-types-treatments

---

What would it be like to have difficulty deriving meaning from the words you hear? If your comprehension problem was severe, what you would experience would be similar to listening to someone speak in a language you had never studied. You would hear the words, but they would have little or no meaning for you. If your comprehension problem was not severe, the experience would be similar to taking a year or two of a foreign language and visiting a country where it is spoken. You would understand some of what you heard, but not all.

Because adults with Wernicke's aphasia have difficulty in deriving meaning from words, they also have difficulty choosing appropriate words to use in their own speech. Without realizing it, they use inappropriate words. In severe cases, almost all of their nouns and verbs are inappropriate. Their speech sounds like a foreign language or jargon. If you read aloud the poem "Jabberwocky," reprinted in Box 5.2, it will give you an idea of what their speech is like.

People who have this type of aphasia tend to be quite fluent because they are not aware of their errors and, consequently, don't revise them. For this reason, Wernicke's aphasia is sometimes referred to as *fluent aphasia*. Can you recall a time in a high school or college foreign language class when you volunteered to translate an English sentence because you thought you knew how to do it but were wrong? Since you were not aware of your error(s) while translating it, you probably were quite fluent—like someone with Wernicke's (receptive) aphasia. This YouTube video shows a patient with Wernicke's aphasia. Go to the website (http://goo.gl/HJtb9X) or scan the code.

Broca's Aphasia–Nonfluent

Broca's aphasia (also called *motor aphasia, expressive aphasia,* and *disfluent aphasia*) is an impairment in the ability to produce speech voluntarily. It usually is caused by a lesion in the part of the left frontal lobe referred to as the **third frontal convolution**. This portion of the frontal lobe is known as Broca's area. Broca, a nineteenth-century neurologist, is credited with being the first to demonstrate a relationship between a lesion in this area and an impairment in motor programming for speech.

Persons with this condition have difficulty moving their **articulators** in the manner required to produce the words they want to say when they want to say them. They know the words they want to say, but cannot say them. In severe cases they may be unable to say any words voluntarily. In mild cases they will be able to say most words voluntarily, but not necessarily fluently. Their speech tends to be slow, labored, and lacking normal inflection. For this reason, Broca's aphasia is sometimes referred to as *disfluent aphasia.*

Persons with Broca's aphasia tend to be more impaired in their ability to produce purposeful "intellectual" speech than in their ability to produce "emotional" speech. If they are upset, they may swear. Persons with Broca's aphasia convey meaning through pragmatics rather than through grammar or vocabulary. If they are angry, for example, the tone of their voice may communicate this. Furthermore, they

---

BOX 5.2   "Jabberwocky" (Carroll, 1871)

What might the language of people with relatively severe receptive aphasia look like? The poem "Jabberwocky" from Lewis Carroll's book *Through the Looking Glass* is close to that which they tend to produce—language that is grammatically correct but, for the most part, meaningless.

> 'Twas brillig and the slithy toves
> Did gyre and gimble in the wabe;
> All mimsy were the borogoves
> And the mome raths outgrabe.

> "Beware the Jabberwock, my son!
> The jaws that bite, the claws that catch!
> Beware the Jubjub bird, and shun
> The frumious Bandersnatch!"

> He took his vorpal sword in hand:
> Long time the manxome foe he sought—
> So rested he by the Tumtum tree,
> and stood awhile in thought.

> And as in the uffish thought he stood,
> The Jabberwock, with eyes of flame,
> Came whiffling through the tulgey wood,
> And burbled as it came!

> One, two! One, two! And through and through
> The vorpal blade went snicker-snack!
> He left it dead and with its head
> He went galumphing back.

> "And has thou slain the Jabberwock?
> Come to my arms, my beamish boy!
> O frabjous day! Callooh, Callay!"
> He chortled in his joy.

> 'Twas brillig and the slithy toves
> Did gyre and gimble in the wabe;
> All mimsy were the borogoves
> And the mome raths outgrabe.

---

are more impaired in their ability to produce voluntary speech than they are in their ability to produce rote speech. They may be able to count from 1 to 10 consecutively but not be able to begin with 3 and count to 10 or repeat a number when asked to do so. This YouTube video shows an individual with Broca's aphasia. Go to the website (http://goo.gl/oxQQlL) or scan the code.

What would it be like to have difficulty programming your articulators to say what you want to say? It would be somewhat similar to what you would experience if you tried to say a tongue-twister rapidly. Try the examples in Box 5.3.

Anomic Aphasia

Anomic aphasia, also a fluent type of aphasia, is a disturbance in word finding, most likely caused by a posterior lesion in the temporal–parietal region. People with this problem have difficulty remembering the names of things even though they recognize the objects. Although most persons who have this condition are senior citizens, it can have its onset during childhood. (See Casby [1992] for a case study of an 11-year-old boy who developed anomic aphasia.)

We have all had the experience of being unable to remember the names of people we know well. We recognize them and are able to remember many things about them, but no matter how hard we try, we cannot think of their names. We say that their names are "on the tip of our tongue." We usually remember them a short time later after we have stopped trying consciously to do so. This is similar to what people with anomic aphasia experience. The main differences are that they are likely to have difficulty finding at least a few words every time they speak, and their problem isn't limited to people's names. If people with anomia are told a word they cannot remember and then are asked to repeat it, they are usually able to do so; however, they may forget it again in a few minutes.

Conductive Aphasia

Conductive aphasia, a type of fluent aphasia that occurs in less than 10% of people with aphasia, results when there is damage to the group of fibers that connects Broca's area to Wernicke's area and the **supramarginal gyrus**. It can also occur when there is damage to the parietal lobe. Individuals with conductive aphasia usually have only a mild impairment in comprehending the speech of others, and their

---

BOX 5.3   **Tongue Twisters**

"Peter Piper picked a peck of pickled peppers."

"Twin-screw steel cruiser."

"Shall he sell sea shells?"

"She sells sea shells by the seashore."

Repeat each rapidly! Does it make you upset to have difficulty doing so? Do you feel compelled to keep working at it? If your answers to these questions are yes, you have a glimpse into what it feels like to have Broca's aphasia.

spontaneous speech is usually fluent, but their ability to repeat what they hear is more impaired.

The primary speech difficulty with conduction aphasia is in **phoneme** sequencing. People with conduction aphasia may distort words by adding syllables or sounds to words or they may transpose sounds in a word (i.e., **paraphasia**). People with conduction aphasia produce more paraphasias when they are trying to repeat. Although they can repeat some short utterances, they are unable to repeat multisyllabic words or syntactically complex utterances. These patients often try to correct their errors by saying a word over and over.

Transcortical Aphasia

Transcortical aphasia, another fluent aphasia, is caused by damage to the cerebral cortex surrounding Broca's area or Wernicke's area. Transcortical aphasias usually occur in older people because they result from a gradual deterioration of the blood supply to arteries. Two types occur, depending on where the lesion is located:

1. *Transcortical sensory aphasia*, a relatively rare fluent aphasia, is characterized by comprehension difficulties. Both reading and writing are affected. Verbal output is relatively fluent (although it may include jargon), and repetition is relatively good.
2. *Transcortical motor aphasia*, a nonfluent type of aphasia, is characterized by expressive language difficulties. Comprehension and repetition may be very good, but there is little spontaneous speech output. The patient can read but not write.

Global Aphasia

Global aphasia (also called *mixed aphasia*) occurs when the damage to the left hemisphere is extensive, covering a wide area of the cortex involved in language functioning. Because such a wide area of cortex has been affected, there is no discernible speech or language pattern that characterizes this type of aphasia. In the most severe forms of global aphasia, patients may be unable to utter more than one or two words (if any at all) in response to any kind of communication. They may also use gestures that are unrelated to their communicative intent.

Other Characteristics of Left-Hemisphere Damage

Extreme Fatigue

Individuals with aphasia often experience periods of extreme fatigue. The National Stroke Association (2014b) states that poststroke fatigue affects between 40% and

70% of individuals who have had a stroke. They point out that fatigue is different from feeling tired for two reasons. First, fatigue can occur without warning and, second, rest may not help. Individuals who experience poststroke fatigue often have difficulty concentrating and remembering. Because of this, therapy sessions for some individuals with aphasia are relatively short.

Seizures

The National Stroke Association (2014c) explains that predicting which stroke survivors will have a seizure is difficult, but they emphasize that seizures can be more serious if they occur shortly after a person has a stroke. Hemorrhagic strokes are more likely to be followed by a seizure than other types of stroke; and if people have a seizure within 24 hours of having a stroke, they have a higher mortality rate (National Stroke Association, 2014c). Their website has a detailed description of the types of seizures and their symptoms (2014c).

Visual Field Disturbances

Individuals with aphasia may also have a **visual field disturbance**. People with this impairment are partially blind. If, for example, they look straight ahead, they may be able to see objects to the left of their bodies but not to the right. Loss of vision in either the right or left half of the visual field in each eye is called **hemianopia**: Strokes in the left hemisphere can result in disturbances to the right visual field of each eye, and strokes in the right hemisphere can impair the left visual field of each eye (National Stroke Association, 2014d).

Perseveration

The inability to stop doing something is known as **perseveration**. An individual with aphasia who shows perseveration may repeat the same word over and over regardless of whether doing it is appropriate. For example, if a person who has this condition is shown a comb and says "comb," he or she may also respond "comb" if shown a pencil or some other object.

Abstract–Concrete Imbalance

People with aphasia who have an **abstract–concrete imbalance** have less than normal ability to categorize. For example, they may remember only some of the attributes that cause an object to be categorized as an animal and therefore may categorize dogs, but not cats or pigs, as animals. Their lack of normal ability to categorize can contribute significantly to the severity of their speech comprehension, speech formulation, and reading and writing problems. It can also contribute significantly to their problems with mathematics. This imbalance also shows in the individual's ability to use figurative language in order to understand idioms, proverbs, similes, and metaphors.

Catastrophic Reaction

Individuals who have severe aphasia may have a **catastrophic reaction** if too many demands are placed on them or when they become aware of the severity of their communication difficulties. For example, being asked by a spouse to say "thank you" for a delivered meal tray may cause an expressive person with aphasia to throw it. Other signs of a catastrophic reaction include aggressive behavior, crying or laughing uncontrollably, screaming, anxiety, and stubbornness (National Health Service Choices, 2014).

This type of reaction can be looked upon as a form of nonverbal communication. Viewed in this way, it should be possible to eliminate it by providing the person with aphasia with a more socially acceptable way to communicate anger or frustration, perhaps by pointing to line drawings on a communication board that convey these feelings.

Depression

It is not surprising that many people with aphasia experience depression. National Health Service Choices (2014), in the United Kingdom, estimates that 80% of people with aphasia will experience depression at least once. Some are suicidal or cry frequently. Others show a lack of energy or appetite, weight loss, withdrawal from others, sleep problems, and little interest in speech–language therapy (National Health Service Choices, 2014).

Altered Relationships

Because people with aphasia have lost the ability to communicate normally, their relationships with family members, friends, and coworkers are likely to change in highly undesirable ways. These changes can be more disabling to them than their language deficits. Vickers (2010) found that when individuals with aphasia participate in aphasia support or therapy groups, they feel more socially connected and less isolated.

When an individual has aphasia, the entire family is affected and can benefit from learning about their loved one's condition and needs, and from learning a variety of coping strategies. ASHA (2014k) offers a detailed list of strategies to help families cope with the serious emotional upheaval of a loved one's aphasia. Here's a YouTube video of a man who had a stroke. He and his wife talk about their life after his stroke. Go to the website (http://goo.gl/x6Gt4P) or scan the code.

Right-Hemisphere Deficits

Damage to the right half of the cerebral cortex results in right-hemisphere deficits. There are several types of right-hemisphere deficits, including those associated with loss of visuospatial and musical skills. These disorders of perception and orientation can underlie language problems. In addition, more subtle language abilities may be affected.

Clients who have right-hemisphere damage are often referred to SLPs for assessment and treatment. The types of disorders of perception and orientation that people with right-hemisphere damage exhibit include the following:

- *Anosognosia.* **A** condition in which an individual is not aware of having a difficulty or condition. For example, William O. Douglas, a former Associate Justice of the United States Supreme Court had **anosognosia**; following a stroke that damaged his right hemisphere and weakened his left arm, he insisted that his arm was injured in a fall.
- *Left neglect.* Individuals with right-hemisphere brain damage often fail to notice the left halves of objects, faces, or their own face or body.
- *Deficits in the recognition of objects or faces.* People who have this deficit may have difficulty identifying objects visually. They may, for example, put cigarette ashes in a sugar bowl (Shallice, 1987). They may also experience **prosopagnosia**, or face blindness. Furthermore, they may see faces where there are none, or vice versa. One patient who had such a deficit looked around for his hat and tugged his wife's head, thinking it was his hat (Sacks, 1985).
- *Deficits in the recognition of spatial relationships between objects.* Persons with such a deficit may experience difficulties dressing themselves. Or they may have difficulty finding their way around by reading maps, remembering familiar routes, or learning new ones.
- *Auditory dysfunctions.* These are usually related to the recognition and processing of music. Such dysfunctions are sometimes labeled *amusica*.

I mentioned earlier that people with right-hemisphere brain damage can have more subtle language problems because of their inability to interpret emotion in faces, scenes, or the tone of utterances. They can also have difficulty understanding idioms, jokes, parables, sarcasm, and irony, and they can struggle with understanding the narrative arc or stories or the logical sequencing of expository discourse.

Causes of Right-Hemisphere Deficits

Although right-hemisphere deficits occur after a right-hemisphere stroke, dementia and traumatic brain injury (TBI) can also produce right-hemisphere deficits.

Dementia

Dementia is a chronic, progressive syndrome characterized by problems with memory, thinking, behavior, and the ability to perform everyday activities (World Health Organization, 2014a). It affects individuals' ability to understand and use language, learn new things, and make appropriate judgments.

Worldwide, dementia from all causes affects between 5% and 7% of adults age 60 years and older (Prince et al., 2013). About 65% of dementia is of the Alzheimer's type. While **Alzheimer's disease** is more prevalent in older adults, it can appear in middle age and on rare occasions can affect people younger than 25. This progressive, **degenerative** disease usually begins with forgetfulness and disorientation and, over a period of 6 to 12 years, progresses to severe memory impairment (e.g., family not recognized), lack of responsiveness to speech, and mutism.

People who have Alzheimer's disease and other types of dementia tend to exhibit disturbances in language functioning. One of the most frequently mentioned is difficulty naming objects. However, the reason for their difficulty does not appear to be the same as for people with aphasia. Whereas the person with aphasia recognizes the object but cannot remember what it is called, the person with dementia fails to recognize the object in the first place.

All dementia results from brain damage. The specific type of damage is a function of the condition that is responsible for the dementia. In Alzheimer's disease, for example, the impairment seems to result from abnormalities known as **senile plaques** and **neurofibrillary tangles** that develop in the brain. Other conditions that can damage the brain to produce dementia include viruses and multiple strokes.

Traumatic Brain Injury

I described TBI in the previous chapter on language development. To review, brain trauma can occur whenever the head sustains a blow or wound that causes the brain to twist, turn, stop or start suddenly (as in a car accident), or be pushed against the skull. Brain injuries can affect many different parts of the brain, regardless of which part sustains the blow or wound. For instance, when the head strikes a hard object in a car accident, the skull hits the brain on the side of the impact, which forces the brain to bounce off the other side of the skull. The result is damage to both sides of the brain. In addition, hemorrhages that arise as a result of the injury can form a **hematoma**, which puts pressure on the brain.

The severity of the head wound or injury depends on the force of the impact and how much brain tissue is affected. The weaker the force and the less tissue that is damaged, the more likely it is that the resulting effects on motor, cognitive, and communication functions will be mild. Greater force and more brain tissue involvement make it more likely that the resulting effects on these functions will be severe.

Assessment and Intervention

Assessment

The assessment process for a person with aphasia involves three phases:

1. observation and interviews begun in-hospital with the individual and family members (includes providing and collecting informal information regarding communication);

2. a thorough examination of the peripheral speech mechanism (lips, tongue, palate, muscles), because apraxia is frequently associated with aphasia, and an informal and, if necessary, a formal evaluation of **hearing**; and

3. more formal assessment after the initial period of spontaneous recovery (usually several days during which the individual maintains a stable level on simple speech and language tasks).

Initial Observations and Interviews

During the first several visits, the SLP needs to observe the individual's speech, language, and communicative comprehension and usage, looking for what the individual communicates, the language forms and content used to communicate, and how the individual communicates. Can the individual understand what is said? Can the individual find the words to say? Is speech intelligible? Does the individual use single words? Phrases? Sentences? What is the individual's intonation; does it match the emotion she or he is trying to communicate? Can the individual read? Write? Recognize family members? Recite the letters of the alphabet? Can she or he hear noises in the environment? Voices?

Family members can provide valuable information about the individual prior to the stroke, including general mood, communication patterns and abilities, interests and habits, and level of support outside the family. It is important to remember, though, that family members may be traumatized and need counseling and support before they can begin to participate in an interview. The University of Michigan Aphasia Program (2014) offers an extensive curriculum for living with persons with aphasia.

Examination of the Peripheral Speech Mechanism and Hearing

Much of what the SLP needs to know about the speech mechanism can be observed while the individual is engaged in routine tasks, such as eating, drinking, and speaking or attempting to speak. However, the SLP will also want to examine the oral speech mechanism, which involves two steps:

1. determining the structural integrity of the oral, lingual, resonanatory, laryngeal, and respiratory structures (teeth and occlusion, hard and soft palates, tongue, face, nose, and mouth, neck and shoulders, postures, respiratory system) and

2. determining the functional adequacy of these structures for speech and nonspeech purposes (breathing to support speaking, swallowing, producing speech sounds, producing voice).

The SLP can obtain a general overview of the individual's hearing by checking for:

- the individual's awareness of and response to sounds in the environment;
- the individual's awareness of and response to others' speech; and
- if the individual produces sound or speech, the appropriateness of its volume.

Formal Speech and Language Assessment

Once the individual has stabilized from the initial consequences of the stroke, the SLP can begin more formal testing to assess the individual's communication system in its entirety, which includes assessing receptive and expressive communication in both oral and written forms and assessing the individual's language across pragmatics, syntax, semantics, phonology and morphology, nonverbal language, and various forms of discourse. Several standardized instruments are available to measure different aspects of the individual's communication functioning, and all require the SLP to determine which offer the most efficient and effective way to assess each particular individual.

Intervention

The primary goal of the SLP for adults with aphasia is to maximize effective use of communication in order to participate fully in their everyday lives. That is, the SLP's goal is to enable them to communicate more effectively in everyday conversational exchanges and to minimize the extent to which their condition limits their activities. Of prime importance is that the SLP treat each individual with respect, remembering that each is a person, not a disorder. In communicating with the individual, the SLP needs to adjust her or his language to meet that person's comprehension and processing abilities. The SLP must take into account the fear and uncertainty the person most likely feels at becoming aphasic and respond appropriately. The intervention the SLP provides flows directly from the relationship she or he has established with the individual.

Two general approaches are used for improving the ability of people with aphasia to communicate. One is to reduce the severity of their impairment in understanding speech, formulating speech, reading, writing, and calculating. The other is to augment their residual communication abilities through the use of gestures, communication boards, or electronic devices. You can see an example of a basic-needs communication board in Figure 5.2.

The first approach, to decrease deficits in affected language abilities, is most likely to be successful during the first 6 months posttrauma, while spontaneous recovery is still occurring. The SLP attempts to manipulate the environment to maximize spontaneous recovery. One way that he or she does this is to arrange for the person to have frequent opportunities for impaired language abilities to be stimulated. The SLP may do some stimulation in the therapy room, and some may be done by encouraging the person to interact frequently with other people outside the family. This may involve encouraging him or her to participate in a therapy group, a stroke support group, or a "golden age" club. Usually, the more communicating practice the person with aphasia gets (i.e., the more the impaired language abilities are stimulated), the more he or she is likely to improve during the spontaneous recovery period.

The second approach, to augment the client's residual communication abilities, is used both during and after the spontaneous recovery period. The goal is to

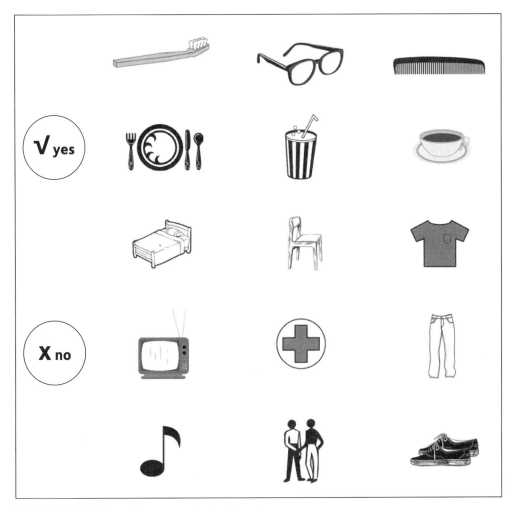

FIGURE 5.2. Basic-needs communication board.

augment the client's existing communication abilities so they will be adequate for meeting his or her communication needs. These could range in complexity from being able to communicate feelings to family and friends, describe physical needs to doctors and nurses during a period of hospitalization, or use professional language necessary to return to his or her job. Although the prognosis for improving communication using the first approach tends to be poor beyond the period of spontaneous recovery, this is not necessarily true with the second approach. For example, although it may not be possible to improve the speech of a client who has severe Broca's aphasia, it may be possible to improve the client's ability to communicate by teaching the client to use a mobile device that can generate speech.

The SLP can help clients continue to communicate by teaching the family to minimize the client's specific communication deficits and, consequently, maximize his or her ability to communicate with them. Family and friends are often willing to learn strategies for coping with the individual's unique set of communication difficulties. The Internet Stroke Center (2014) provides a detailed list of communication strategies families can employ to help the individual communicate to the best of her or his abilities.

Augmentative and Alternative Communication

In Chapter 4 I cited ASHA's definition of augmentative and alternative communication (AAC): any form of communication other than speech to articulate thoughts, needs, wants, observations, and feelings. Most of us use means other than speech—text messages, video messaging, photograph messaging, tweeting, posting on Facebook, making a YouTube video, e-mailing—as a matter of course in our communications with others. Still, for the majority of people, speech remains the primary way in which we communicate on a daily basis.

For people with disabilities that limit or prevent speech production, AAC is a way to maintain the ability to convey their messages. The SLP's job is to assist clients in achieving what the AAC Institute (2014) states are the two most important goals of people who rely on AAC: "saying exactly what they want to say, and saying it as fast as they can" (para. 2). Current AAC technology is moving toward mobile devices with apps that allow them to act as "multi-function devices that can offer options for not only communication, but also Internet access, education, social interaction, entertainment, gaming, and information access" (Light & McNaughton, 2012, p. 200).

Up to 40% of individuals with aphasia have language impairments that are considered to be severe (Beukelman et al., 2007). Most of these individuals will not recover sufficient language ability to be able to communicate successfully enough to participate fully in their everyday lives without compensatory support, which AAC offers. However, some individuals with severe language impairment may fear that using AAC will hinder the restoration of their natural language system and thus will refuse to use it, especially those systems that generate speech. Two types of AAC systems are used by individuals with limited speaking abilities: unaided and aided.

Unaided AAC Systems

Unaided AAC systems involve no external equipment or device but rely instead on the individual's body to communicate. Examples include gestures or postures to convey information; sign language, which, because it has its own syntactic structure and morphology, allows the individual to communicate more complicated and nuanced messages; or fingerspelling, which is slower than signing but useful when the individual's sign vocabulary is small.

Unaided AAC systems require the individual to have sufficient motor ability to produce gestures, postures, fingerspelling, or signs. In addition, because many individuals with aphasia have some degree of language impairment, learning to fingerspell or sign may be too difficult. An additional problem is that most adults with aphasia do not have communication partners fluent in fingerspelling or sign.

Aided AAC Systems

According to Beukelman et al. (2007), low-technology AAC systems (communication boards and books, drawing, photo books, word boards) have been in use for almost 30 years. However, in medical settings, most low-tech systems are impersonal (i.e., generic) and limited to the medical context. Outside of medical settings, SLPs often design personal communication boards and books for their clients with aphasia, changing them as the client's communication develops poststroke. Using personalized systems allows the SLP to include items that let the individual communicate to maintain relationships with family and friends, tell listeners new ideas or thoughts, and use the polite forms that punctuate conversations.

High-tech systems currently available include computer software that displays icons the individual can manipulate to communicate more extensive and complex ideas. Some include visual scenes the individual can use to establish the context for what she or he wants to talk about. Speech-synthesizing technology allows an individual to generate sentences. However, many such devices produce speech that is difficult for listeners to understand. Perhaps the most famous person using speech synthesis is Stephen Hawking, a renowned theoretical physicist who is known for his work on general relativity and black holes.

The most common speech-generating devices (SGDs) are those that use digitized recordings of natural speech, which allows the user to choose among a stored database of sentences, and those that actually synthesize speech, which allows the user to speak novel sentences. Both systems rely on a database of vocabulary based on the user's needs and the contexts in which he or she will be using the device. The exact words, how they're organized, and how they're updated depend on each user. The output of SGDs is slower than natural speech, which places a burden on the listener.

Working With Bilingual Clients With Aphasia

According to Faroqi-Shah, Frymark, Mullen, and Wang (2010), half the world's population is bilingual, meaning they use two or more languages or dialects in their daily communications. Consequently, SLPs are providing services to more bilingual adults with aphasia, which raises questions about how to improve the individual's communication in both languages. When the SLP speaks the same first language (L1) as the person with aphasia, intervention poses less of a challenge than if the SLP does not speak the same first language as the client. Perhaps more important, though, is whether to focus on one of the individual's languages or to include both in the intervention process.

Faroqi-Shah et al.'s (2010) evidence-based systematic review examining the language outcomes of intervention using only the individual's second language (L2) showed the following:

1. receptive and expressive language outcomes were positive;
2. cross-language transfer was seen in the majority of individuals studied; and
3. age of acquisition of L2 and whether L1 and L2 are closely related in structure had little effect on the language outcomes of intervention.

What these findings mean clinically is that when the SLP is not bilingual and does not have access to a bilingual translator, conducting intervention using the individual's second language will not impede the client's outcomes. Of course, as I pointed out earlier, the SLP needs to also take into consideration the client's preferences and those of her or his family when designing the intervention plan.

Kiran and Roberts (2009) reported that in individuals who use more than one language, all those languages are active during language processing, which means that intervention using one language will likely transfer to the other language(s) the individual uses. However, if one language is strongly dominant and the intervention occurs in the less dominant language, the individual may experience interference from the dominant language.

The clinical implications of what is currently known about providing intervention to bilingual individuals with aphasia first require the SLP to thoroughly investigate the client's language use before the stroke, including whether the client uses L1 in some contexts and L2 in others, or whether they are used interchangeably. Second, they require the clinician to understand that assessment instruments are limited, even those that have been adapted to multiple languages.

Kiran and Roberts (2009) offer the following conclusions about how to make an informed decision about which language to train during intervention:

1. Using one language is not likely to impede or limit the other language.
2. If only one language can be used during intervention, the best results will come from using the individual's stronger language.
3. Take into account the client's own preferences, including the cultural and sociolinguistic contexts within which intervention is taking place.

They point out, for instance, that if the client wishes to maintain multicultural communication, then providing intervention in both (all) of the client's languages makes sense.

PART 3

Speech Disorders

The chapters in this section address speech disorders. Chapter 6 is devoted to voice production and the disorders associated with the voice. I describe the speech mechanism and how it works to produce voice and then turn to describing the various disorders that affect the voice, and then to assessment and intervention. I also include in this chapter a discussion of providing services to transgender/transsexual individuals.

Chapter 7 focuses on the speech and swallowing disorders associated with dysarthria in both children and adults. I include a discussion of how swallowing works and how to diagnose and treat both swallowing and speech disorders when the muscles of the mouth, face, and respiratory system are weakened or impaired because of neural damage.

In Chapter 8, I discuss the articulation and phonological disorders that affect children. I begin with a description of how speech sounds are produced and follow with a discussion of assessment and intervention strategies.

Chapter 9 addresses fluency disorders. I begin by describing normal versus abnormal fluency and the types of disfluencies people produce during speech. In this chapter I include discussion of theories of fluency disorders and their impact on the design of assessment and intervention.

chapter 6

Voice Production and Disorders

Learning Objectives

Describe the respiratory system and its function in voice production.

Describe the motor system and its role in voice production.

Describe the anatomy and function of the larynx in voice production.

Describe the five major types of voice disorders and their characteristics.

Describe laryngectomy and consequent voice production.

Describe what to include in a voice or resonance evaluation.

Describe the focus of evaluation and treatment when providing transgender or transsexual voice services.

Overview

To understand voice disorders, you'll need to know how the entire **speech** mechanism is structured and how it functions to produce voice. The speech mechanism includes the **respiratory system**, **larynx**, and **vocal tract**. These three sets of structures act in concert to produce voice and the unique resonance patterns characteristic of each individual. The vocal tract is controlled by the **motor system**. Voice production is affected by a variety of factors that can result in a voice disorder, which are assessed and managed with a wide range of tools and techniques. A representation of the speech mechanism is shown in Figure 6.1

The Speech and Voice Mechanism

Respiratory System

The respiratory system produces the raw material—air under pressure—from which speech is generated. The main component of the respiratory system is the **lungs**. Air

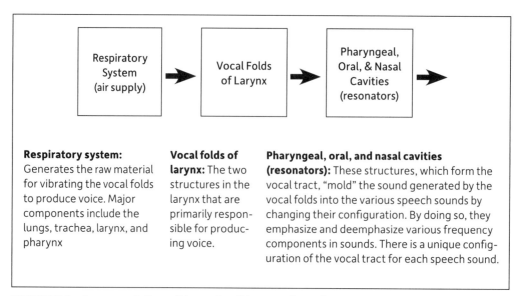

FIGURE 6.1. A representation of the parts of the speech mechanism.

Respiratory system: Generates the raw material for vibrating the vocal folds to produce voice. Major components include the lungs, trachea, larynx, and pharynx

Vocal folds of larynx: The two structures in the larynx that are primarily responsible for producing voice.

Pharyngeal, oral, and nasal cavities (resonators): These structures, which form the vocal tract, "mold" the sound generated by the vocal folds into the various speech sounds by changing their configuration. By doing so, they emphasize and deemphasize various frequency components in sounds. There is a unique configuration of the vocal tract for each speech sound.

from the environment is drawn into the lungs through **inspiration**. Air is stored in the lungs for a short time, during which oxygen is extracted and waste products are sloughed. The air is then expelled from the lungs under pressure through **expiration**.

Air enters the lungs either through the nose, which warms and moistens the air, or through the mouth. From there the air descends through the **oropharynx**, into the **laryngopharyngeal** region to the larynx, then through the larynx and down into the trachea. The trachea divides into two branches, which carry air into the left and right lungs.

Breathing is an automatic process that functions to supply oxygen to our blood and to remove carbon dioxide from our bodies. Various muscle groups act to increase and decrease the volume of the thoracic cavity, which directly affects the volume of the lungs. One of the largest of the respiratory muscles, the **diaphragm** creates the primary force during inspiration. When it contracts it pulls downward and increases the thoracic cavity and the lungs. The **external intercostals**, located between each of the ribs, elevate the rib cage, which further increases the thoracic cavity. The **sternocleidomastoid** muscle, active only during deep breathing, pulls the breastbone and the collarbone upward.

At the end of an inspiration, these muscles relax, which allows the thoracic cavity to decrease, beginning the expiratory phase. At the same time, gravity pulls the ribcage down, while the elasticity of the diaphragm causes it to move upward into its normal, relaxed position. The **internal intercostal muscles**, located between the ribs, depress the ribs, and several abdominal muscles indirectly force the diaphragm upward. All of these factors contribute to expiration.

Phonatory System

During expiration, air under pressure is sent from the lungs to the larynx, which is illustrated in Figure 6.2. The function of the larynx (particularly the **vocal folds**) is to set the molecules of this breath stream into vibration, which results in **phonation**.

As you see in Figure 6.2, the larynx is made up of several cartilages that serve as the base on which various ligaments and muscles attach. The three largest cartilages are the thyroid cartilage, cricoid cartilage, and epiglottis. The thyroid cartilage is what makes up the bump in people's throats, more prominent in men than in women. The cricoid cartilage, which sits on top of the trachea, forms the base of the larynx. The epiglottis, a large, broad, leaf-shaped cartilage, helps prevent food from entering the larynx during swallowing.

The two vocal folds, shown in the schematic in Figure 6.3, are attached at the front to the thyroid cartilage and at the back to the arytenoid cartilages. When we

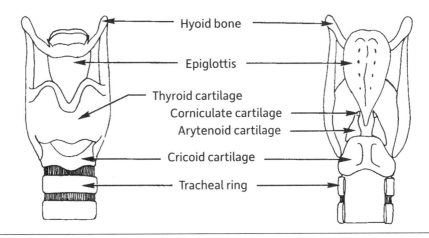

FIGURE 6.2. Anatomy of the larynx.

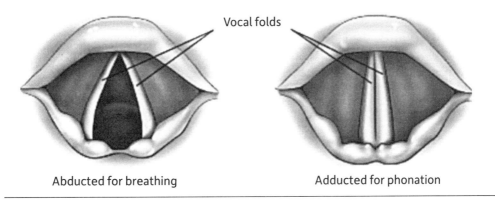

FIGURE 6.3. Vocal folds.

are breathing, they move apart (**abduct**) to allow air to flow freely to and from the lungs, and when we are producing voice, they move together (**adduct**), which constricts the airflow and causes them to vibrate, thus producing phonation.

Each vocal fold has within it a bundle of muscle tissue known as the **thyroarytenoid muscle**. because it attaches to the thyroid cartilage and the arytenoid cartilage. Its function is to relax and shorten the vocal folds to assist in producing low vocal pitch.

Vocal Fold Vibration

The vibration of the vocal folds results from the buildup of air pressure coming up from the lungs. The rate (i.e., frequency) at which the vocal folds vibrate is determined by several factors, including their length, mass, and tension. The thicker they are, the lower the frequency at which they tend to vibrate. This is why the pitch of male voices tends to be lower than that of female ones. The greater the vocal folds' mass (i.e., thickness), the lower the frequency at which they tend to vibrate. Tumors on the vocal folds, for example, increase their mass and result in a lowering of the pitch of the voice. And the less tense they are (for a given length and mass), the lower the frequency at which they tend to vibrate and the lower the pitch of the voice. Therefore, the lowest frequency would occur with someone with long, thick, less tense vocal folds. This YouTube video demonstrates the typical vocal folds of a woman vibrating at various frequency (pitch) levels. You'll notice in the video that, as the woman raises and lowers her pitch, her vocal folds lengthen and shorten. Go to the website (http://goo.gl/rXaOn8) or scan the code.

Opening and Closing the Vocal Folds

When we are breathing and not attempting to speak, the vocal folds are in the abducted position (see Figure 6.3). The folds are widely separated, allowing an unrestricted flow of air from the environment to the lungs and vice versa. They do not vibrate, and air flows continuously through the opening between them. This open space is referred to as the **glottis**.

When we are speaking, the vocal folds adduct (again, see Figure 6.3). During phonation, the vocal folds adduct at the midline of the larynx. Air pressure then builds up below them, causing them to vibrate. Anything that keeps the vocal folds from approximating normally can produce a voice disorder.

Changing Pitch

We vary the pitch of our voice by varying the tension of the vocal folds. We do this by causing the thyroid cartilage—the bottom of which is attached by two joints to the right and left sides of the **cricoid cartilage**—to move in either an anterior or a posterior direction. Because the anterior ends of the vocal folds are attached to the thyroid cartilage, when the cartilage rocks forward, tension on the vocal folds increases. And when it rocks backward, the folds become less tense. Consequently, we raise the pitch of our voice by causing the thyroid cartilage to move in an anterior (i.e., forward) direction.

Looking at the Vocal Folds

To look at the vocal folds (the **laryngoscopic view**), the examiner places a round mirror with a hole in the center over one eye. A light reflected from this head mirror is directed into the patient's mouth and onto the laryngeal mirror, which is placed against the back wall of the patient's pharynx at a 45-degree angle. The light from this mirror is directed into the patient's larynx, allowing an image of the top surface and edges of the vocal folds to be reflected in it. This is called *indirect laryngoscopy.* What you see in Figure 6.4 is a schematic drawing of the laryngoscopic view of the vocal folds.

Vocal Tract and Resonance

The vibration pattern of molecules produced by phonation is complex. The sound produced contains a wide range of frequencies and has a buzzing quality. This sound, called the **laryngeal tone**, is molded into phonemes by the vocal tract.

The vocal tract can be imagined as a box containing three major cavities that mold voice into speech sounds. The vocal tract consists of the **pharyngeal cavity** (i.e., pharynx), **oral cavity**, and **nasal cavity** (as illustrated in Chapter 1 in Figure 1.2). The configuration (i.e., shape) of the vocal tract at any particular moment determines which speech sound will be produced.

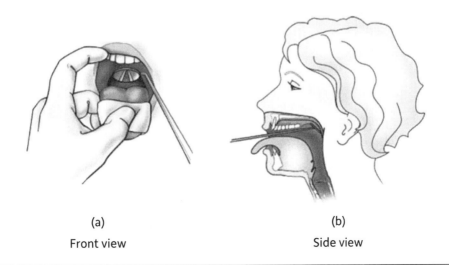

(a)

Front view

(b)

Side view

FIGURE 6.4. Indirect laryngoscopy.

This configuration can be changed by the movement of several structures within it: the tongue, lips, **mandible**, and **velum**, or soft palate. The tongue, lips, and mandible are located in the oral cavity. The velum, which is located in the pharyngeal cavity, controls the influence of the nasal cavity on the remainder of the vocal tract. The velum either stays down to allow the breath stream to flow from the oral cavity into the nasal cavity (to produce the sounds /m/, /n/, and /ŋ/) or lifts up to close the opening into the nasal cavity. When it lifts up and prevents sound from going into the nasal cavity, the oral cavity alone shapes the speech sound.

The components of the vocal tract act as resonators; in this capacity they increase the intensity of certain frequencies in the laryngeal tone and reduce the intensity of others. The configuration of these cavities at any given moment determines which frequencies in the laryngeal tone will be reinforced and which will be damped. That is, the voice **resonates** in particular ways because it passes through, bounces off, and echoes inside the throat (pharynx), the oral cavity (mouth), and the nose (nasal cavity).

Think about how your voice sounds when you have a cold or nasal congestion. The congestion changes the resonating qualities of the nasal cavities, rendering your voice more nasal (i.e., **hyponasal**). Each person's voice quality results in part from his or her own unique resonating characteristics of the vocal tract.

Motor System

The movements produced by all the parts of the vocal tract are controlled by the motor system. You'll remember that these movements change the configuration of the vocal tract, which changes the resonance of the laryngeal tone.

The tongue plays a significant role in changing the vocal tract configuration. The tongue contains muscle fibers that contract to change its shape, thereby changing the configuration of the vocal tract. For example, the contraction of certain muscle fibers within the tongue raises its tip, which produces sounds much different from those that result from the contraction of muscles to raise the back of the tongue: /d/ versus /g/. The contraction of muscle fibers is controlled directly by the peripheral nervous system (PNS) and the central nervous system (CNS), and indirectly by the autonomic nervous system (ANS). Figure 6.5 shows a diagram of the motor system, which I discuss below.

The **pyramidal system**, which originates in the primary motor cortex of the brain, includes the **upper motor neurons** and **lower motor neurons**, and determines which muscles will contract during voluntary movements, such as phonation. To elevate the tongue tip, for example, certain muscle fibers in the tongue have to contract. For this to happen, the upper motor neurons send messages to their lower motor neurons, which cause the lower motor neurons to send electrical signals to the muscle fibers that innervate the tongue, causing those muscles to contract. The pyramidal system is also involved with the inhibition of certain reflexes that can interfere with voluntary movement. If the pyramidal system is not functioning prop-

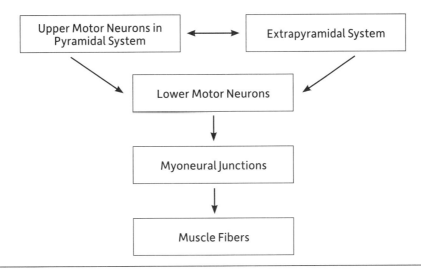

FIGURE 6.5. Diagram of the motor system.

erly, there is both reduced ability to make voluntary movements and hyperactive (i.e., increased) reflexes. Both of these conditions can interfere with the functioning of the speech mechanism.

The **extrapyramidal system** indirectly controls motion movement patterns and is involved in maintaining equilibrium, coordination, posture, muscle tone, and reflexes. It allows movements, such as those involved in speech production, to be made smoothly and accurately at a rapid rate. If the extrapyramidal system is not functioning properly, it may only be possible to make movements at a very slow rate; it may be possible to make rapid movements, but not accurately; or movement patterns may be accompanied by involuntary movements, such as tremors.

People with **Parkinson's disease** have an abnormality in the functioning of the extrapyramidal system. People with Parkinson's disease are unable to make movements rapidly, and they make involuntary movements (i.e., tremors), which can obviously disturb the functioning of the speech mechanism. To learn more about Parkinson's disease, visit the National Institute on Neurological Disorders and Stroke (NINDS; 2015c) webpage.

Lower motor neurons conduct electrical signals to muscle fibers through **myoneural** (i.e., muscle–nerve) **junctions**. Lower motor neurons and muscle fibers do not come into direct contact; rather, there is a thin layer of chemical between them at the myoneural junction. If particular myoneural junctions do not function properly, electrical signals will not reach certain muscle fibers, and the muscles will not contract. This occurs with the partial paralysis that accompanies **myasthenia gravis**, a condition caused by an abnormality in the chemical makeup of the myoneural junctions. This YouTube video shows a young woman with myasthenia gravis. To learn more, visit the NINDS (215b) webpage on myasthenia gravis. Go to the website (http://goo.gl/3g4IWw) or scan the code.

If appropriate electrical signals pass through their myoneural junctions but some of the fibers in a muscle are abnormal, the muscle will not contract. One disease with this characteristic is **muscular dystrophy**. (To learn more, visit the NINDS, 2015a, webpage on muscular dystrophy.)

Emotional states, particularly anxiety, can influence motor functioning through the activity of the autonomic nervous system (ANS). The activity of this system affects the functioning of both the pyramidal and extrapyramidal systems. The speech mechanism appears to be particularly susceptible to disturbance by anxiety. People tend to repeat sounds and syllables when they are highly anxious—for instance, when experiencing stage fright.

Voice and Resonance Disorders

There are five major types of voice disorders: disorders that can be related to (1) trauma, (2) problems that have an unknown cause, (3) **congenital** problems, (4) disorders of the brain or nervous system, and (5) vocal resonance.

Trauma-Related Disorders

There are three primary causes of trauma to the larynx. Behavioral trauma involves overuse of the voice (i.e., hyperfunction). Mechanical trauma is physical injury from sources either external or internal. Trauma from burns may also cause a voice disorder.

Behavioral Traumas

Either vocal abuse or vocal misuse can cause behavioral trauma to the larynx. Table 6.1 lists some common ways people abuse or misuse their larynges and the possible side effects on the voice. Figure 6.6 shows four types of vocal fold growths. The most common of these is vocal nodules, which are caused by behavioral trauma.

Mechanical Traumas

Mechanical traumas to the larynx can come from either external or internal sources. External injuries to the larynx occur in several ways. The most common cause of an external injury to the larynx is an automobile accident in which the neck and larynx come into contact with the steering wheel or other part of the car. An external injury to the larynx can also come from other blunt objects striking the larynx with great force, for instance, a child hitting the handlebars of a bicycle, falling on a curb or step, running into a wire, or being hit with a baseball bat.

External injuries that penetrate the larynx usually are caused by a gunshot, a knife wound, or an automobile accident. Malpositioning of a **tracheostomy** tube during an emergency procedure, especially in children because of their incompletely developed laryngeal structures, may cause injury to the larynx.

TABLE 6.1. Possible Side Effects of Vocal Misuse and Abuse

Vocal misuse and abuse	Possible side effect
Yelling, screaming, cheering (which cause vocal folds to adduct with great force)	• Hematomas • Vocal nodules • Breathy, hoarse, or harsh voice
Strained vocalizations (e.g., children mimicking machine noises or vocalizations made when lifting heavy objects) that cause vocal folds to adduct tightly to trap air	• Vocal fold irritation • Breathy, hoarse, or harsh voice
Excessive talking	• Vocal fold irritation • Hoarse or harsh voice
Frequent use of hard glottal attack (adducting the vocal folds, building up air, and releasing it in an explosion)	• Hoarse, harsh, or breathy voice • Chronic laryngitis • Vocal nodules • Vocal polyps • Contact ulcers
Throat clearing and coughing	• Hoarse voice • Contact ulcers
Inhaling dust, cigarette smoke, and other pollutants	• Vocal edemas • Carcinoma • Vocal polyps
Singing with poor technique (too loud, at an inappropriate pitch, or with hard glottal attack)	• Vocal fold irritation • Vocal nodules • Hoarse, harsh, or breathy voice
Talking with an inappropriately low pitch	• Contact ulcers
Talking with an inappropriately high pitch	• Vocal nodules • Breathy, hoarse, or harsh voice
Alcohol overuse	• Vocal edemas
Untreated infection	• Acute laryngitis

Injuries to the larynx caused by internal sources include (1) an endoscopic examination performed improperly, (2) an **endotracheal intubation** during surgery that irritates the mucus membrane, or (3) a **nasogastric tube** that causes laryngeal irritation during swallowing, resulting in hoarseness or laryngeal pain.

The most severe form of mechanical trauma is when one or both of the vocal folds are removed surgically in a procedure called a **laryngectomy**. If the vocal folds aren't present, they can't vibrate! The primary reason for this type of surgery is cancer of the larynx. The entire larynx may be removed (total laryngectomy), or only the tumor and the tissue surrounding it may be removed (partial laryngectomy). People who have had a laryngectomy usually can have the ability to speak through the use of an **artificial larynx**, or through being taught to utilize the musculature of the **esophagus** or trachea to set molecules of air into vibration.

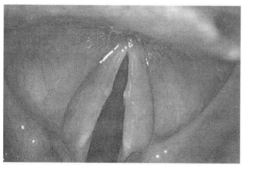

Vocal Nodules

Typically on the anterior third of the vocal folds

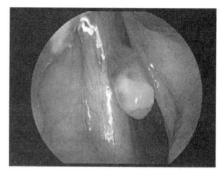

Vocal Polyp

Typically on one vocal fold but can form on both

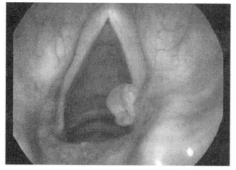

Contact Ulcer

Typically on the posterior third of the vocal folds

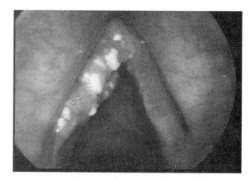

Laryngeal Cancer (carcinoma)

Typically on the edges of the vocal folds

FIGURE 6.6. Laryngoscopic views of four types of vocal fold growths.

Trauma Caused by Burns

Burns to the larynx are either thermal or chemical. Thermal burns, which are seen most often in firefighters and members of rescue teams, may be caused by inhaling hot air or gas. Thermal burns may also be caused by swallowing hot foods or liquids. Thermal burns are painful and cause a hoarse voice; however, if treatment is begun immediately, healing is usually rapid.

Chemical burns to the larynx occur most frequently in children who have swallowed a dangerous substance. These burns are frequently serious and are accompanied by burns of the esophagus and upper pharynx. Some people may lose their voices altogether, while others may have a hoarse, breathy voice. Because scarring is common, voice quality may not improve with healing.

Voice Disorders of Unknown Cause

Some voice disorders are caused by faulty approximation of the vocal folds that does not result from any known organic cause. Vocal folds can be either overly tense and hyperadducted (held tightly together) or lax and hypoadducted (held somewhat apart). These disorders can range in severity from complete **aphonia** to continuous use of a high pitch.

Ventricular Dysphonia (False Vocal Fold Phonation)

Ventricular dysphonia, a rare voice disorder, occurs when an individual uses the **ventricular (vestibular) folds** (i.e., false vocal folds) to produce voice. Sometimes, a person will hold the true vocal folds slightly apart (i.e., hypoadducted) and use the ventricular folds for phonation. Often, the voice that results is lower in frequency than that produced with the true vocal folds.

Voice Disorders Related to Stress or Psychological Conditions

When a person loses all or part of her or his phonatory ability because of stress, emotional distress, or a psychological problem, the resulting condition is called a *conversion disorder*. These disorders, which are relatively uncommon, include complete mutism, in which the individual makes no attempt to phonate. They also include functional aphonia, in which the person can whisper but the vocal folds do not vibrate, and **dysphonia**, in which the individual exhibits varying degrees of hoarseness. These disorders may continue until the individual has engaged in a counseling process that resolves the psychological aspects associated with the voice disorder.

Puberphonia (Mutational Falsetto)

Puberphonia is the continued use after puberty of the higher-pitched voice used before puberty, in spite of a larynx that is physically capable of producing the normal lower pitch of adults. This disorder affects both boys and girls, although it is more noticeable in boys because their prepubescent voice is about one octave higher than the postpubescent voice. (For girls the difference is only three to four semitones.) Vocal quality is characterized by a high pitch, low intensity (soft voice), and breathiness. Postpubescent boys and men who use falsetto voice often suffer social consequences, which vary from **culture** to culture.

Spasmodic Dysphonia (SD)/Laryngeal Dystonia

Spasmodic dysphonia, a form of **dystonia**, stems from either hyperadduction or hypoadduction of the vocal folds or a combination of the two. In the hyperadducted form, the vocal folds are so tightly closed that they cannot vibrate for any length of time; in the hypoadducted form, the vocal folds periodically move apart, producing a severely breathy voice. Spasmodic dysphonia is considered a neurological disorder and is thought to be caused by abnormal functioning in the **basal ganglia** (National Institute on Deafness and Other Communication Disorders, 2014c). Spasmodic dysphonia affects slightly more women than men and usually begins in middle adulthood. This YouTube video shows voice samples from four people with spasmodic dysphonia. Go to the website (http://goo.gl/2m33oS) or scan the code.

Vocal Fold Dysfunction

Vocal fold dysfunction (VCD), also called *paradoxical vocal fold motion*, is a closing of the vocal folds even when the person is inhaling, resulting in an airway obstruction. This disorder is chronic and is sometimes mistaken for asthma, although in VCD the tightening that restricts breathing occurs in the vocal folds rather than in the bronchial tubes. Adding to the difficulty in distinguishing VCD from asthma is that many people who have asthma also have VCD. There is no consensus regarding its cause, although most recent studies suggest multiple causes, including respiratory infections, exercise, acid reflux, secondhand tobacco smoke, and stress. VCD produces several nonphonatory symptoms, including tightness in the throat and chest, wheezing, coughing, and shortness of breath. The voice is often breathy or hoarse.

Congenital Conditions Resulting in Voice Disorders

Congenital dysphonias

Congenital dysphonias occur as a consequence of certain congenital anomalies of the larynx, including airway obstructions. These obstructions cause respiratory difficulties, hoarseness, a weak cry, and dysphagia. These congenital abnormalities, which are usually identified in children, are usually treated medically before the **speech–language pathologist (SLP)** becomes involved. One congenital condition that can result in dysphonia is laryngeal papillomatosis, which appears as a mass lesion of the vocal folds that is caused by an **HPV (human papillomavirus)** infection.

Congenital Mass Lesions of the Larynx

Mass lesions of the larynx include tumors and viral growths, both of which may produce voice symptoms. Although neither type of lesion typically results in voice problems themselves, the most common voice symptom that does occur is hoarseness that appears following the surgical removal of the lesion.

Congenital Structural Anomalies of the Larynx

Sometimes infants have insufficient or delayed calcium depositing in the larynx, which can cause nonphonatory problems. However, a tracheostomy may be performed to allow time for the symptoms to disappear. Because the child is unable to produce voice until the tracheostomy has been closed, the SLP may need to monitor the child's developing **language** and provide alternative communication forms if necessary.

Children with Cri du Chat syndrome, a chromosomal **anomaly** in which there is a partial deletion of chromosome number 5, have voices that sound like a kitten mewing. Children with this syndrome also have other characteristics, including developmental disability, small-size head, widely spaced and downward-slanting eyes, asymmetrical eye movements, and speech and language delays.

Congenital Laryngeal Webs

A laryngeal web is connective tissue that **occludes** the larynx, either partially or totally. While relatively rare, total laryngeal webs are usually treated immediately at birth in order for the infant to be able to breathe. Laryngeal webs are caused by the failure of the vocal-fold tissue to develop during the first trimester of pregnancy. If the web is located at the level of the glottis, the voice can be hoarse, aphonic, or elevated in pitch. Figure 6.7 provides a picture of a laryngeal web.

Disorders of the Brain or Nervous System

Dysarthrias, or motor speech disorders, are neurogenic dysphonias that result from impairments in the innervation of the respiratory, resonatory, or phonatory muscles used to produce voice; impairments of muscle function; or impairments of motor planning at the neurologic level. The type of disorder and its severity depend on which area of the nervous system has been affected. Many conditions can result in dysarthria, including brain injury or tumor, cerebral palsy, multiple sclerosis, muscular dystrophy, Parkinson's disease, myasthenia gravis, and Lyme disease, among others. The speech of people with dysarthria can be slow and slurred; rapid, produced only in a whisper; or with nasal, strained, or hoarse voice quality. In addition, these individuals may have difficulty controlling their facial muscles and chewing, swallowing, and controlling the tongue (Healthline, 2014).

The most common way to classify dysarthria is based on a system, still used today, devised by Darley, Aronson, and Brown (1975). Their system describes six types of dysarthria. Table 6.2 summarizes the types of dysarthria and their voice characteristics.

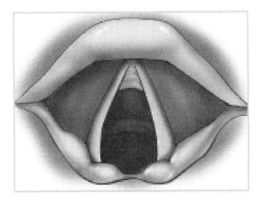

FIGURE 6.7. Laryngeal web.

TABLE 6.2. Dysarthrias and Their Voice Characteristics

Dysarthria classification	Location of damage	Possible causes	Possible voice characteristics
Ataxic	Cerebellum	Degenerative diseases, strokes, TBI, tumors, lead or mercury poisoning	• Harsh • Loud • Irregular intonation and long pauses • Vowel distortions and inaccurate consonant production
Flaccid	Nerves that enervate the speech musculature	Muscular dystrophy, myasthenia gravis, ALS, polio, infections secondary to AIDS, surgical trauma	• Weak voice • Hypernasal • Breathy • Monoloud • Monopitch
Spastic	Damage to both the pyramidal and extrapyramidal systems	Stroke, ALS, TBI, brainstem tumor, cerebral anoxia, viral or bacterial infection, multiple sclerosis	• Strained • Harsh • Low pitched • Hypernasal • Bursts of loudness
Hyperkinetic	Extrapyramidal system (basal ganglia)	Essential tremor syndrome, Huntington's disease, dystonia	• Harsh • Strained • Voice stoppages • Hypernasal
Hypokinetic	Extrapyramidal system	Parkinson's disease, Alzheimer's, stroke, TBI, tumors, drug toxicity	• Hoarse • Low volume • Hypernasal • Monotonous • Monoloud
Mixed	Combination of 2 or more dysarthria types	ALS, multiple sclerosis	• Varies based on neurological conditions

Apraxia of Speech

Apraxia of speech is a motor system planning disorder. Unlike the various types of dysarthria, apraxia does not result from damage to speech muscles or from weakness in the muscles used to produce speech. Rather, it stems from difficulty retrieving the motor speech patterns required to produce fluent speech. The results are greatly increased effort to speak, groping for the position(s) needed to produce sounds, abnormal stress and intonation patterns, altered speech rhythm and prosody, and inconsistent articulation errors.

Apraxia of speech often coexists with aphasia, but because apraxia of speech is a motor speech disorder and aphasia is a language disorder, intervention must target both conditions.

Disorders of Vocal Resonance

Languages vary in the amount of nasality their consonants use. In English speech, **nasality** is used to produce only three phonemes: /m/, /n/, and / ŋ /. All other English consonants are produced using **orality**, although some nasality is also present. Other languages (e.g., French) use more nasality than English, and some United States dialects incorporate a more nasal "twang" than others.

Oral resonance is shaped by the oral cavity. The size and resiliency of the pharynx and the postures of the tongue, palate, and lips combine to shape the oral cavity. At the same time the velum and the nasopharyngeal wall close against each other to seal the oral cavity so that little or no air escapes into the nasal cavity.

To produce nasality, the velum drops down and the pharynx relaxes. This allows air and voice to flow into the nasal cavity to be shaped by their various structures. The resulting voice sounds more nasal than the voice produced when there is no resonance in the nasal cavity.

Hypernasality

Excessive nasal resonance results in **hypernasality**, which usually occurs because the velum (soft palate) has not made sufficient closure between the oral and nasal cavities. Sometimes a structural defect makes it difficult or impossible for the soft palate to seal the oral cavity. This can happen with a cleft palate, a short velum, or surgical or accidental injury to the velum.

Hyponasality

Hyponasality occurs when an individual cannot produce any nasal resonance. The resulting voice sounds like the person has a stuffy nose. Hyponasality almost always stems from an organic disorder causing an obstruction in the nasal cavities or nasopharyngeal area (e.g., a chronic sinus infection).

Assimilative Nasality

Assimilative nasality occurs when the nasality of a consonant "leaks" over to a vowel nearby. It is usually associated with an inability to move the **velopharyngeal port** quickly enough or far enough to create closure.

Faulty Tongue Postures

Resonance problems can occur if the tongue is habitually held high and to the front (i.e., anterior) of the mouth, or deep in the back (i.e., posterior) of the mouth. Because habitual anterior tongue posture is almost always a habit and not the result of any organic condition, it is more likely to be changeable through intervention than the posterior tongue position. Organically based tongue postures are much more resistant to change than those that are not organic.

Stridency

Strident resonance occurs when the pharynx is shortened, which raises the larynx and increases the reflective properties of the pharynx. A strident voice is usually harsh, shrill, and strained. Because it is the result of habit rather than an organic condition, stridency can be reduced through learning to relax the pharyngeal musculature.

Assessment

Evaluating a voice disorder involves three main processes: taking a case history from the person with the disorder, evaluating the person's voice and its characteristics, and evaluating the motor and sensory function of the speech musculature. The primary goals of the SLP in evaluating the individual's voice are to ascertain whether there is a significant problem and whether it warrants intervention. The voice evaluation pinpoints which functions are impaired and how severely, which leads directly to making a prognosis and designing intervention goals that are targeted specifically to the individual's specific needs

Case History

One of the main purposes of a case history is to determine the individual's overall communication patterns and how he or she is affected by the disorder. The case history can be obtained from the individual, a family member, or a caregiver. The SLP gathers basic biographical information, including any occupation, activity, or event that has affected the person's voice. Table 6.3 shows the specific biographical information to be collected in the case history. In addition to biographical information, the SLP will want a complete health history, as shown in Table 6.4.

TABLE 6.3. Biographical Information for the Voice Disorder Case History

1. Vocal hygiene (e.g., water intake, caffeine intake, daily alcohol, daily smoking)
2. Daily vocal activities (e.g., talking on the telephone; talking in noisy environments; talking to groups; yelling or shouting; throat clearing; coughing; talking while exercising; singing)
3. Environmental factors affecting the voice (e.g., smoke, chemicals, temperature swings, allergens)
4. History of reflux (e.g., gastroesophageal reflux, laryngopharyngeal reflux)
5. History of vocal performance, including solo or accompanied and type of music performed

TABLE 6.4. Health Information for the Voice Disorder Case History

1. The client's description of his or her voice disorder
2. The client's description of other people's reactions to the voice disorder
3. The effects of the voice disorder on his or her life
4. What she or he believes caused the disorder
5. When the disorder began and how it has progressed
6. Presence of a tracheostomy or tracheotomy
7. Presence of mechanical ventilation

Voice Evaluation

In most instances, individuals with voice disorders will have seen a medical professional and will be able to provide the SLP with the results of any diagnostic procedures that have been done, particularly assessment of vocal fold structure and function. The evaluation conducted by the SLP includes analysis of respiration, glottal closure, pitch characteristics, loudness and vocal quality, and areas of hyperfunction. Table 6.5 provides more detail about each of these aspects of the voice evaluation.

TABLE 6.5. The Voice Evaluation

Focus of evaluation	Assessment of . . .
Respiration	• Lung volume • Type of breathing (clavicular, thoracic, abdominal–diaphragmatic) • Respiratory efficiency for phonation • Extraneous respiratory noises (may be indicative of concomitant conditions such as asthma, neoplasms, vocal fold paralysis, or laryngeal web)
Glottal closure	• Ability to adduct the vocal folds completely; inability to do so may indicate neuromuscular weakness
Various measures of pitch	• Pitch range, lowest to highest • Optimal pitch (e.g., the pitch level at which the voice is produced most efficiently) • Habitual pitch (e.g., the pitch level the individual uses most often in everyday speech) • Abnormal variations in pitch (unlike vibrato, trill, and trillo, which are all normal, controlled pitch variations that are cultivated by vocal performers) • Special pitch problems (e.g., falsetto, diplophonia [two distinct pitches])
Various measures of loudness	• Hearing acuity to determine whether the individual has a hearing loss that is contributing to the voice disorder • Vocal loudness that is too high (person is talking too loud) • Vocal loudness that is too low (person's voice is hard to hear) • Person's ability to vary loudness
Voice quality: breathiness, harshness, hoarseness, vocal/glottal fry, hypernasality, hyponasality	• During informal conversation • While reading a standard paragraph (e.g., "The Rainbow Passage" [Fairbanks, 1960]) • Phonating while exerting (which forces the vocal folds to close if they can)
Vocal endurance	• Ability to count rapidly to 200 without losing phonation, increasing breathiness or hypernasality, or losing precision in articulating
Site(s) of vocal hyperfunction	• Excessive laryngeal tension (usually accompanied by excessive tension in the muscles of the neck and face) • Glottal attack (too hard means heightened tension) • Complaints of laryngeal pain or discomfort

Motor and Sensory Evaluation of the Speech Musculature

An evaluation of motor and sensory abilities during speech and nonspeech (e.g., sticking out the tongue, pretending to lick an ice-cream cone) can reveal problems that are related to dysarthria or apraxia. These abilities can be assessed during the **oral peripheral exam** (also called *oral mechanism exam*). Table 6.6 shows the areas addressed during an oral peripheral exam.

Intervention

Intervention with voice disorders depends on a variety of factors, including the etiology of the disorder (organic or nonorganic, neurological or muscular, congenital or acquired); whether there is medical information available, and if so, how detailed it is; the client's perception of her or his disorder and commitment to change; and the support available to the client (family and friends). Intervention usually involves a team of professionals that includes an **otolaryngologist** and an SLP. If the client has or had cancer, an **oncologist** will also be part of the team, and if the client is experi-

TABLE 6.6. The Oral Peripheral Exam

Structure	Assess/look for/ask client to
Face	• Facial symmetry at rest • Tremors, grimaces, tics • Gaze upward, then downward • Puff out cheeks • Repeat "ooo eee ooo eee" for 15 seconds • Mouth breathing
Lips	• Pucker lips • Smile: normal range of motion and symmetry? • Repeat "puh" for 10 seconds
Tongue	• Symmetrical protrusion of the tongue • Repeat "tuh" for 10 seconds • Repeat "kuh" for 10 seconds • Move tongue tip to right and left, then rapidly alternate
Teeth	• Occlusion: normal, overbite, underbite • All teeth present • Hygiene
Soft palate & uvula	• Symmetrical position of both at rest • Uvula moves symmetrically when saying "ahhhhh" • Voice exhibits no hypernasality during phonation
Jaw	• Slowly lower and raise the jaw • Repeat "jah jah jah" for 10 seconds
Larynx	• Sustain the vowel /ɑ/ for as long as possible with even phonation • Cough sharply with no breathiness • Produce /ɑ/ alternately at high, then low, pitch

encing stress or psychological manifestations, the team will also include a **psychiatrist** or **psychologist**.

The first goal in the process of voice rehabilitation is to restore the condition of the vocal folds to normal or, if this is not possible, compensate for whatever abnormality is present. The primary goal of voice rehabilitation following a laryngectomy is providing the person with an alternative means for communicating, which I describe below.

Voice Disorders Unrelated to Laryngectomy

For people whose voice disorder is unrelated to laryngectomy, the main objective of intervention is to help them produce the best voice possible or prevent a recurrence of the laryngeal pathology. In many situations, this involves teaching the client strategies for maintaining vocal hygiene, as outlined in Table 6.7.

Sometimes surgery is part of voice management. If the vocal folds are unable to approximate because they are either paralyzed or absent, it may be possible to compensate for the abnormality through surgery. If, for example, one vocal fold functions normally and the other is paralyzed at a position other than the midline of the larynx, the paralyzed vocal fold may be moved to the midline so that the normal one can approximate against it. If a growth between the vocal folds is keeping them from approximating or a laryngeal web is keeping them from vibrating along their full length, it will be removed surgically. If there is a growth or other lesion on the vocal folds that can be eliminated through surgery or vocal rest, either or both processes will be undertaken.

The prognosis in some voice disorder cases is poor because the client may not perceive the disorder as needing change, the client may not be motivated to change, or the client may not have the familial support to carry out the necessary procedures involved in changing vocal habits and patterns. In children, the conditions leading to the voice disorder may not be under their control. The SLP may need to include the family in the intervention process to ensure that any necessary environmental and situational changes can be made and the child can benefit from intervention.

Families also play a major role in the intervention process with adults. Without support and contributions from family members, many adults with voice disorders are unable to follow through on the commitment necessary to effect permanent changes in their voice.

Voice Disorders Related to Laryngectomy

If a client has had a total laryngectomy, he or she could use several strategies to set the molecules of air in the oral and nasal cavities into vibration. One involves the use of an instrument known as an artificial larynx, which is pictured in Figure 6.8. The instrument pictured is a small, battery-operated device that can be held in one hand and has a surface that vibrates. When the device is turned on and this

TABLE 6.7. Vocal Hygiene Information: Medications and Voice

Drug/medication	Effects	Recommendation
Tobacco (cigarettes, pipes, cigars, chewing tobacco, snuff, e-cigarettes)	Dries and irritates the voice; can cause cancer	Quit or reduce consumption
Marijuana	Dries and irritates the voice	Quit or reduce consumption
Cocaine	Dries and irritates the voice; constricts blood vessels	Do not use
Caffeine	Dries; is a diuretic so you lose fluids	Balance caffeine use with plenty of water
Alcohol	Dries; is a mild diuretic; can cause stomach acids to back up into the pharynx and oropharynx	Use sparingly; increase water consumption
Antihistamines	Dry the voice; thicken mucous	Use with caution
Cough medicines	Dry the voice; thicken mucous	Use with caution
Pain relievers (except acetaminophen)	May cause vocal folds to bleed	Check with your physician if you have any throat pain; do not yell or scream if you're taking pain relievers
Sleeping pills containing antihistamines	Dry; thicken mucous	Use with caution
Prescription oral inhalers	Dry; steroids can cause dysphonia	Use with caution
Diuretics	Dry; thicken mucous	Use with caution
Blood pressure medications	ACE inhibitors can cause coughing	Use with caution
Female hormones	Can permanently lower pitch level	Use with caution
Antidepressants	Dry	Use with caution

Things to do	Things to avoid
• Drink lots of water and natural juices • Keep dust and smoke out of your home • Keep your home humid if possible • Keep your home environment quiet • Talk with people by going to the same room rather than shouting • Take care of any allergies, colds, or congestion as soon as possible • Manage your stress as well as you can • Get adequate sleep • Watch your diet • Use your easiest voice in as many situations as possible • Rest your voice periodically throughout each day	• Caffeine, soda • Smoking • Highly spiced foods, especially late at night • Dry, dusty, or smoky environments • Yelling or trying to talk over loud noise • A loud home environment (e.g., TV, computers, music at high volume; people talking from room to room) • Over-the-counter medications for colds • Excessive coughing or throat clearing • Heavy vocal use (cheering or yelling) • High-stress situations • Forcing your voice to do things it doesn't want to do (e.g., singing out of your natural range)

Note. Adapted from *Manual of Voice Therapy, Second Edition* (pp. 299–300), by J. F. Deem and L. Miller, 2000, Austin, TX: PRO-ED. Copyright 2000 by PRO-ED, Inc. Adapted with permission.

surface is not in contact with anything solid (only in contact with air), it produces a relatively low-pitched buzzing sound. This particular device has the capability of producing a range of tones that the user controls with a thumb button, resulting in speech that sounds less machine-like and more realistic.

To set the molecules of air in the oral and nasal cavities into vibration, the vibrating surface of the Electrolarynx is pressed against the neck. This causes the skin and underlying structures (e.g., muscle fibers) in the neck to vibrate, which in turn causes molecules of air in the oral and nasal cavities to vibrate. The person then forms speech sounds in the usual way by moving structures in the speech musculature. You can see a video of a man demonstrating two types of artificial larynges here. Go to the website (http://goo.gl/YJ1po4) or scan the code.

Another approach that can be used to set the molecules of air in the oral cavities into vibration is ingesting air into the esophagus and expelling it in a controlled way. Speech produced in this way is known as **esophageal speech**. Inside the esophagus is a structure, the upper esophageal sphincter, that functions as a valve to prevent the contents of the stomach from being expelled into the oral cavity. This valve opens and closes in a manner somewhat similar to the vocal folds and is used to control the airflow of esophageal speech.

To get air into the esophagus, the person opens the esophageal sphincter and ingests (i.e., swallows) air. To produce voice, the person then expels this air through the closed sphincter. This action sets the sphincter's edges into vibration, which in

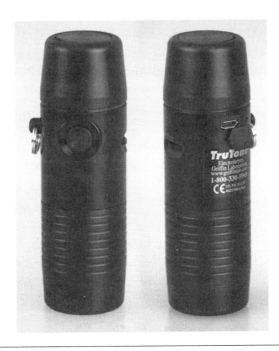

FIGURE 6.8. A TruTone Plus Electrolarynx, manufactured by Griffin Laboratories, Inc., Temecula, CA. Photo used with permission.

turn sets the molecules of air above it (in the oral cavity) into vibration. The person then forms speech sounds in the usual way. In this video, a man demonstrates his successful use of esophageal speech. Go to the website (http://goo.gl/EMVgiO) or scan the code.

Augmentative and Alternative Communication Devices

In addition to artificial larynges, two other types of augmentative and alternative options exist for people who have had a total laryngectomy. One is the surgical insertion of a vocal prosthesis during the total laryngectomy. The prosthesis, usually made of silicone, is fitted into a puncture made between the esophagus and the trachea—a tracheoesophageal puncture—and allows the individual to speak using air from the lungs, which requires that he or she also occlude (close) the stoma (the opening in the trachea through which the person breathes after the laryngectomy).

The second type of augmentative and alternative communication, which is less often used with people who have had a laryngectomy, is electronic speech generation using computer keyboards on which the individual types sentences that are spoken electronically; communication boards using pictures or words (I described these in more detail in Chapter 5); and tablets (e.g., iPads) containing software with speech-generating capabilities.

Transgender and Transsexual Voice Services

Both female-to-male and male-to-female individuals undergo a voice transition during gender reassignment and often seek the services of SLPs. Although each individual's voice is of primary concern, a major part of evaluation and treatment focuses on pragmatics (social communication), prosody (intonation, stress patterns, rhythm, and intensity), nonverbal communication (body postures, facial expressions, body movements and gestures), and articulation to ensure that the client is successful in acquiring the speech, language, and voice patterns typical of his or her gender. Here is a video of a voice therapy session with a male-to-female woman learning to use her more feminine voice. Go the website (http://goo.gl/X7Bqi1) or scan the code.

Although individuals undergoing a female-to-male transition are administered androgens as part of their transition, their voices may not sound as masculine as they wish until they have been receiving testosterone for at least one year (Scheidt, Kob, Willmes, & Neuschaefer-Rube, 2004). Especially for people who use their voices in high-demand settings, voice therapy can help them learn how to use their voice more efficiently and eliminate vocal behaviors that can harm their voice (e.g., straining to speak at a lower pitch or putting excess pressure on the vocal folds to make the voice sound harsh or coarse). In addition, voice therapy can focus on the gendered use of gestures, body postures and movements, and facial expressions.

chapter 7

Speech and Swallowing Disorders Associated With Dysarthria

Learning Objectives

Describe the major speech characteristics of dysarthria and apraxia in children.

Describe the major speech characteristics of dysarthria and apraxia in adults.

Describe cerebral palsy and its relationship to dysarthria in children.

Describe the management of dysarthria in children.

Describe the management of dysarthria in adults.

Describe dysphagia and how swallowing works.

Describe the management of dysphagia in both children and adults.

Overview

In Chapter 6, I described the types of voice disorders associated with various types of **dysarthria.** Some of the same disease processes that cause dysarthria can also affect swallowing and speech. In this chapter, I address dysarthria in children and adults and feeding and swallowing disorders (dysphagia) in both populations. The most common cause of dysarthria in children is **cerebral palsy (CP)**. In adults, dysarthria is most frequently associated with neurological disease, cerebrovascular disease, and trauma. Dysphagia affects both children and adults, and **speech–language pathologists (SLPs)** usually work on a team of medical professionals and therapists to assist individuals with dysphagia.

Dysarthria

As you will recall from Chapter 6, dysarthrias are neuromuscular disorders that prevent structures within the vocal tract, particularly the oral cavity, from moving properly to produce speech sounds. In their most severe form, they result in paralysis. More often, they keep movement from occurring in a well-coordinated manner.

The specific type of movement disturbance that results from dysarthria is determined by the site of the damage. Predictable sets of symptoms are associated with lesions at various sites in the central and peripheral nervous systems. Consequently, all conditions that damage a particular site will have similar symptomatologies—that is, all of them will result in similar disturbances in the functioning of the **articulators**.

Flaccidity, for example, is the symptom associated with damage to the muscle fibers, **myoneural junctions**, or **lower motor neurons**. A number of conditions can cause such a lesion. The condition responsible most often for damaging muscle fibers is **muscular dystrophy**, which I described in Chapter 6. This condition usually begins during childhood, appears to be hereditary, and is characterized by a chronic, progressive deterioration of muscle fibers.

The condition most often responsible for damaging the myoneural junctions is **myasthenia gravis** (or grave muscle weakness). This condition usually has its onset during adulthood, is progressive in nature, and tends to produce weakness of muscle contractions rather than paralysis. The musculature of the **velum** is particularly susceptible. In fact, one of the first symptoms a person with this condition is likely to show is **hypernasality**. Medication that augments the functioning of the myoneural junctions can often improve the nasality of persons with myasthenia gravis.

Several conditions can damage the lower motor neurons. One is **trauma**, which can occur during certain surgeries. For instance, the tongue may become paralyzed following an accidental cut to a nerve during heart surgery. Another condition that can damage the lower motor neurons is a viral disease such as **polio**, in which the functioning of the soft palate is frequently affected.

Spasticity is associated with a lesion in the **pyramidal** and **extrapyramidal systems**. Such a disturbance in the control of voluntary movement and reflex activity can limit the extent of an articulatory movement (e.g., elevation of the tongue tip). The range of movement possible may be so limited that the person cannot produce the movement at all. A number of conditions can cause spasticity, including **anoxia** and stroke. Audio Clip 7.1 (http://goo.gl/RwpY6K or scan the code) provides a sample of dysarthria caused by relatively mild spasticity.

Anoxia is an insufficient flow of oxygen to the brain. If this occurs either before, during, or immediately following birth and the pyramidal system is damaged, the person will be diagnosed as having spastic cerebral palsy.

Another condition that can cause spasticity is a stroke. Some strokes damage the pyramidal system on only one side of the brain (right or left), which produces spasticity on the opposite side of the body (i.e., **hemiplegia**). Damage to the pyramidal system on the left side of the brain produces spasticity on the right side of the body.

Dysarthria in Children

Most dysarthrias in children are the result of cerebral palsy, which is the result of an incident that causes anoxia. The lack of oxygen usually occurs **prenatally**, **perinatally**, or **postnatally**. The resulting damage to the developing brain causes abnormal movements and postures of various muscles, including those involved in respiration, phonation, resonance, and articulation. Cerebral palsy is not progressive, and it is not reversible. It can range in severity from mild to severe, and it can affect one or more parts of the body.

Categories of Cerebral Palsy

Cerebral palsy is categorized in two ways—one to describe the effects and one to describe the types. The three most typical categories for describing the effects of CP follow:

1. *Hemiplegia*, which affects one side (left or right) of the body.
2. *Paraplegia*, which affects only the legs and lower trunk.
3. *Quadriplegia*, which affects all four limbs.

Cerebral palsy is usually described by type, which is related to the neurological system(s) involved. Most professionals describe four main types of cerebral palsy:

1. *Spastic cerebral palsy*, which is characterized by slow, stiff, and abrupt movements; increased muscle tone; and rigidity of the muscles.
2. *Athetoid cerebral palsy*, which is characterized by involuntary, uncontrolled, slow, and writhing movements.
3. *Ataxic cerebral palsy*, which is characterized by a disturbed sense of balance and depth perception, awkward gait, and uncoordinated movements.
4. *Mixed cerebral palsy*, which is a combination of these types in a person.

Speech Problems Associated With Cerebral Palsy

The speech problems associated with CP depend on severity, which parts of the body are affected, and whether there are any associated conditions, such as cognitive disabilities. Because the motor system is impaired in CP, children's speech development will be affected by the resulting weakness and incoordination. Children with CP typically have problems with articulation because it requires rapid, coordinated movements and adjustments in numerous muscles. These children often have poor respiratory control, are unable to coordinate respiration with phonation, and produce weak voices. Their ability to produce coordinated speech sounds may be so impaired that their speech is relatively **unintelligible** unless their listener knows the topic. Children with CP have the most difficulty producing the sounds that develop latest in typically developing children and often experience difficulties into adulthood.

Impaired **prosody** of speech, shortened utterance length, and hypernasality also contribute to lowered intelligibility of speech in persons with CP. Impaired prosody results in a monotonic speech pattern, robbing it of the nuances carried by the melody and intonation associated with various meanings. Children with CP also tend to produce shorter utterances because they do not have the respiratory support for longer sustained phonation. Their speech can also be hypernasal because of an inability to coordinate the muscles of the **velum** and pharynx to seal the oral cavity from the nasal cavities.

Management of Childhood Dysarthria

Assessment of dysarthria in children involves evaluating the child's respiratory function; ability to sustain phonation, nasal, and oral resonance; soft palate and uvular movement; voice production; and articulation. Specifically, the SLP is observing speech that is

- slower than expected for the child's age;
- forced because of coordinating breathing with speaking;
- imprecise articulation;
- phonation that is too loud or too soft or varies unpredictably between loud and soft;
- irregular pitch;
- intonation patterns that do not match the meaning intended;
- any indication of hoarseness, hypernasality, or breathiness;
- drooling; and
- difficulty chewing or swallowing.

Treatment for childhood dysarthria involves increasing muscle tone and strength through structured activities and repetition. The goal is to increase speech intelligibility through decreasing rate of speech and improving range and rate of motion. The initial goal for a child with dysarthria may be to develop a stable respiratory pattern to support speech. Once the child has learned to phonate using the stable breathing pattern, the SLP teaches various movements of the articulators that are basic to producing consonants (e.g., closing the lips, blowing, putting the upper teeth on the lower lip). From here, articulation of consonants and vowels is gradually differentiated. The SLP may also elect to teach caregivers, family members, and teachers how to elicit more successful communication from children with dysarthria.

Children whose intelligibility cannot be improved enough for successful communication via speech often learn alternative means for communicating. These may include augmentative and alternative devices, such as computers or communication boards that use pictures or words.

Dysarthria in Adults (Acquired Dysarthria)

Dysarthrias in adults are speech disorders emanating from neurological problems that cause impaired muscular control of the speech mechanism. Impaired control may include incoordination, weakness, or paralysis. Either the central nervous system or the peripheral nervous system may be involved.

Dysarthria in adults differs from dysarthria in children in two important ways. First, the adult has developed speech and **language** in a relatively normal fashion, while the child with CP experiences speech and language difficulties throughout the developmental process. Second, children with CP suffer damage to the motor system early in development, while adults with dysarthria develop motor system damage later in life. Some of the most common causes of dysarthria in adults are **Parkinson's disease**, **Huntington's disease**, **amyotrophic lateral sclerosis (ALS)**, **multiple sclerosis (MS)**, and stroke (**cerebrovascular accident**). Dysarthrias can also result from the toxic effects of alcohol and drugs, or encephalitis.

Speech Problems Associated With Acquired Dysarthria

Dysarthria in adults can be categorized into six types, based on the muscle dysfunction that characterizes the disorder. Table 7.1 summarizes the types of dysarthria and their speech characteristics.

Management of Dysarthria in Adults

The evaluation of dysarthria in adults focuses on the same factors as in children with dysarthria. The primary goal is to discover which particular aspect of communication is in greatest need of intervention: respiration, phonation, resonance, articulation, or a combination. Refer back to Chapter 6. The process used for assessing dysarthria is the same as for evaluating a voice disorder.

Because the speech disorders related to dysarthria in adults vary considerably, treatment includes a wide range of techniques, including focus on respiration, phonation, resonance, articulation, or any combination of these processes. Respiration must be sufficient for sustained phonation; phonation must be sustained and of high enough quality to support the production of speech sounds. Resonance must be primarily oral so that the voice and speech do not sound hypernasal. Treatment of articulation includes focus on the muscles used in producing phonemes and modifying speaking rate, prosody, pitch, and loudness.

More specifically, the SLP will assist the individual in learning strategies for slowing speech, improving the volume or clarity of her or his speech, and increasing communicative effectiveness. For instance, the **American Speech-Language-Hearing**

TABLE 7.1. Dysarthrias and Their Speech Characteristics

Dysarthria classification	Location of damage	Possible causes	Speech characteristics
Ataxic	Cerebellum	Degenerative diseases, strokes, TBI, tumors, lead or mercury poisoning	• Slurred and slow • Elongated phoneme and syllable production • Imprecise consonants • Distorted vowels • "Drunken" sounding
Flaccid	Nerves that enervate the speech musculature	Muscular dystrophy, myasthenia gravis, ALS, polio, infections secondary to AIDS, surgical trauma	• Slowed rate • Imprecise consonants • Short phrases
Spastic	Damage to both the pyramidal and extrapyramidal systems	Stroke, ALS, TBI, brainstem tumor, cerebral anoxia, viral or bacterial infection, multiple sclerosis	• Imprecise consonants • Distorted vowels • Short phrases • Slowed rate
Hyperkinetic	Extrapyramidal system (basal ganglia)	Essential tremor syndrome, Huntington's disease, dystonia	• Imprecise articulation • Short phrases • Speech flow breakdowns
Hypokinetic	Extrapyramidal system	Parkinson's disease, Alzheimer's, stroke, TBI, tumors, drug toxicity	• Imprecise consonants • Phoneme repetition • Slowed rate • Moments of freezing
Mixed	Combination of 2 or more dysarthria types	ALS, multiple sclerosis	• Range from barely noticeable to completely unintelligible

Association (ASHA; 2014h) lists five tips for the person with dysarthria to improve communication with others:

1. Before beginning to speak in complete sentences, introduce the topic with one word or a short phrase.
2. Check with your listener(s) to make sure they're following what you're saying.
3. Slow your speech down, and pause frequently.
4. If you're tired, limit your conversations because you won't be as clear.
5. If you get frustrated, try other strategies, such as gesturing, pointing, or asking to try again later after you've been able to rest.

Dysphagia

Dysphagia, pronounced /dɪsˈfɑʒə/, is an inability to swallow or difficulty in swallowing. Some people with dysphagia also experience pain when swallowing. Because swallowing is an automatic process, most of us swallow without thinking about how we do it. However, swallowing is a complex process involving 50 or so pairs of muscles and numerous nerves, all coordinated in order to carry food or liquid from the mouth, through the throat, and into the stomach (American Board of Swallowing and Swallowing Disorders, 2014). When individuals have a condition that affects swallowing, they can experience a range of problems. One serious medical problem that can result is that a person may become undernourished or dehydrated. Perhaps more serious, though, is that the individual may develop aspiration pneumonia, because the trachea doesn't get closed off during swallowing, and food or liquid enters the lungs and causes an infection.

Eating plays an important role in the social fabric of every **culture**. Difficulties with swallowing effectively prevent people from participating in family rituals and social events. Furthermore, a swallowing disorder removes a person's pleasure in eating and can instead turn eating into an unpleasant and frightening experience.

How Swallowing Works

Swallowing involves three phases. Whenever we eat or drink, the mouth collects and controls either the food or the liquid. Chewing makes the food the right size to swallow and helps to mix the food with saliva. Saliva softens and moistens the food, which makes the food easier to swallow. The food is then formed into the **bolus**, which can be swallowed (the oral phase).

During the second phase, the tongue pushes the bolus to the back of the mouth, This triggers the swallowing reflex that causes the food to pass through the **pharyngeal cavity** to the entrance of the **esophagus**. Also, the **larynx** elevates under the base of the tongue, and the **epiglottis** closes tightly over the airway to prevent **aspiration**.

During the third phase, the esophageal phase, the bolus enters the esophagus, where wave-like contractions convey the food or liquid downwards toward the stomach. Passage of the bolus through the esophagus usually takes about 3 seconds, depending on the texture and consistency of the material. See Figure 7.1 for an illustration of the swallow.

Dysphagia in Children

Dysphagia in children typically involves both feeding and swallowing. To get food into the mouth, children have to be able to grasp the food, get it to their mouths, and then completely close their lips to keep the food in the mouth. After the food is inside the mouth, the child then sucks or chews it, moves it to the back of the mouth, and begins the second phase of the swallow.

Any condition that weakens or damages the nerves of muscles involved in feeding or swallowing can cause dysphagia in children. Swallowing requires adequate neural control and tongue, cheek, pharyngeal, and esophageal muscles that are

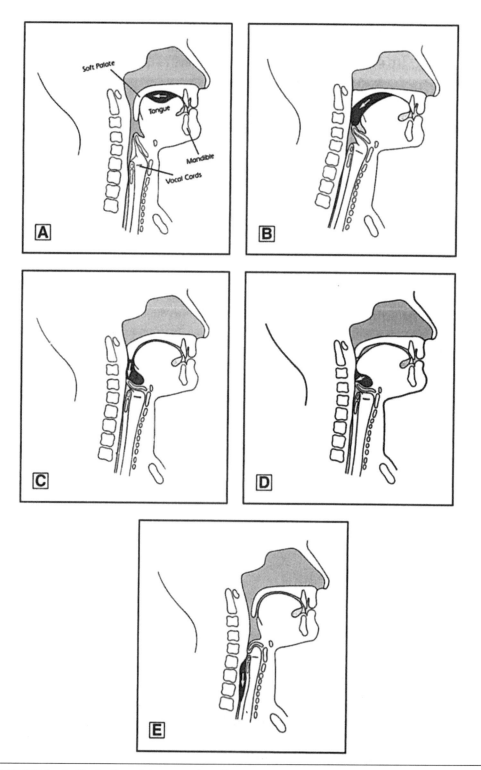

FIGURE 7.1. An illustration of the normal swallow.

Note. From *Evaluation and Treatment of Swallowing Disorders* (2nd ed., p. 28), by J. A. Logemann, 1998, Austin, TX: PRO-ED. Copyright 1998 by PRO-ED, Inc. Reprinted with permission.

capable of moving in concert throughout the three phases of swallowing. Box 7.1 lists the most common causes of dysphagia in children.

ASHA (2014l, para. 5) lists 15 possible symptoms of dysphagia in very young children, including refusing food or liquid, difficulty breast-feeding or chewing, extremely long feeding time, frequent spitting up or vomiting, recurring pneumonia or respiratory infections, and lower-than-expected weight gain or growth. SLPs who specialize in treating children with dysphagia typically work as part of a feeding team with medical personnel and other therapists. The team can assess the child's feeding and swallowing history and current functioning and perform any necessary special swallowing tests, such as a **modified barium swallow** or an **endoscopic assessment**. Members of these teams evaluate and modify child positioning for feeding, provide adapted feeding equipment (e.g., specialized cups and spoons), and recommend optimal food textures.

In addition to treating children who have been diagnosed with feeding impairments, SLPs also treat children who appear to be at risk for developing dysphagia. These are children whose birth and developmental histories suggest that they have a neurological deficit that could result in an oral-motor impairment. Suggestions would be made to parents for improving the strength and functioning of the child's oral musculature.

Tongue thrust is a swallowing pattern that is common in infancy but usually disappears by age 6. When it does not disappear, it is considered an **orofacial myofunctional disorder** that thrusts the tongue forward in an exaggerated way. During a tongue-thrust swallow, the tongue either pushes against the upper front **incisors** or protrudes between the upper and lower incisors. (During the normal swallow,

---

BOX 7.1   **Causes of Dysphagia in Children**

The American Speech-Language-Hearing Association (2014l, sec. 6) lists the following causes of dysphagia in children:

- nervous system disorders (e.g., cerebral palsy, meningitis, encephalopathy)
- gastrointestinal conditions (e.g., reflux, "short gut" syndrome)
- prematurity or low birth weight
- heart disease
- cleft lip, cleft palate, or cleft lip and cleft palate
- conditions affecting the airway
- autism
- head and neck abnormalities
- muscle weakness in the face and neck
- multiple medical problems
- respiratory difficulties
- medications that may cause lethargy or decreased appetite
- problems with parent–child interactions at mealtimes

the tongue moves up and back in the mouth.) The average person swallows 600 to 2,000 times a day, and each tongue-thrust swallow exerts a pressure on the incisors. Consequently, it is not particularly surprising that a tongue-thrust swallow can be a contributing factor to dental problems (e.g., the upper incisors being pushed forward, resulting possibly in an anterior open bite) or malformations of the jaw.

A number of conditions can contribute to the development or maintenance of a tongue-thrust swallow. They include thumb sucking; enlarged tonsils or adenoids; allergies; and a high, narrow palate.

A malocclusion that is due, at least in part, to a tongue-thrust swallow may be corrected by an orthodontist. However, the problem is likely to recur if the tongue-thrust swallow is not eliminated and, consequently, many orthodontists refer their patients to SLPs to have it eliminated. Although it is desirable to eliminate a tongue-thrust swallow before any orthodontic work is done, SLPs often receive referrals from orthodontists for **myofunctional therapy** after they have completed their work.

The goal of myofunctional therapy is to retrain the muscles involved in swallowing and eliminate the tongue thrust. Adolescent or adult clients have swallowed incorrectly millions of times. Consequently, the tongue-thrust swallow is a strong habit and requires a real effort to be eliminated. To be successful, a client must be willing to make myofunctional therapy a priority almost every day, for 3 or 4 months.

Dysphagia in Adults

In dysphagia, weak cheek or tongue muscles can make it harder to move food around in the mouth for chewing, so at least some of the pieces remain too large for swallowing. Pieces of food too large for swallowing can also enter the pharynx, block the pharynx, and block the passage of air through the **larynx** into the lungs. In addition to this life-threatening risk, other problems that can result in dysphagia include the following:

- The inability to start the swallowing reflex because of a stroke or other nervous system disorder
- Weak pharyngeal muscles that cannot move all the food to the entrance of the esophagus

The American Board of Swallowing and Swallowing Disorders lists three main causes of swallowing disorders in adults: neurological, mechanical, and psychogenic, including stroke, traumatic brain injury, multiple sclerosis, Parkinson's disease, dementia, and side effects of certain prescription drugs. Box 7.2 shows a more specific list of causes of dysphagia in adults.

Dysphagia in adults can cause several problems. One, of course, is an inability to take in a sufficient amount of nourishing food. Another is food or liquid entering the lungs (i.e., aspiration) through the larynx that coughing or throat clearing

---

BOX 7.2   **Causes of Dysphagia in Adults**

The American Speech-Language-Hearing Association (2014u) lists the following as causes of dysphagia in adults:

Damage to the nervous system, such as:
- stroke
- brain injury
- spinal cord injury
- Parkinson's disease
- multiple sclerosis
- amyotrophic lateral sclerosis (ALS, or Lou Gehrig's disease)
- muscular dystrophy
- cerebral palsy
- Alzheimer's disease

Problems affecting the head and neck, including:
- cancer in the mouth, throat, or esophagus
- injury or surgery involving the head and neck
- decayed or missing teeth, or poorly fitting dentures (sec. 6)

---

cannot dislodge. Such material remaining in the lungs can cause a serious bacterial infection.

Dysphagia in adults can occur at any of the three phases involved in swallowing. Disorders in the *oral phase* involve problems with chewing because of reduced tongue movement, reduced range of jaw movement, poor alignment of upper and lower jaw, and reduced tension in the mouth. Disorders in forming the bolus may occur because the tongue has difficulty moving in a posterior direction, or caused by collecting food residue, premature swallowing or aspiration before the swallow, tongue thrust, reduced strength of the oral musculature, and reduced range of tongue movement.

Disorders in the *pharyngeal phase* are related to the act of swallowing and may be caused by a delayed or absent swallow reflex, food that is in the nasal cavities or trachea, aspiration before and after the swallow, pharyngeal paralysis or reduced ability to contract the pharyngeal musculature, reduced ability of the base of the tongue to move, and inadequate closure of the trachea.

Disorders in the *esophageal phase* of swallowing, when the bolus has moved into the esophagus, result from problems with musculature that is not under voluntary control. People may have difficulties during this phase because food has moved back up from the esophagus to the pharynx (i.e., backflow), the esophagus cannot contract enough to move the food through, the esophagus may be obstructed (e.g., by a tumor), an abnormal pouch that collects food may be present, or there may be a hole in the esophagus.

Diagnosis and Treatment

Dysphagia treatment includes medical procedures, compensatory therapy, and facilitating therapy. SLPs provide both compensatory and facilitating therapy but are not involved in the medical procedures used to treat dysphagia. Compensatory therapy for clients who have dysphagia includes evaluating the ability to eat and drink and teaching new ways to swallow. It may also involve teaching the client to eat with the body positioned in a way that facilitates the swallowing process (e.g., with the head turned to one side) or teaching caregivers how to prepare food to facilitate it being swallowed (e.g., a thickener may have to be added to some liquids).

Facilitating therapy is focused on improving muscle strength throughout the three phases of swallowing. Treatment may include exercises to strengthen weak muscles or improve coordination between the various muscles that contribute to swallowing, including those of the lips, tongue, palate, pharynx, larynx (to close the airway), and jaw. Also, treatment can include stimulating the swallow reflex.

In recent years, SLPs have become increasingly involved in providing services to clients with tracheostomies and **ventilator dependence**. These SLPs typically work as part of a team that includes a variety of health-care practitioners, including physicians, nurses, **respiratory therapists**, registered dieticians, and **social workers**, among others.

The type of services provided by SLPs varies from facility to facility. Although assessment and management are highly individualized because of the wide range of conditions presented by clients, certain knowledge and skills are necessary regardless of client or facility. Dikeman and Kazandijan (2004) listed these four areas:

- Knowledge of both vocal and nonvocal communication methods.
- Knowledge of posttracheostomy anatomy and the potential impact on swallowing of the tracheostomy and ventilator dependence.
- An awareness of other conditions that can affect swallowing function.
- Skills with dysphagia assessment, including clinical approaches and instrument management.

End-of-Life Issues

Many patients nearing the end of life have feeding or swallowing issues that benefit from the services of an SLP. The goal of intervention for these individuals is to develop compensatory strategies that will allow them to eat orally for as long as possible (ASHA, 2014i). In other words, intervention shifts from a focus on rehabilitation to a focus on quality of life.

To do this work, the SLP needs to recognize the emotional and psychological aspects associated with end of life and to understand that cultural groups vary significantly in their beliefs and ability to deal with dying and death. What is best clinically for a particular client may not be best for that client's quality of life (ASHA, 2014i). For a detailed discussion of what SLPs need to know about end-of-life care for adults, read the thoughtful essay by Mary Ann Toner and Barbara B. Shadden (Toner & Shadden, 2012).

chapter 8

Articulation and Phonological Disorders

Learning Objectives

Explain how phonemes are formed.

Explain how speech sounds are classified.

Explain how articulation and phonological disorders are similar or different.

List some possible causes of articulation disorders.

Describe the management for articulation and phonological disorders.

Describe the management for dysarthria.

Overview

People who have articulation disorders do not produce **speech** sounds as accurately as most other people their age. Although children often make mistakes in pronunciation, mistakes that continue past a certain age are considered to be disorders of articulation. Children with **phonological disorders** have difficulty with the rules for the sound system rather than with the production of speech sounds. Most often, the difficulty shows up as a pattern of sound errors, such as eliminating certain sounds or substituting one type of sound for another (e.g., using front-of-mouth consonants for all back-of-mouth consonants) or eliminating one of the initial sounds in words that begin with two consonants (e.g., /bokən/ for "broken").

To understand why speech sound errors occur, it will help you to understand, at least intuitively, how the speech mechanism—specifically, the **vocal tract**—molds air particles flowing from the lungs into the **phonemes** of a **language**. Articulation errors result when this physical mechanism does not function as it should.

Speech–language pathologists (SLPs) have been working with clients on articulation skills since the early years of the profession. Box 8.1 provides a list of terms used to describe articulation disorders during that time period. Phonological disorders are a more recent diagnosis that evolved with greater understanding of **phonology** as a rule-based system that governs the use of speech sounds in a language.

Production of Speech Sounds

You will recall from Chapter 1 that air from the lungs is molded into phonemes by the vocal tract (pharyngeal cavity, oral cavity, and nasal cavity), which extends from the glottis to the lips and nose.

All vowels and most consonants are produced by vibration of the vocal folds. Some consonants, however, are produced solely by air that is set into vibration in the oral cavity; these are called *voiceless consonants*. During the production of /f/, for example, air is set into vibration by being forced to exit through the narrow passage

---

BOX 8.1   **Historical Terms Used to Describe Articulation Disorders (Robbins, 1948)**

Seventy-five years ago, all students of speech–language pathology were required to master long lists of Greek and Latin names for speech disorders. Such a name could make a disorder appear to be more debilitating than it was. These terms are rarely used today. The following types of dyslalia (i.e., articulation disorders) were recognized by the Nomenclature Committee of the American Academy of Speech Correction during the 1940s.

- *Asapholalia:* Mumbled speech, in which the patient can usually produce each vowel and consonant correctly by itself, or a consonant with a vowel, but speaks so rapidly—or moves his lips, tongue, or jaw so little—that he sounds as though he were talking with a full mouth.
- *Atelalalia:* Delayed development of speech.
- *Barbaralalia:* Foreign dialect.
- *Bradylalia:* Abnormal slowness of speech.
- *Dialectolalia:* Provincial dialect.
- *Embololalia:* Adding speech sounds or syllables that do not belong to the word.
- *Idiolalia:* Invented language in which the patient uses a language all his own.
- *Leipolalia:* Omission of speech sounds or syllables that belong to the word.
- *Metalalia:* Transposition of speech sounds, such as "er" for "re."
- *Paralalia:* Mispronunciation or substitution of one speech sound for another.
- *Pedolalia:* Baby-talk; a syndrome composed of sound omissions, sound substitutions, and the omission of articles, prepositions, conjunctions, and many pronouns.
- *Rhinolalia aperta* (*hyperrhinolalia*): Functional-cleft-palate type of speech that includes nasality, nasal fricatives, and the substitution of glottal click or nasals for plosives.
- *Rhinolalia clausa* (*hyporhinolalia*): Hypernasality; sounds like speech with a plugged nose.
- *Tachylalia:* Abnormally rapid speech without mumbling.

between the upper **incisors** and lower lip. The production of /s/ is accomplished by pushing air between the tongue and the **alveolar ridge**.

The configuration (i.e., shape) of the cavities in the vocal tract at a particular moment determines which phoneme will be produced. Each phoneme has a unique configuration. Because during every second of conversational speech as many as 14 phonemes are produced (Darley, Aronson, & Brown, 1975), the configuration of the vocal tract is continually in a state of transformation.

The oral cavity is the most important component of the vocal tract for determining which phoneme will be produced because it significantly affects the production of all but one English speech sound (/h/, as in *hat*). The nasal cavity, on the other hand, only affects the production of three English speech sounds: /m/ as in "*mat*"; /n/ as in "*no*"; and /ŋ/ as in "si*ng*."

The structures in the oral cavity that affect the configuration of the vocal tract are the tongue, teeth, lips, **mandible**, **hard palate**, and **velum**. These structures are referred to as the **articulators**.

The tongue is one of the most important structures in the oral cavity for determining the configuration of the vocal tract. Either the back or tip of the tongue is involved in the production of most consonant sounds. Those in which the back is active include /k/ and /g/. Examples of those in which the tip is active are /s/, /z/, /t/, /d/, /n/, /l/, and /r/.

The most important teeth for the production of speech are the two central and two lateral incisors—the four front ones in each jaw. They are used with the lower lip to create a constriction for /f/ and /v/. They are also used with the tongue to create a constriction for the two "th" sounds, the ones in "*think*" (/θɪnk/) and "*the*" (/ðə/).

Some phonemes are shaped by the lips. For example, closure of the lips is one of the main features of three English speech sounds: /p/, /b/, and /m/. During the production of /u/ (as in *boot*) and /w/, the lips protrude.

The mandible plays an active role in the production of most English speech sounds. It brings together and separates the upper and lower lip and the upper and lower teeth. Consequently, it is active during the production of all speech sounds that involve these structures, including /f/, /v/, /s/, and /z/, /ʃ/, /ʒ /. It also plays an active role during the production of speech sounds in which the mouth is open, such as /ɑ/ as in "*father*" and /k/ as in "*king*."

The hard palate forms the anterior portion of the roof of the mouth. The anterior three-fourths of the hard palate are a part of the same bone that forms the **maxilla**. Along with the velum, the hard palate separates the oral cavity from the nasal cavity. The alveolar ridge, a ridged shelf, is just behind the upper teeth. The action of the tongue tip in relation to the alveolar ridge contributes to the production of many speech sounds, including /t/, /d/, and /n/.

The velum forms the posterior portion of the roof of the mouth. When the velum is not elevated, an opening is present in the roof of the mouth and air can flow from the oral cavity into the nasal cavity. When the velum is elevated, it contacts the posterior wall of the pharynx. As a result, the opening in the roof of the mouth is closed, and no air flows from the oral cavity into the nasal cavity. This **velopharyngeal closure** occurs to some degree during the production of all English speech sounds, except /m/, /n/, and /ŋ/.

Classification of Speech Sounds

English contains approximately 44 phonemes, which are classified according to whether they are vowels or consonants. Vowels are produced by voice flowing fairly freely through the mouth, while consonants are produced with either partial or complete closure of the vocal tract.

Vowels

Vowels are described according to the position of the tongue and where in the mouth they are formed. So, for example, when you say the word *eat*, the vowel sound at the beginning, /i/, is formed in the front of the mouth with the tongue held high. You produce front vowels with your lips spread. When you say "ought" /ɔt/, however, you form the vowel in the back of the mouth with your tongue held relatively low. You say back vowels with your lips rounded. Table 8.1 is a schematic showing vowel production according to tongue position on the vertical axis and placement in the mouth on the horizontal axis.

Consonants

Consonants are classified based on three categories: voicing, place of articulation, and manner of articulation.

Voicing

All speech sounds can be classified as either **voiced**, **voiceless**, or **nasal**. All the vowel sounds in English are voiced, but some consonants are voiced, some are voiceless,

TABLE 8.1. Vowels of English

	Front	Central	Back
High	i		u
	ɪ		ʊ
Mid	e	ʌ, ə	o
	ɛ	ɚ, ɝ	ɔ
Low	æ		
	ɑ		

and three are nasal. An example of a voiced consonant sound is /z/, and an example of a voiceless consonant is /s/. The only difference in the configuration of the vocal tract for these sounds is that while /z/ is being produced the vocal folds are approximated, and while /s/ is being produced they are separated.

You can feel the presence of voicing by touching the front of your neck at the level of the **larynx** and producing the voiced and voiceless members of a pair. For example, first produce a sustained /z/ and then a sustained /s/. You should feel vibration during the production of /z/, but not during that of /s/.

The three nasal consonants in English are /m/, /n/, and /ŋ/. As I described above, these three consonants are produced when the velum is open enough for some of the voice and breath to enter the nasal passages, which produce the nasality associated with these sounds. Table 8.2 shows English voiced consonants, voiceless consonants, and nasal consonants.

Place of Articulation

Place of articulation refers to where in the vocal tract consonants are formed or where articulatory contact is made: lips, teeth and alveolar ridge, and the hard and soft palates. The following terms are used to classify consonant phonemes according to their place of articulation: **bilabials**, **labio dentals**, **lingua dentals**, **lingua alveolars**, **palatals**, **velars**, and **glottals**.

Manner of Articulation

Manner of articulation refers to how consonants are produced. *Plosives,* or *stops,* are small "explosions" that occur because the airflow out of the mouth is stopped, followed by a sudden release. For instance, if you put your hand in front of your mouth as you say the word "pin," the *p* produces a puff of air—thus, the plosive. *Fricatives* are hissing sounds, such as the *s* in "silk," produced by air that is forced through a relatively narrow constriction in the mouth—in this case, between the tongue and the alveolar ridge and upper teeth. *Affricates* combine the qualities of plosives and fricatives, as, for example, the /tʃ/ in "*ch*air" and the /dʒ/ in "*j*ump." I described the

TABLE 8.2. Voiced and Voiceless Consonant Pairs, Nasal Consonants

Voiced consonants	Voiceless consonants	Nasal consonants
/z/ zebra	/s/ sit	/m/ man
/b/ big	/p/ pig	/n/ now
/d/ dog	/t/ toy	/ŋ/ bang
/g/ girl	/k/ kick	
/dʒ/ judge	/tʃ/ church	
/v/ vine	/f/ fin	
/w/ why	/hw/ who	
/ʒ/ treasure	/ʃ/ ship	
/ð/ this	/θ/ thin	

nasals earlier: /m/ ("*m*ud"), /n/ ("*n*o"), and /ŋ/ ("ri*ng*"). The *laterals* result when the air flows out of the mouth alongside the tongue (e.g., the two *l* sounds in "lollygag"). *Glides*, or *semivowels*, are produced by movement rather than stoppage or constriction of the air. Examples are the *y*-sound /j/ in "yellow" and the *w*-sound /w/ in "will." Table 8.3 shows place and manner of articulation of English consonants.

Each language has its own unique phonemic system. The native-language phonemic system of an individual learning English as a second language may influence how that individual produces phonemes in English. The **American Speech-Language-Hearing Association** (ASHA, 2014q) has compiled a list of phonemic inventories for English and 16 other languages, as well as a list of resources for SLPs working with individuals whose native language is not English.

TABLE 8.3. Place and Manner of Articulation of Consonants

Place of Articulation		
Lips	**Teeth/Alveolar ridge**	**Hard/Soft palate**
/p/ pig	/t/ tin	/k/ cat
/b/ big	/d/ dog	/g/ goat
/f/ fin	/s/ sit	/ʃ/ ship
/v/ van	/z/ zebra	/ʒ/ azure
/w/ why	/θ/ thin	/tʃ/ church
/m/ man	/ð/ then	/dʒ/ judge
	/n/ now	/j/ yes
	/l/ log	/r/ rip
		/ŋ/ sing

Manner of Articulation		
Plosives/Stops	**Fricatives**	**Affricates**
/p/ pop	/f/ fin	/tʃ/ church
/b/ bob	/v/ vine	/dʒ/ judge
/d/ dog	/θ/ thin	
/t/ tin	/ð/ this	
/g/ goat	/s/ sing	
/k/ coat	/z/ zebra	
	/ʃ/ shine	
	/ʒ/ azure	
Nasals	**Laterals**	**Glides/Semivowels**
/m/ man	/l/ lateral	/j/ yes
/n/ now		/r/ rock
/ŋ/ sing		/h/ hello
		/w/ where

Speech Sound Disorders

In the fifth edition of the *Diagnostic and Statistical Manual of Mental Disorders* (DSM-5), the American Psychiatric Association (2013) describes speech sound disorders as including both articulation disorders and phonological disorders. Articulation disorders occur when a child has difficulty producing the specific sounds that are expected at her or his age—that is, the child has difficulty with the motor movements required to actually produce the sounds. A phonological disorder, on the other hand, occurs when a child has difficulty learning the rules of language that govern the sound system. The child may be perfectly capable of making the motor movements required to produce specific sounds but tends to use a highly limited number of sounds, has difficulty combining specific sounds, and has problems adding morphological markers, such as past tense and plurals.

Phonological Disorders

Many children make multiple speech sound errors for which there appears to be no organic cause. The structure and function of their peripheral speech mechanism seem normal, and there is no evidence of a **hearing** loss or developmental disability. Such children usually are diagnosed as having a phonological disorder. Strictly speaking, **phonological disorders** are language-based disorders rather than speech disorders. It is assumed that their speech sound errors are caused by faulty learning on the phonological level of language. Because it is important to differentiate between a phonological disorder and an articulation disorder, I discuss phonological disorders here rather than in the chapter on child language disorders.

From a phonological perspective, spoken English consists of ordered sequences of phonemes that are segmented into words. Phonemes are represented by a notational system called the International Phonetic Alphabet (IPA), which is used to transcribe speech when diagnosing various types of speech disorders and which I've used to indicate specific speech sounds throughout what you've read so far. Box 8.2 shows some typical words and how they are represented by the IPA.

In English, the phrase "I love you" is perceived as an ordered sequence of six phonemes—/ɑi l ʌ v j u/—segmented into three words. By producing this sequence you are following the rules English phonology requires, something you most likely learned at a very young age. Failure to produce multiple phonemes correctly, in appropriate sequences, by an age at which most peers can produce them is classified as a phonological language disorder, unless it is caused by some abnormality in the structure or function of the peripheral speech mechanism (e.g., **dysarthria**).

Recall from Chapter 3 that phonological language learning involves two interrelated tasks: learning to produce the various phonemes of one's language (articulation) and learning the rules that dictate how they can be combined into words, phrases, and sentences (phonology).

BOX 8.2 **IPA Transcriptions of Selected Words**

shadow	ʃædo	aphasia	ə'feʒə
church	'tʃɝtʃ	judge	'dʒʌdʒ
yesterday	j'ɛstɚde	pinch	'pɪntʃ
satisfy	'sædɪsfaɪ	yellow	'jɛlo
speech	'spitʃ	pathology	pæθ'ɔlədʒi
audiology	ɔdi'ɔlədʒi	stuttering	'stʌdɚɪŋ
communication	kəmjunɪ'keʃən	science	'saɪənts
disorders	dɪs'ordɚz	language	'læŋgwɪdʒ

Many of the words produced by typically developing children who are learning to speak do not sound like the adult pronunciations of those same words. Children simplify them, for example, by omitting phonemes they have trouble producing or substituting other phonemes they are better able to produce. As their ability to produce speech sounds improves, their simplifications decrease, and their speech becomes more like adults'.

When children simplify the production of words, their simplifications are predictable and universal across languages. These simplifications have been observed in the speech of young children in many countries. SLPs refer to these simplifications as **phonological processes**. Children with phonological disorders exhibit many phonological processes (several common ones are shown in Table 8.4), but by the age of 6 most typically developing children have stopped using them. To learn more about phonological processes, see Heidi Hanks's discussion and complete list on her website (Hanks, 2014).

Williams (2006) described error patterns in terms of **phoneme collapse**, which occurs when a child substitutes one phoneme for many different phonemes (e.g., /t/ is used as the initial consonant in "call," "ball," "fall," and "tall"). Using a small number of different phonemes rather than the full set used by age peers makes a child's speech highly **unintelligible**.

A child who simplifies the production of words more than same-age peers is likely to be regarded as having a phonological disorder. Children with articulation or phonological disorders constitute the largest subgroup of clients served by SLPs (ASHA, 2012). Although most preschool children with a moderate-to-severe phonological disorder will improve their speech-sound-production abilities dramatically by the later elementary grades, manifestations of communication disabilities persist for many of these individuals throughout childhood and adolescence, and sometimes even beyond (Felsenfeld, Broen, & McGue, 1992).

TABLE 8.4. Five Common Phonological Processes Used by Children

Process	Definition	Examples
Weak syllable deletion	The child deletes the weak syllable in a word	/bæ/ for *basket*; /tɛfon/ for *telephone*
Final consonant deletion	Child deletes the final consonant in a word	/fɪ/ for *fish*; /hæ/ for *hat*
Velar fronting	Child substitutes /t/ and /d/ for /g/	/do/ for *go*; /tuti/ for *cookie*
Cluster reduction	Child deletes 1 or both consonants in a consonant cluster	/nek/ for *snake*; /bo/ for *boats*
Gliding	Child substitutes /j/ (*yellow*) or /w/ for another sound	/jɑɪt/ for *light*; /wop/ for *rope*
Fronting	Child replaces a back consonant with a front consonant	/tæt/ for *cat*
Reduplicating	Child repeats a complete or incomplete syllable	/bɑbɑ/ for *bottle*

Articulation Disorders

Individuals (mostly children) who have an articulation disorder make more speech sound errors than their age peers. They may omit speech sounds (e.g., they may say "leap" when they wish to say "sleep"). They may substitute one speech sound for another (e.g., substituting /w/ for /r/ and say "wed" for "red"). Or they may produce a speech sound in a distorted manner (e.g., producing /s/ in a manner that sounds like a whistle). Most people with articulation disorders make some combination of these types of errors. Errors rarely occur on vowel sounds, partly because vowels require less precise movements of the articulators than consonant sounds. Audio Clip 8.1 (go to link http://goo.gl/aAU9pQ or scan code) is an example of a sound omission.

The majority of people diagnosed with an articulation disorder are children, but not all children who make articulation errors have a disorder. Most preschool children, particularly those below the age of 3, make articulation errors. Acquisition of the ability to produce the various consonant sounds correctly tends to follow a predictable developmental sequence, which is summarized in Table 8.5. We ordinarily would not be concerned about a child's inability to produce a particular consonant correctly unless his or her chronological age exceeded the upper age limit given in the table. For example, the failure to produce /g/ correctly would not ordinarily be of concern in children below the age of 4.

The extent to which articulation errors interfere with communication depends on several factors. One factor is the number of errors. The greater the number of articulation errors in a person's speech, the more difficulty listeners are likely to have understanding it. A second factor is the type of error. Sound omissions are more

TABLE 8.5. Age at Which 75% of Children Produce English Consonant Phonemes Correctly

Age	Phoneme
3 years	/m/ mother /n/ no /ŋ/ sing /p/ pan /f/ fan /h/ hot /w/ won
4 years	/b/ ball /d/ dog /g/ girl /r/ run
4.5 years	/s/ sun /ʃ/ shoe /tʃ/ church
6 years	/t/ tall /v/ van /l/ lamp /θ/ thumb
7 years	/ð/ the /z/ zoo /ʒ/ azure /dʒ/ jump

Note. From *Certain Language Skills in Children: Their Development and Interrelations* (Child Welfare Monograph Series No. 26), by M. C. Templin, 1957, Minneapolis: The University of Minnesota Press. Copyright 1957 by the University of Minnesota Press. Reprinted with permission.

likely than sound distortions to interfere with others' comprehension. A third factor is which phonemes are produced in error. Some phonemes occur more often in English than others and, consequently, producing them incorrectly will result in a greater number of errors. For example, a defective /s/ in English is likely to result in more errors than a defective /w/.

Causes of Speech Sound Disorders

Most speech sound disorders have no known cause and are considered functional disorders. However, a number of different conditions can result in speech sound disorders. Some are caused by the improper functioning of structures within the vocal tract because of developmental disorders, hearing loss, illness, or **cerebral palsy**, while others result from genetic conditions, such as Down syndrome. In addition, if children have experienced frequent ear infections accompanied by hearing loss, even temporary, they are at increased risk for speech sound disorders.

Structural Irregularities

If the size, shape, or alignment of one or more of the structures within the vocal tract is abnormal or if one of these structures is incomplete or missing, it may not be possible for the vocal tract to assume the configuration required for the production of a particular phoneme. Depending on the structure affected and the extent of the anomaly, the result could be anything from a minor sound distortion to a complete inability to produce a particular phoneme. Following are some examples of structural anomalies that can cause articulation errors.

Glossectomy

Because the tongue (particularly the tip) influences the configuration of the vocal tract for most consonant sounds, a **glossectomy** will almost always cause articulation errors. In spite of this, speech may remain fairly intelligible. The impact of a glossectomy on speech intelligibility is largely a function of the amount of tissue removed (excised) and its location. The greater the amount of tissue excised, particularly from the tongue tip, the poorer speech intelligibility is likely to be. Excision of tissue at the back of the tongue tends to affect the production of vowels more than consonants, and excision at the tongue tip affects consonants more than vowels (Leonard, Goodrich, McMenamin, & Donald, 1992). Here are two YouTube videos of a young woman (Elliot, 2011), the first 4 days following a partial glossectomy surgery. Go to the website (http://goo.gl/VtTm6a) or scan the code.

The second is a YouTube video from 1 year later (Elliot, 2012). Go to the website (http://goo.gl/Mlrbgn) or scan the code.

Some patients who have had only a partial glossectomy can be helped to improve the intelligibility of their speech. A **prosthodontist**, for example, could make an appliance that attaches to the hard palate and provides a surface with which the tongue stub could make contact. This would enable the person to more closely approximate the vocal tract configuration required for such speech sounds as /t/ and /d/, for which contact between the tongue tip and hard palate is essential. Another possibility would be to surgically increase the length of the tongue stub. Both of these approaches partially compensate for the shortening of the tongue and thereby increase intelligibility.

Acquired Structural Deficits Other Than Glossectomies

Acquired structural deficits ordinarily result from trauma to oral cavity structures or **ablative surgery**. Ablative surgery can involve partial or total removal of the mandible, the lips, or the palate (hard or soft). The impact on articulation often can be reduced by reconstructing the affected structure(s) surgically or by means of a **prosthesis**.

Dental Anomalies

The teeth, particularly the lateral and central incisors, play an important role in configuring the vocal tract for a few consonant sounds, especially /s/ and /z/. If these teeth are missing, the tongue may protrude through the opening and the person will substitute /θ/ for /s/. This sound substitution, which is referred to as a *frontal lisp*, also can occur if there is an **anterior open bite**.

You will recall from the discussion in Chapter 7 on tongue thrust that some people exhibit anterior movement of the tongue during speech; that is, they "thrust" their tongue against their anterior incisors while swallowing and talking. They may also press their tongue against their incisors when they are not speaking or swallowing. This pressure of the tongue on the incisors can cause the teeth to protrude and can result in articulation errors. The speech sound most likely to be affected is /s/.

A dental **anomaly** such as missing incisors or an open bite will not necessarily cause articulation errors. Some people with dental anomalies produce all the speech sounds correctly (Bernthal, Bankson, & Flipson, 2012). They compensate by positioning their articulators, particularly their tongue, a little differently than do most people when saying certain sounds.

Cleft Palate

A **cleft palate**, shown in a photograph in Figure 8.1, is a **congenital** opening between the oral cavity and the nasal cavity. It results in an abnormal configuration of the

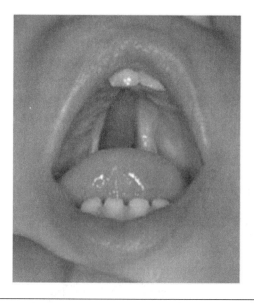

FIGURE 8.1. Cleft of the hard palate.

vocal tract for all but three English speech sounds: /m/, /n/, and /ŋ/. (These are the only ones for which there is normally a flow of air through the nasal cavity.) An unrepaired or partially repaired cleft palate is highly likely to result in at least a few articulation errors (it also usually adversely affects vocal resonance). It may, in fact, result in so many errors that the person's speech is unintelligible.

Childhood Apraxia of Speech/Verbal Apraxia

Verbal apraxia, unlike dysarthria, results from difficulty programming the speech mechanism to produce certain speech sounds and is thus a motor speech disorder. Also unlike dysarthria, in verbal apraxia, there is no weakness, paralysis, or incoordination of the oral musculature while it is being used for manipulating food in the mouth, chewing, and swallowing. A child with apraxia of speech (CAS) usually knows what she or he wants to say but cannot coordinate the muscle movements required.

Young children with CAS often begin talking late and use only a restricted set of vowels and consonants; they have difficulty combining sounds and pause between sounds. They may also have difficulty eating. Older children with CAS understand language much better than they speak, make inconsistent sound errors that are unrelated to maturity, have problems speaking longer words or phrases with clarity, and often use irregular intonation patterns.

Hearing Loss

To produce speech sounds correctly, speakers have to be able to hear and monitor their speech to know whether they are producing speech sounds correctly. When a child develops a severe hearing loss before beginning to speak, he or she may not be able to learn to produce at least some speech sounds without special training. This is why children who are deaf at birth do not learn to speak in the usual way. If a person develops a severe hearing loss after learning to speak, the ability to produce at least some speech sounds may deteriorate.

A **sensorineural hearing loss** is more likely than a **conductive hearing loss** to cause articulation errors, for two reasons. First, sensorineural hearing losses tend to interfere more than conductive losses with self-monitoring of speech. People who have sensorineural hearing losses tend to hear their own speech as relatively soft, while those who have conductive hearing losses tend to hear it as relatively loud. Second, sensorineural hearing losses can be more severe than conductive hearing losses. (Conductive hearing losses cannot cause deafness). The more severe a hearing loss, the more likely it is to interfere with monitoring speech auditorily. I discuss hearing loss in more detail in Chapter 10.

In this video clip, Rachel Kolb (2013) gives a TEDx presentation describing how she navigates deafness in a hearing world. Go to the website (http://goo.gl/JpC15D) or scan the code.

Cognitive Disabilities

The acquisition of speech sounds tends to follow a predictable developmental sequence (refer back to Table 8.5) that is related to intellectual development. Children usually do not learn to produce specific speech sounds until they achieve a certain level of mental maturity. Consequently, children who have a **cognitive disability** usually do not produce the various speech sounds by the ages most children learn to produce them, which means they tend to make more articulation errors than most children their age.

Assessment of Speech Sound Disorders

Speech sound disorders are typically diagnosed by an SLP. As part of the assessment, the SLP will perform an **oral peripheral exam** (which I described in Chapter 6), listen to the individual's speech, collect a spontaneous speech sample for later analysis, and evaluate the individual's intelligibility in various communication environments, and may administer a formal articulation test. If the individual's hearing has not previously been screened or evaluated, the SLP will also arrange for a hearing screening to ensure that the speech sound problems are not related to hearing loss.

According to the World Health Organization (WHO; 2001), the three goals of the assessment of speech sound disorders are to identify and describe

1. underlying structural or functional strengths and weaknesses (deficits) that affect speech sound production sufficiently to affect communication;
2. the effects of speech sound disorders on an individual's ability to participate in everyday communication activities; and
3. the factors that enhance or impede successful communication.

To these three goals I add a fourth, which is to monitor the individual's progress over time. This means that assessment is ongoing throughout the intervention phase and acts as a guide to the SLP in designing the most effective and appropriate intervention strategies.

Assessment of a speech sound disorder typically results in

- a diagnosis—in this case, of a speech sound disorder, including CAS;
- a thorough clinical description of the individual's speech sound abilities, including intelligibility, the ability to discriminate among speech sounds, the presence of any developmental phonological processes, the ability to produce phonemes in various linguistic contexts, and phonemic awareness;

- a prognosis for expected change;
- recommendations for intervention and support services; and
- referral to other services if indicated.

As with other types of **communication disorders**, most SLPs will take a case history as one of their first steps in assessing an individual's speech sound system. Box 8.3 lists some of the areas that should be included in the case history.

Once the case history has been obtained, the SLP can take a speech sample to use to analyze intelligibility, typical speech sound patterns, and a speech sound inventory (for articulation problems) or a phonological process analysis (for phonological processing problems).

Intelligibility can be assessed informally using an intelligibility rubric (see Figure 8.2) or more objectively using an intelligibility formula, shown in Box 8.4.

The result of using this formula allows the SLP to describe the individual's intelligibility as a percentage of words understood by an unfamiliar listener (usually another SLP) listening to a taped sample of the individual's speech during conversation.

The analysis of the individual's speech sound system, either through analyzing a spontaneous speech sample or through using a standardized instrument, such as the *Goldman-Fristoe Test of Articulation, Second Edition* (GFTA-2; Goldman & Fristoe,

---

BOX 8.3　　　　　**Speech Sound Disorder Case History**

Taking a case history for an individual with a speech sound disorder usually includes information regarding:

- the language(s) spoken in the individual's home;
- the individual's primary language;
- the family's perceptions of the individual's intelligibility;
- history of middle ear infections;
- history of speech, language, or literacy difficulties in the individual or family;
- how the individual's speech has developed thus far;
- the degree to which the individual or family are concerned; and
- the individual's willingness to engage in the intervention process.

---

1. Completely intelligible in conversation
2. Mostly intelligible in conversation
3. Somewhat intelligible in conversation
4. Intelligible only with careful listening in conversation
5. Mostly unintelligible in conversation, even with careful listening
6. Completely unintelligible in conversation, even with careful listening

FIGURE 8.2. A rubric for assessing speech intelligibility.

BOX 8.4   Formula for Calculating Speech Intelligibility

$$\text{Percentage of intelligible words} = \frac{\text{Number of intelligible words} \times 100}{\text{Total number of words}}$$

2000), allows the SLP to determine which phonemes the individual uses most commonly and in which contexts (i.e., the beginning, end, or middle of words; the beginning, end, or middle of sentences).

For a speech sound disorder involving articulation, the next step is to take an inventory of the sounds the individual misarticulates, again through analysis of a speech sample or through using a standardized assessment instrument. Most analyses focus on errors of **substitution**, **omission**, **distortion**, and **addition** in syllable and word positions.

For a phonological processing disorder, the SLP will analyze the individual's phonological processes, either through an informal analysis or using a standardized instrument, such as the *Khan-Lewis Phonological Analysis, Second Edition* (KLPA-2; Khan & Lewis, 2002) or the *Hodson Assessment of Phonological Patterns-3* (HAPP-3; Hodson, 2004). The aim of this analysis is to identify whether the individual is using patterns of sound errors that have persisted beyond what is expected for the individual's age. For instance, a 3-year-old child using a voiceless consonant for a voiced consonant at the end of a word (e.g., /bɪk/ for "big") is exhibiting a phonological process known as *final consonant devoicing*. Another example is a 4-year-old using an affricate instead of a nonaffricate (e.g., /dʒɔr/ for "door"). To learn more about speech sound disorders, see Flahive and Hodson (2013).

Management of Speech Sound Disorders

The long-term goal for individuals with speech sound disorders depends on the etiology and severity of the disorder, each individual's commitment to changing her or his speech, and support at home. For some individuals, the goal may be to completely correct the disorder, while for others it may be to increase intelligibility or augment their ability to communicate.

Deciding on which phonemes or phonological processes to focus on in intervention usually rests on the SLP's analysis of the intelligibility and pattern of phonological processes. In most instances, the SLP will begin with error phonemes that appear more frequently in English (assuming the intervention is in English) rather than phonemes that occur rarely. For instance, the phoneme used least frequently in English is /ʒ/ (as in "azure"), while another frequently misarticulated phoneme, /ð/ (as in "there"), is much more frequently used. Consequently, the SLP would choose to begin focusing on /ð/ rather than /ʒ/. Targeting a high-frequency phoneme first will be more likely to increase the individual's intelligibility than focusing on a low-frequency phoneme.

The same logic applies to selecting which phonological processes to focus on during intervention. The processes that impact intelligibility the most are the ones the SLP will target first because their remediation will be more likely to increase the child's intelligibility. The SLP will also take into account which phonological process patterns the child produces consistently and frequently, and can, with support, change relatively easily.

Intervention for Phonological Disorders

When a child's speech errors are classified as a phonological disorder, remediation focuses on target patterns to be acquired rather than on isolated phonemes. Several different approaches may be followed when remediating phonological disorders.

Hodson (2006) designed the Cycles Phonological Pattern Approach (CPPA), a word-based approach in which error patterns are identified and treated and individual phonemes are targeted as a means to achieving the end goal (i.e., producing the patterns). For example, the final consonant deletion error pattern may be targeted with word-final /t/ words (e.g., *boat, hat, boot, dot*) during one cycle and word-final /p/ words (e.g., *cup, pipe, rope, mop*) in a subsequent cycle, rather than teaching each sound the child deletes.

Williams (2006) recommended the use of multiple contrastive word pairs for children who have moderate to severe speech sound disorders that result in a one-to-many phoneme collapse of several adult target sounds into one substitution or omission. For example, it is not uncommon for children to substitute /t/ for several adult targets, such as /k, s, ʃ, tʃ/ and clusters, such as /st, tr, kl, kr/. This error substitute results in a 1:8 phoneme collapse of adult target phonemes and clusters. As a result, the child produces words with these different target sounds as homonyms, such as /tu/ for all these words: *two, coo, Sue, shoes, chew, stew, true, clue,* and *crew*. A multiple oppositions approach would direct intervention across the entire phoneme collapse, or rule set, by training up to four target sounds in contrast to the child's error substitute. For example, a multiple oppositions approach could target /t/ in contrast with /k, s, kl, tr/ to induce multiple phonemic splits by directing the child's learning across the multiple homonymous forms that exist as a result of the phoneme collapse.

Intervention for Articulation Disorders

For children whose articulation errors do not have an organic cause, the goal of intervention is to correct the errors. Most of these children do not have a hearing loss, nor do they have a developmental disability. In addition, there is no dysarthria, verbal apraxia, or structural abnormality that affects the functioning of their vocal tracts. They simply have not learned to produce the sound(s) correctly. Adults can also learn to correct their errors. However, they usually need a higher level of motivation than do children because they have a longer history of making their errors and the stronger habit is hard to overcome.

Correcting the errors would also be the goal for children whose articulation errors appear to have an organic etiology that can be either corrected or compensated for. These include some dental anomalies, short lingual frenums, cleft palates, and hearing losses.

Several strategies are used for getting clients to produce speech sounds correctly. One is a drill approach in which the client is asked to simply imitate the clinician. The clinician makes the sound, and the client imitates it. Another is teaching them how to configure the vocal tract for making the sound. This could involve a straightforward description of where to place the articulators. For example, a client with a lateral lisp (an /s/ distortion in which the air flows between the side teeth rather than the incisors) would be told where to place the tongue so that air will flow between the incisors. An indirect strategy could also be used for getting clients to configure the vocal tract appropriately. For example, if a client has a lateral lisp, he or she could be told to make the voiceless /s/ while keeping the tongue behind the teeth (rather than placing it between them). Most persons who follow this instruction will produce a fairly normal /s/.

Another strategy that is used for getting clients to produce speech sounds correctly involves the use of **biofeedback**. For example, an adult who was unable to learn to produce /r/ correctly through other approaches may be taught to produce /r/ by speaking into a microphone attached to a device containing a computer. Graphic information is displayed on the computer screen, which allows the speaker to judge the correctness of the productions (Schuster, Ruscello, & Smith, 1992). For more information on biofeedback, visit the Arizona Behavioral Health Associates (2005) web page describing biofeedback.

After the client has learned to produce a misarticulated speech sound correctly in isolation, he or she is taught to produce it in syllables, words, sentences, and finally, conversational speech. Once the client is able to produce a sound correctly during conversational speech in the therapy room, the SLP works to generalize the correct production to situations outside of the therapy room.

Intervention With Apraxia and Dysarthria

For individuals whose errors are caused by disorders such as dysarthria or verbal apraxia, correcting their articulation errors is not the primary goal because the prognosis for correcting articulation errors with these etiologies is usually not good. If it is not possible to correct the client's articulation errors either because the vocal tract cannot be made to function normally or it is not possible to compensate for all the abnormalities, the clinician will attempt to increase the intelligibility of the client's speech. The goal will be to make a client's speech understandable to conversational partners.

One approach is to improve the functioning of the vocal tract as much as possible. For example, a client might be encouraged to take a medication if it reduces the severity of dysarthria. Increasing the intelligibility of a client's speech could also involve teaching the client to speak in a way that differs somewhat from his or her habitual manner. For example, if a client who has dysarthria is able to speak but the speech is difficult to understand, it may be possible to improve intelligibility by teaching the client to speak at a slower rate.

Some children with severe CAS benefit from a program called *Dynamic Temporal and Tactile Cueing (DTTC) for Speech Motor Learning* (Strand, Stoeckel, & Baas, 2006). This program uses a hierarchy of steps, beginning with either the child imitating the SLP or, if that is not possible, having the child

- produce prolonged vowels with the SLP;
- reduce vowel length, increasing the rate of speech to a normal rate;
- produce the sounds while the SLP reduces his or her voice until it disappears;
- directly imitate the SLP on targeted phonemes or words;
- produce the targeted phoneme or word after a 2-second delay; and
- spontaneously produce the target phoneme or word.

For children with dysarthria, intervention focuses on improving intelligibility and voice (pitch, quality, loudness) to the extent possible. In addition, the SLP may help children learn specific communication strategies that can assist listeners in understanding their speech. Some examples are teaching children to look directly at the person they're conversing with; take a breath before speaking in order to have adequate breath to support the voice throughout their utterance; slow their rate of speech; and speak in short utterances with pauses between (Bowen, 2013). Bowen further recommends assisting the child's conversational partners—family, friends, schoolmates, and teachers—to learn to stop and take time to listen attentively, ask the child what he or she wants, and give feedback to the child about what is unclear in their speaking.

In some instances, individuals may not be able to speak with enough clarity to be understood and would benefit from using an augmentative and alternative communication system, such as those I described in Chapter 5.

chapter 9

Fluency Disorders

Learning Objectives

Describe normal fluency.

Describe the difference between normal and abnormal speech fluency.

Describe stuttering and its speech characteristics.

Describe the physiological and psychological symptoms of stuttering.

Identify the primary theories of what causes stuttering.

Discuss the relationship between pragmatics and stuttering.

Describe the two primary goals for managing stuttering.

Discuss the difficulty faced by SLPs designing intervention for people who clutter.

Overview

Fluency is the term used to describe the effortless and smooth production of **speech**. However, the ability to speak fluently does not mean one's speech is entirely free of **disfluencies**. If you listen carefully to how people speak, you will notice that almost everyone experiences some interruptions in their speech flow. In fact, if you listen to your own speech, you may be surprised at how many interruptions are present.

The Stuttering Foundation (2014b) estimates that, worldwide, about 1% of the world population (a little more than 68 million people) stutters, and in the United Sates more than 3 million people stutter. The foundation reports that approximately 5% of children will go through a period of stuttering lasting 6 months or longer. Of these children, 75% will recover by late childhood (Stuttering Foundation, 2014b). This video offers a good introduction to **stuttering**, its incidence, and what it feels like to live with stuttering (CBS, 2011). Go to the website (http://goo .gl/e23MQt) or scan the code

Recall Van Riper and Erickson's (1996) definition of a **communication disorder** from Chapter 2, in which they described a communication disorder as having at least one of the following three aspects:

1. There is a perception by others that the person's communication deviates enough from normal **hearing**, speech, or **language** that it interferes with communication.
2. The person's communication calls adverse attention to him or her.
3. It causes the person to be self-conscious about it.

When a person's speech flow deviates from what is considered "normal," when it calls adverse attention to itself, or when it causes the person to be self-conscious or maladjusted, it can be considered to be outside the realm of normal fluency. In the following sections I discuss normal and abnormal speech fluency, and then I describe stuttering and related disfluencies.

Normal Versus Abnormal Speech Fluency

Hesitations are a normal part of speaking. Most people hesitate frequently while they are speaking. Box 9.1 lists the types of things we all do occasionally when we speak, particularly when we are tense.

If everyone has moments of disfluency while speaking, when is the disfluency abnormal—that is, when is it symptomatic of a speech disorder? This question is not an easy one to answer. Considerable research has attempted to identify differences between normal disfluency behaviors and those resulting from fluency disorders. No one knows definitely whether or not normal disfluencies and those categorized as stuttering share the same neurology, motor production sequences, or the brain mechanisms used in formulating and producing spontaneous language. As you will see, there is considerable overlap in the speech of people with disfluencies and people with normal speech.

BOX 9.1 **Characteristics of Normal Speaking**

- Repeating sounds, syllables, words, and phrases
- Interjecting sounds and syllables between words (e.g., "um")
- Leaving abnormally long pauses between words
- Prolonging speech sounds, particularly the initial sounds of words
- Stopping to correct errors of pronunciation, syntax, and word usage

---

Frequency of Occurrence

One of the first areas investigators analyzed for differences between normal and abnormal disfluency behaviors was frequency of occurrence. They thought that although all speakers exhibit such behaviors, those who have fluency disorders may exhibit them more often than those who do not have a fluency disorder. The findings of these studies indicated that while some persons who have fluency disorders are disfluent more often than normal speakers, overlap (sometimes considerable) occurs between the groups. Consequently, there are normal speakers who are disfluent as often as some of those who have a fluency disorder. This overlap between groups appears to be greater for preschool-age children than for adults.

Duration of Individual Moments of Disfluency

If amount of disfluency does not sharply differentiate people who have fluency disorders from those who do not, perhaps the duration of their individual moments of disfluency does. That is, perhaps individual moments of disfluency of people with fluency disorders tend to last longer. Most studies comparing the durations of normal speakers' moments of disfluency to those of persons who have a fluency disorder found the durations to be similar to those for frequency of disfluency. So, while the moments of disfluency of some persons who have a fluency disorder tend to last longer than those of persons who do not have one, there is overlap between the groups. Some normal speakers can have moments of disfluency that last as long as those of some persons who have a fluency disorder. Again, this overlap between groups appears to be greater for preschool-age children than for adults.

Amount of Tension Present

A third attribute of moments of disfluency that investigators have looked at in an attempt to differentiate normal from abnormal disfluency behavior is the amount of tension present. Normal disfluencies tend to be relatively free from tension or struggle and are rarely accompanied by facial grimaces or other signs of tension. Almost all people whose moments of disfluency are accompanied by audible or visible signs of tension are considered to have a fluency disorder. However, some individuals who have a fluency disorder do not show such signs, especially preschool children.

Speakers' Awareness of and Attitude Toward Moments of Disfluency

A fourth attribute of moments of disfluency that has been investigated is the speakers' awareness of them. Disfluencies are more likely to be labeled abnormal if the speaker appears embarrassed by them. Embarrassment is often communicated nonverbally (e.g., staring at the floor, blushing). Having a negative attitude about being disfluent can handicap a person in other ways. For example, it can cause him or her to avoid talking. A person who avoids talking is being handicapped by being disfluent regardless of his or her amount of disfluency. While those who are highly aware of their moments of disfluency tend to be individuals who have a fluency disorder, many do not exhibit such awareness.

Distribution in the Speech Sequence

A fifth attribute of moments of disfluency that has been investigated is their distribution in the speech sequence. Does the distribution tend to be random, or do moments of disfluency tend to occur more often than would be expected by chance on (or adjacent to) words having certain characteristics? The findings of most studies suggest the latter.

Moments of disfluency tend to be more likely to occur, for example, on words having certain grammatical functions. However, this attribute does not differentiate normal from abnormal disfluency behavior. People who stutter, for example, tend to do so on words having the same grammatical functions as those on which normal speakers tend to be disfluent.

In summary, the findings of most studies that have compared audible and visible attributes of moments of disfluency in the speech of typical speakers with those of persons who have a fluency disorder suggest that they have much in common. In fact, the disfluency behaviors of some people who have a fluency disorder seem similar both quantitatively and qualitatively to those of typical speakers. The age group for which this similarity has been reported most often is preschool-age children. However, the relationship between normal and abnormal speech disfluency is not a settled issue, and research on it is ongoing.

A number of protocols have been developed for helping speech–language pathologists (SLPs) decide whether disfluency is abnormal. Most of them consist of criteria for differentiating beginning stuttering from the normal disfluency of preschool children. For descriptions of several of these protocols, see Gordon and Luper (1992a, 1992b) and Onslow (1992).

Types of Disfluencies

All children and adults are disfluent occasionally. Both psycholinguists and SLPs have conducted considerable research on what happens when this occurs. The psycholinguistic literature refers to such investigations as research on *hesitation phenomena,* and the speech–language pathology literature refers to it as research on *disfluency behaviors.* In the next paragraphs I summarize some of the findings of this research to provide you with a basis for differentiating normal from abnormal disfluency behavior, particularly in young children.

Eight types of behaviors may occur in the speech of children and adults while they are being disfluent:

1. **Part-word repetitions** occur when a person repeats sounds or syllables in words. This phenomenon usually occurs at the beginning of words and almost never at the end of them. Though the number of times a particular sound or syllable is repeated can be quite high, it is usually only once or twice.

2. **Word repetitions** are repetitions of entire words, most often single-syllable words. Although a word may be repeated a relatively large number of times, it is usually repeated only once or twice.

3. **Phrase repetitions** are repetitions of phrases consisting of two or more words. Phrases are usually repeated only once or twice.

4. **Interjections** are sounds, syllables, words, or phrases that are added between words. They do not usually perform a linguistic function in messages—that is, their presence does not usually affect the denotative meanings of messages. Examples are *um* and *you know*.

5. The **revision-incomplete phrase** category includes instances in which the speaker becomes aware of making an error and corrects it. The error may be in how a word was pronounced or it may be related to the meaning of the word that was said. Also included are instances in which the speaker begins an utterance but obviously does not complete it.

6. **Dysrhythmic phonations** are disturbances in the normal rhythms of words. The disturbance may be attributable to a prolonged sound, an accent or timing that is notably unusual, an improper stress, a break (usually between syllables), or any other speaking behavior that occurs within words and is not compatible with fluent speech.

7. **Tense pauses** are phenomena that occur between words, part-words, and interjections. They consist of pauses during which there are barely audible manifestations of heavy breathing or muscle tightening. The same phenomena within words would be classified as dysrhythmic phonations.

8. **Unfilled pauses** are abnormally long pauses between words. Although the existence of such pauses is acknowledged by all investigators of speech disfluency, they have not been studied as much as the other seven types because they are difficult to identify reliably. Investigators disagree about how long a pause between words has to be before it can be classified as abnormal.

In this video, produced by the Stuttering Foundation (2011), *Stuttering: For Kids, By Kids*, a group of children and adolescents describe what stuttering is, how they feel about stuttering, how to converse with someone who stutters, what to do if they get teased, and how speech therapy helped them. You'll notice examples of each of the eight types of disfluency, sometimes in the same sentence. Go to the website (http://goo.gl/8e5quL) or scan the code.

Fluency Disorders

There are three types of fluency disorders: cluttering, neurogenic stuttering, and developmental stuttering, which is the most common of the three.

Cluttering

People who study fluency disorders generally agree that people who have a cluttering disorder are unusually disfluent because they do not monitor their speech adequately and are usually unaware of their disfluency or the fact that they are talking rapidly. To reduce their speaking rate and disfluency, therefore, it is necessary to get them to monitor their speech more carefully.

One problem that is frequently encountered when working with people who clutter is lack of motivation because many do not believe their speech is difficult to understand. Almost all are seen by SLPs because someone (usually a parent, teacher, or employer) insists that they need therapy. The prognosis for reducing their speaking rate and disfluency will, of course, be poor if they do not take therapy seriously.

Differentiating cluttering from stuttering is often difficult, even for experienced SLPs. Box 9.2 lists some of the common characteristics of cluttering.

According to the International Cluttering Society (2014), other conditions that frequently coexist with cluttering include the following:

- difficulty formulating language
- disordered thought processes
- sound-specific articulation disorders
- problems with motor speech coordination
- ADHD
- auditory processing disorders
- Asperger's syndrome
- apraxia

Neurogenic Stuttering

Neurogenic stuttering usually occurs because of some neurological incident, disease, or trauma. People who acquire neurogenic stuttering almost always have had

---

BOX 9.2   Common Characteristics of Cluttering (International Cluttering Society, 2014)

- Abnormally rapid or irregular rate of speech
- High number of disfluencies, most of which are not typical of people who stutter
- Frequent use of pauses and prosodic patterns unrelated to the semantic content or syntactic structure of what the person is saying
- Collapsing of syllables in multisyllabic words (e.g., "sgetti" for "sphagetti")

no history of stuttering, and the sudden onset of stuttering is associated with a neurological event, such as strokes, head traumas, and tumors. Their disorder is referred to most often as *neurogenic acquired stuttering*. Other terms used are *neurogenic stuttering, acquired stuttering, neurological disfluency, cortical stuttering,* and *stuttering of sudden onset.* The types of abnormal disfluency behaviors observed in the speech of people with this disorder include repetitions or dysrhythmic phonations. The specific symptomatology is determined, in part, by the neurological condition with which the disorder is associated.

Neurogenic acquired stuttering appears to differ from ordinary stuttering and cluttering in several ways. First, most people with this type of fluency problem develop it as an adult rather than as a child. The development of stutter-like hesitations in an adult who has been a normal speaker can be an early symptom of a neurological condition.

A second way in which neurogenic acquired stuttering differs from ordinary stuttering and cluttering is that it varies little (if at all) across situations—the amount of disfluency is approximately the same in all situations. People with this disorder, for example, are quite disfluent even when they read in unison with someone, while almost all people who stutter are completely fluent under this condition. There may be no condition under which people with neurogenic acquired stuttering are normally fluent. To learn more about neurogenic acquired stuttering, visit Judith Kuster's (2005b) website describing neurogenic acquired stuttering. (Note: she also describes the disfluencies associated with Tourette syndrome and spasmodic dysphonia.)

Stuttering

Stuttering is the most common disorder of fluency. Although its onset usually occurs between the ages of 3 and 5, it can begin at any age, even during adulthood. More males than females stutter—the ratio between males and females is somewhere between 3:1 and 5:1. The disorder tends to run in families, but no one has yet been able to pinpoint exactly what genetic factors contribute to stuttering. The effect, however, is that individuals who stutter have a reduced ability to produce the coordinated and complex muscle movements required to fluently produce multiword sentences.

Because stuttering usually begins in early childhood, some physicians counsel parents to wait to see if their child outgrows it. However, children who receive intervention when they are young experience far fewer disfluencies than if they did not receive intervention at this age (Stuttering Foundation, 2015). The Stuttering Foundation (2014b) emphasizes that early intervention is particularly effective, not only in reducing disfluencies but also in preventing the child from developing negative emotional reactions to stuttering.

Characteristics of Stuttering

In addition to the speech characteristics of stuttering I described previously, individuals who stutter may also appear out of breath while speaking. Some individuals become completely blocked in the middle of a word or sentence, unable to speak even though their mouth is poised to produce the next sound. Others rearrange words to avoid having to say a word they fear will cause them to stutter, or they may pretend to forget what they wanted to say in order to "buy" time to get through the stuttering. They may yawn—or pretend to—over and over because they can speak fluently while they're yawning.

No person who stutters does so on every word he or she says. In fact, few stutter on more than half their words. Both frequency and duration tend to vary on a situational basis. Most people who stutter tend to be relatively fluent in these situations:

- Reading in unison with another person, even another person who stutters
- Speaking to an infant or an animal
- Singing
- Swearing or openly expressing anger
- Speaking in any nonhabitual manner (e.g., in an overly loud voice, with objects in the mouth, at a very slow rate) or while engaging in rhythmic physical activity, such as dancing, walking, or swinging the arms

However, in high-demand situations, individuals who stutter usually stutter more, especially when they fear they will stutter. High-demand situations for most people who stutter include

- talking on the telephone;
- speaking to an authority figure;
- speaking in a situation in which they wish to avoid stuttering;
- speaking to people who react adversely (e.g., laughing, being impatient, viewing the speaker as childlike or cognitively delayed); and
- desiring to communicate quickly (e.g., when giving an order to a waitress, answering the question "What is your name?," or experiencing difficulty securing talking time in the midst of a conversational "crossfire").

The frequency and duration of moments of stuttering vary not only on a situational basis but also on a day-to-day basis. People who stutter tend to have "good" and "bad" days with respect to the amount they stutter, and the amount they stutter in any given situation is likely to vary considerably from day to day.

The frequency and duration of moments of stuttering are also influenced by certain word characteristics. Those who stutter are more likely to stutter on words they stuttered on previously. This phenomenon is known as the **consistency effect**. They also show a greater-than-chance tendency to stutter on words that are nouns, verbs, adverbs, or adjectives; begin with consonant sounds; are relatively long; or occur at the beginnings of sentences.

Most persons who stutter develop strategies to avoid stuttering, although many of these strategies cause them to lose more than they gain. One such strategy is not talking when they expect to stutter. Obviously, they will not stutter if they do not talk. Many school-age children who stutter, for example, refrain from asking or voluntarily answering questions in class. Although this strategy will allow a person who stutters to avoid some stuttering, it also is likely to have another effect—that is, to impede the person's ability to give and receive information and to express feelings. The use of this strategy can be more handicapping than the stuttering it is intended to eliminate.

A second avoidance strategy is to substitute words they do not expect to cause stuttering for those that do. Most adults and some children are able to accurately predict many of the words on which they are going to stutter. This ability is referred to as the **expectancy phenomenon**. Sometimes the words they substitute are not entirely appropriate, which can interfere with their ability to communicate.

A third strategy that individuals who stutter use to avoid a moment of disfluency is **secondary behaviors** (i.e., *secondaries;* also called *accessory behaviors*). Secondary behaviors include speaking in a nonhabitual manner, using interjections, increasing vocal pitch, or a making a movement of some type. For example, people who stutter may speak at an abnormally slow rate or with an accent, or they may use **starters**. Persons who stutter believe that by using starters they can give their speech mechanism a "running start." An example of a starter is a person who wants to say, "I like coffee with cream" but says, "I mean I was going to say I like coffee with cream." Movements that a person may make to avoid a moment of disfluency include looking away from the listener, making jerking movements of the head, blinking the eyes, and facial contortions.

Why do secondary behaviors accompany moments of stuttering? The most widely held explanation is that they began as devices for avoiding disfluencies or reducing their severity. A person who stutters and anticipates stuttering on a word may attempt to avoid it by doing something prior to saying the word. Or a person who begins to stutter on a word may attempt to do something to reduce the duration of the disfluency. A person who stutters is likely to continue using the device until he or she no longer believes that doing so will keep disfluencies from occurring or reduce their duration. By this time, the behavior has become a learned component of the moment of disfluency. Thus, such behaviors may accompany stuttering either because they are currently being used as devices for coping with stuttering, or they are behaviors that were used for this purpose in the past but no longer "work" and have become habitual. Judith Kuster's website provides a rich resource of information about stuttering (Kuster, 2005b).

What Causes Stuttering?

For centuries, people have proposed theories about what causes stuttering. Although genetic factors play a role, no one knows its exact cause. For most people who stutter, there is no family history of the disorder or any other apparent cause. Brain imaging studies in adults who stutter show definite anomalies in how the brain functions during speech (Fox et al., 1996; Fox et al., 2000; Sommer, Koch, Paulus, Weiller, &

Buchel, 2002). Most experts believe that these anomalies reflect a deficit in the sensorimotor integration required to regulate the rapid muscle movements that produce fluent speech.

The onset of stuttering in most children begins between the ages of 3 and 5, when they are engaged in the intense process of developing more complex and demanding speech and language skills. During that time, their utterances undergo tremendous change—from two words to multiword sentences with more elaborate structural frameworks. As they attempt to produce these more complicated grammatical structures, their disfluencies become more apparent.

Over the hundreds of years people have attempted to explain what causes stuttering, many theories have been generated. Some focus on psychological factors (e.g., stuttering is a symptom of some deeper, unconscious neurosis); others argue that stuttering is a learned behavior (e.g., when parents overreact to the child's disfluencies, the child learns to avoid the disfluencies and develops a stutter).

More recently, however, researchers using sophisticated technologies (e.g., functional magnetic resonance imaging, or fMRI; positron emission tomography, or PET) and advances in knowledge about the brain and genomes are finding that there is, in fact, a genetic basis for stuttering that affects both the sensory and the motor areas of the brain in nonobvious ways. Furthermore, this research shows that stuttering can be affected by psychological and environmental influences (Ambrose, 2004). Reviewing the results of current work, Ambrose concluded that stuttering is most likely a combination of several disorders: motor, motor speech, language, genetics, psychological, and learned behavior.

A series of studies by Weber-Fox (2005) corroborates Ambrose's conclusion. Weber-Fox's findings support what she terms a multifactorial model of stuttering in which stuttering in adults is seen to arise from the complex interactions among genetics, speech motor control, language processing, and emotion or social aspects. Weber-Fox et al. (2013) reported that the preschool children in their study who stuttered had speech motor control systems that were different from those of their typically fluent peers. Specifically, the children who stuttered showed electrophysiological differences related to language processing compared to their typically fluent peers even during speaking conditions that were undemanding. In addition, when compared with typically fluent peers, the speech motor control systems of preschool children who stutter are susceptible to breakdowns and unusual variability under high-demand speaking conditions (McPherson & Smith, 2013), further supporting the multifactorial model.

Relationship Between Pragmatics and Stuttering

As I mentioned earlier, some clinicians believe that because the period of greatest language development (i.e., ages 3 to 5) is also the period of greatest risk for developing stuttering, stuttering should be considered within the context of a child's language development (see Bloom & Cooperman, 1999), specifically pragmatics.

Disfluencies disrupt both the rhythm of the person's speech and his or her ability to keep up with the pace of taking turns with conversational partners. For instance, disfluencies add to the time required to complete an utterance or phrase. Because turn taking in conversations is partly based on the amount of time each person takes per turn, the person who stutters is perceived as taking longer turns and slowing the pace of the conversation. In addition, his or her conversational partners must alter their pacing in order to accommodate the person's elongated turns. Individuals who stutter may perceive that their conversational partners are interrupting—beginning to speak before they have finished their turn. The quick give-and-take of multiple turns gives way to a slower conversation with fewer turns.

Some people who stutter have developed habits during speaking that interfere with their ability to monitor their conversational partners' understanding and participation. For example, if individuals who stutter close their eyes or look at the floor during a disfluency, they are unable to see how their conversational partners are responding. Bloom and Cooperman (1999) teach their young clients how to wait for their turn before talking, listen to what the other person is saying, and maintain the topic the other person is talking about.

Several people who study stuttering have discovered that one of the factors affecting how children maintain fluency is the degree of conversational demand required (Weiss, 2004). Weiss gives the example of asking children who stutter different types of choice questions, such as "Do you want macaroni or peanut butter and jelly?" or "What do you want for lunch?" The latter question carries a higher conversational demand because it requires the child to decide not only what she or he wants for lunch but also how to construct a sentence to express that desire. However, the first question requires only that the child select one of the two choices on offer, which doesn't carry the responsibility of providing a unique answer constructed from a large number of possibilities. Thus, the conversational demand is lower for the first question than for the second.

Assessment

In young children, the primary purpose of assessment is to determine whether they have a disfluency disorder, which is not always as easy as it sounds. As I described earlier, most children produce normal developmental disfluencies. Between 18 months and 3 years of age, typical disfluencies are repetitions of sounds, syllables, and words, usually at the beginnings of sentences. Most children cycle through these phases of disfluencies fairly frequently.

After they reach 3 years of age, most children's sound and syllable repetitions diminish, but they may repeat whole words and phrases, and they use interjections such as "uh" or "um." These types of disfluencies are more obvious when children are tired, upset, excited, or eager to speak. As in younger children, children over age 3 also cycle through phases of disfluencies (Stuttering Foundation, 2014a).

Children who stutter often exhibit the same sound, syllable, and word repetitions as children with normal disfluencies, but their repetitions are more frequent and more frequently repeated within each instance. Children who stutter also occasionally prolong sounds, tense their mouths, look to the side, or blink or close their eyes (Stuttering Foundation, 2014a).

Some children will exhibit severe stuttering, which typically includes physical struggle and tension and involves disfluencies in almost every phrase or sentence. Severe stuttering usually persists, especially if the child has been stuttering for a long period of time, and the child will usually become frustrated and embarrassed enough about speaking to fear talking (Stuttering Foundation, 2014a).

An evaluation for stuttering includes a case history, during which the SLP will ask about a family history of stuttering; how long the child's stuttering has been going on; whether there might be other speech or language disorders; and whether anyone (including family members) have fears or concerns about the child's stuttering.

In addition to the case history, the SLP will gather information about

- the number and types of disfluencies the child produces and in which specific speaking situations;
- the child's rate of speech;
- the prosodic characteristics of the child's speech; and
- the presence of secondary symptoms, and if present, a description.

In older children and adults, the purpose of assessment no longer focuses on whether a fluency disorder exists. Evaluation for these individuals consists of interviews, observations, and tests to assess the severity of the disorder and the impact of the disorder on the individual's life (ASHA, 2014u). Box 9.3 lists various types of evaluation instruments and methods used to assess stuttering.

Intervention

Intervention with young children usually emphasizes reducing disfluencies through teaching parents how to support their child's production of fluent speech. Box 9.4 lists some of the strategies parents are taught to use.

Designing intervention for older children and adults involves teaching them to speak more fluently, communicate more effectively, and participate more fully in daily life (ASHA, 2014u). More specifically, the goals for therapy include

- reducing stuttering frequency;
- reducing articulatory tension;
- easing the onset of voicing, first with vowels and later with consonants;
- decreasing tension and struggle during stuttering;
- decreasing word or situation avoidance; and
- preparing for a school project or job interview (Stuttering Foundation, 2014b).

BOX 9.3   **Checklists and Instruments for Assessing Stuttering**

Tool	Purpose
Real-Time Analysis of Speech Fluency (Yaruss, 1998)	Assesses frequency, duration, types, and severity of disfluency in spontaneous speech. All ages.
Fluency Severity Rating Scale	Five-point scale, ranging from *Mild* to *Severe*, rating frequency of blocks; stuttered words/minute; duration; and secondary characteristics. All ages.
Stuttering Severity Rating Scales	Various scales that measure the individual's stuttering in different contexts and times of day and week.
Situational Fears/Avoidance Checklist	The individual checks the speech situations that cause the most stuttering, those she or he wishes to avoid, and ranks them from most to least difficult.
Behavior Assessment Battery for School-Age Children Who Stutter (Brutten & Vanryckeghem, 2006)	Assesses individuals' emotional reaction to their speech in different situations, their coping strategies for dealing with disfluency, and their attitudes toward their speech. All ages.
Test of Childhood Stuttering (TOCS; Gillam, Logan, & Pearson, 2009)	Differentiates stuttering from nonstuttering, determines the severity of stuttering, documents changes in a child's fluency over time. Ages 4 through 12.
Stuttering Severity Instrument-Fourth Edition (SSI-4; Riley, 2009)	Measures stuttering frequency, duration, physical concomitants, and naturalness of the individual's speech. Ages 2 and older.
Overall Assessment of the Speaker's Experience of Stuttering (OASES; Yaruss & Quesal, 2010)	Assesses the individual's reaction to stuttering, communication in daily situations, and quality of life.

BOX 9.4   **Strategies Parents Can Use to Encourage Fluent Speech in Their Young Child**

- Set aside a relaxed time to talk when they can listen attentively to what the child is saying and the child has multiple opportunities to talk.
- Reduce their own speech rate to model a relaxed manner.
- Allow the child ample time to speak without pressuring her or him to answer or respond.
- Allow the child to finish sentences—do not finish sentences or interrupt.
- If the child asks about the stuttering, talk about it openly and honestly.

Some individuals who stutter benefit from using an altered auditory feedback (AAF) device, which plays the person's voice back after a slight delay (delayed auditory feedback), or with a slight alteration in pitch (frequency-shifted auditory feedback), or both. Some devices fit into or around the ear like hearing aids; others are cell-phone-size and include an ear set and microphone. In addition to special devices that produce AAF, there are AAF apps available for use on iPhones and Android phones, as well as AAF software for computers. The effect of AAF is to slow the individual's speech rate while maintaining the length of pauses between syllables and words. The result is a decrease in disfluency.

For older children and adults, reducing or eliminating stuttering may not be feasible, in which case they can benefit from learning stuttering modification techniques. Charles Van Riper, one of the early pioneers in the field of communication sciences and disorders, described four techniques that have evolved into effective therapeutic strategies (Van Riper, 1973): identification, desensitization, modification, and stabilization. These four strategies are meant to be undertaken sequentially.

1. *Identification*—Working with an SLP, the individual learns to identify the primary and secondary characteristics of her or his stuttering, along with the feelings and attitudes that accompany it.
2. *Desensitization*—The individual learns to accept that she or he stutters; to prolong moments of stuttering so that they lose their emotional charge, and to stutter voluntarily to learn how to remain calm during stuttering.
3. *Modification*—The individual learns three stages of "easy" or "fluent" stuttering:
   - *cancellations*—when stuttering, the individual stops, pauses, and says the word again slowly, with reduced articulatory pressure.
   - *pull-outs*—After mastering cancellations, the individual uses "easy" stuttering while in a stutter in order to pull out of the stutter and say the word fluently.
   - *preparatory sets*—After mastering pull-outs, the individual looks ahead for words on which she or he is likely to stutter and use "easy" stuttering on those words.
4. *Stabilization*—The individual seeks to automatize preparatory sets and pull-outs and to begin thinking of her- or himself as a person who speaks fluently most of the time and only occasionally stutters mildly.

In this video, Megan Washington, an Australian singer/songwriter, talks about her stuttering and its effect on her life (Washington, 2014). Go to the website (http://goo.gl/vlfTlg) or scan the code.

PART 4

Hearing Disorders

Chapter 10 addresses hearing and hearing disorders. The first part of the chapter lays the foundation necessary for understanding hearing disorders: how sounds are produced and differentiated from each other; the anatomy and physiology of the hearing mechanism and how sounds are transmitted from the ear to the brain; and the types and causes of hearing and auditory disorders. In the next sections, I describe the relationship between hearing loss and cognitive decline, and I discuss deafness and Deaf culture. In the last part of the chapter, I describe the specifics of assessing and managing hearing disorders in children and adults. I include a description of the major types of hearing testing and an overview of the primary approaches used to help people with hearing disorders regain some or all of their hearing, capitalize on their residual hearing, and learn alternative methods for communicating.

chapter 10

Hearing
and Hearing Disorders

Learning Objectives

Describe how sound is generated.

Identify the characteristic waveform associated with different types of sounds.

Define the common terminology associated with sound production and hearing.

Describe the anatomy of the outer, middle, and inner ear.

Describe how sound is conducted from the ear to the brain.

Describe the etiology and characteristics of a conductive hearing loss.

Describe the etiology and characteristics of a sensorineural hearing loss.

Describe a mixed hearing loss.

Describe hearing difficulties associated with central auditory disturbances.

Describe the relationship between hearing loss and cognitive decline.

Discuss the impact of Deaf culture on how deafness is viewed.

Describe the primary goals of assessment.

Describe three types of treatment used with hearing disorders.

Describe when aural rehabilitation is used.

Overview

A **hearing** loss is the partial or complete inability to hear and can be caused by a variety of factors, such as aging, genetic conditions, noise exposure, physical trauma, certain illnesses, or exposure to chemicals. If not treated early, hearing loss in children can result in significant difficulties in developing **language** and in learning. In adults, hearing loss can result in difficulties communicating with family and friends, challenges at work, and depression or social isolation.

The Hearing Health Foundation (2014) reported the following:

- In the United States, close to 50 million individuals have hearing loss in at least one ear.
- One in five teenagers has a hearing loss.
- Sixty percent of soldiers returning from Iraq and Afghanistan experience hearing loss and **tinnitus**.
- A greater number of men than women have hearing loss.
- Three out of every 1,000 children in the United States are born deaf or hard of hearing.
- The incidence of hearing loss increases with age.
- Loud noise at work or during leisure activities accounts for hearing loss in approximately 26 million Americans between 20 and 69 years of age.
- Individuals with mild hearing loss are twice as likely as hearing individuals to develop dementia; this risk increases with the severity of the loss.

Hearing loss can have a significant impact on children's ability to develop spoken language at the same rate and to the same degree as hearing age-peers. However, Deaf[1] children born to deaf families who are fluent in **American Sign Language** **(ASL)** develop ASL at the same rate that hearing children acquire spoken language (Gallaudet University Laurent Clerc National Deaf Education Center, 2014).

In approximately 30% of babies with hearing loss, the loss is related to a syndrome, which often causes other problems as well. Over 400 genetic syndromes have been identified that can cause hearing loss (Toriello, Reardon, & Gorlin, 2004), some of which affect both hearing and vision. Box 10.1 lists some of the most common genetic syndromes that affect hearing.

Sound

Sound is generated by the movement of air molecules, which produces sound waves. They are invisible to the human eye but can be detected by various types of instruments, and they can be displayed graphically. Sound travels not only through air but also through other mediums, such as water, steel, space, and planets. To understand sound, music, and hearing, you need to understand the physics of waves.

Waves and Waveforms

Sound waves begin with a source. Think of someone producing a single note on a piano, which creates a vibration that then disturbs the air. Or think of a singer producing different tones, each of which disturbs the air in a different way, which

---

[1]People who identify with the Deaf community use the uppercase *D*. The condition of having a hearing loss is referred to as *deafness*, using the lowercase *d*.

BOX 10.1   **Examples of Genetic Syndromes
That Can Cause Hearing Loss**

Down syndrome–caused by an extra copy of chromosome 21.

Usher syndrome—a condition resulting in hearing loss and retinitis pigmentosa, an eye disorder of the retina causing night blindness and loss of peripheral vision.

Treacher Collins syndrome—a condition affecting the development of bones and other tissues of the face, the ear canal, and the bones of the middle ear.

Crouzon syndrome—a condition resulting in premature fusion of the skull bones, impairment of the bones of the middle ear, absence of ear canals, and lack of development of the inner ear.

Alport syndrome—a condition characterized by kidney disease, eye disease, and hearing loss related to abnormal cochlea development.

Waardenburg syndrome—a group of genetic conditions, among them sensorineural hearing loss.

---

we perceive as a melody. When you speak, the vibrations of your vocal folds create sound waves your listeners perceive as **speech**. Each sound has a unique movement pattern, called a **waveform**. As you can see in Figure 10.1, the waveform for the vowel /ɑ/ differs considerably from that for middle C played on a piano and the noise produced by an electric motor. Furthermore, the waveform for the vowel /ɑ/ differs from that for every other vowel and consonant sound.

The movements of particles of air that cause sounds to be generated can be classified as either simple or complex. Those classified as simple—which are referred to as **pure tones**—produce a waveform known as a **sine wave** and a tone containing acoustic energy at a single frequency (hence, one that is "pure"). The waveform at the top of Figure 10.2 (labeled 100 Hz) depicts a single sine wave (also known as a single cycle), and the two in the middle (labeled 300 Hz and 500 Hz) depict a series (or a number of cycles or replications) of sine waves. The number of sine waves (or the number of cycles) that occur each second determines the pitch of a pure tone—the larger the number, the higher the pitch. This number is designated in a unit of measurement known as **hertz (Hz)**. A 500-Hz pure tone has more cycles per second and consequently a higher pitch than a 300-Hz tone (see Figure 10.2). Tuning forks are one of the few instruments that can generate pure tones. The size (i.e., mass) of the fork, rather than the force used to strike it, determines the pitch of the tone.

Almost all the sounds we hear are complex because particles of air in the real world rarely vibrate at a single frequency and therefore do not have the waveform of a single sine wave. Complex sounds are of two types: periodic and aperiodic. The waveforms for individual cycles for periodic sounds are complex but repeat themselves. Complex periodic tones consist of combinations of pure tones. The waveform at the bottom of Figure 10.2 illustrates how pure tones combine to produce complex

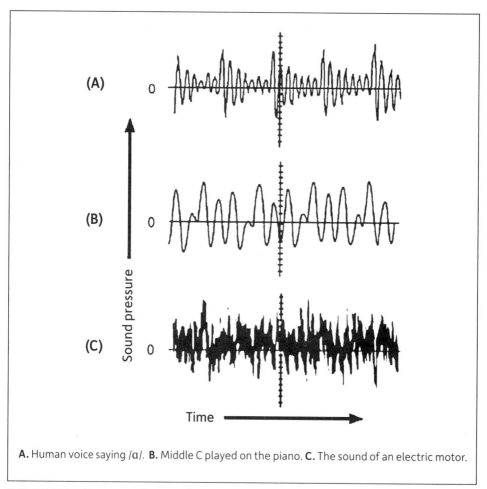

A. Human voice saying /a/. **B.** Middle C played on the piano. **C.** The sound of an electric motor.

FIGURE 10.1. Three complex waveforms.

periodic tones. The waveforms for all three sounds displayed in Figure 10.1 are complex periodic ones, as are those for all vowel sounds.

Many sounds (e.g., those produced by a book dropping or production of the consonant /s/) are complex in that they consist of more than one frequency, but they are aperiodic because their waveforms over time do not consistently (i.e., periodically) repeat themselves.

Intensity (Loudness)

Sounds are differentiated from each other not only by the nature and periodicity of their waveform, but also by the height (i.e., amplitude) of the waveform. The amplitude of a waveform determines the relative intensity (i.e., loudness) of the sound it generates. The unit of measurement for the loudness of sounds is the **decibel (dB)**. The louder a sound (i.e., the higher its number on the decibel scale), the greater the

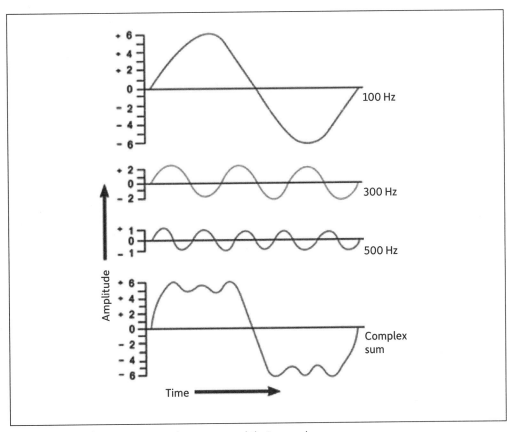

FIGURE 10.2. Three pure-tone sine waves and their complex sum.

amplitude of the waveform that produced it. The amplitude of the waveform for the 300-Hz tone in Figure 10.2 is greater than that for the 500-Hz one. Consequently, people with normal hearing would perceive the 300-Hz tone depicted in this figure as being louder than the 500-Hz one. If you'd like to learn more about the physics of sound, The Physics Classroom (2014) offers a useful tutorial.

Anatomy and Physiology of the Auditory System

Almost all hearing disorders are caused by damage (on one side or both sides) to the outer ear, middle ear, inner ear, **auditory nerve**, or brain—specifically that part of the brain referred to as the **central auditory nervous system (CANS)**. The functions of these structures are represented in Figure 10.3. To understand why damage to these structures results in a predictable type of hearing deficit, you have to know something about their functions, or physiology. When one or more of these structures functions abnormally, the result is a problem with hearing. The specific type

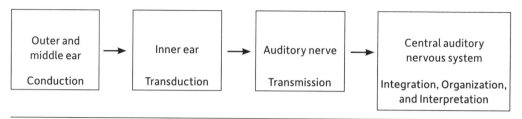

FIGURE 10.3. A model of the auditory system.

of problem is determined by the anatomical location of the damage rather than its cause (i.e., etiology). All conditions that damage a particular structure in the ear, auditory nerve, or CANS produce the same type of hearing problem (i.e., all exhibit the same symptomatology). Figure 10.4 illustrates the anatomy of the ear. I briefly describe the outer ear, the middle ear, and the inner ear in the following sections.

Outer Ear

The largely cartilaginous external portion of the outer ear is referred to as the **auricle** (see Site 1 in Figure 10.4). This is the only part of the ear we can fully observe without using instruments. The auricle acts like a funnel to direct sound-induced vibration of air particles into the **external auditory meatus** (see Site 2 in Figure 10.4). On the inner surface of this tubelike structure there are small hairs called **cilia**, and **ceruminous glands** that secrete **cerumen**. Cilia and cerumen help to protect the **tympanic membrane** (see Site 3 in Figure 10.4), which is situated at the end of this canal, from being damaged by dirt, insects, or other foreign objects. The tympanic membrane separates the outer ear from the middle ear. It is conical in shape, with the tip of the cone facing inward into the head.

Middle Ear

The middle ear consists of a small, air-filled cavity containing a chain of three tiny bones—the **malleus** (i.e., hammer), the **incus** (i.e., anvil), and the **stapes** (i.e., stirrup)—known as the **ossicles** (see Site 4 in Figure 10.4). The size of the cavity is about that of a garden pea. The stapes is the smallest bone in the human body, about the size of a grain of rice. The malleus is attached to the tympanic membrane. When the tympanic membrane vibrates, it causes the malleus to vibrate, which causes the incus to vibrate, which, in turn, causes the stapes to vibrate. The stapes is attached to a membrane known as the **oval window** (see Site 5 in Figure 10.4). The oval window is located in the bony wall that separates the middle ear from the inner ear.

The middle ear is connected to the nasopharynx (in the back wall of the throat) by a hollow structure that is referred to as the **eustachian tube** (Site 7 in Figure 10.4). Its function is to aerate the middle ear so that the air pressure behind the tympanic membrane equals that in front of it. Equal air pressure is necessary for the mem-

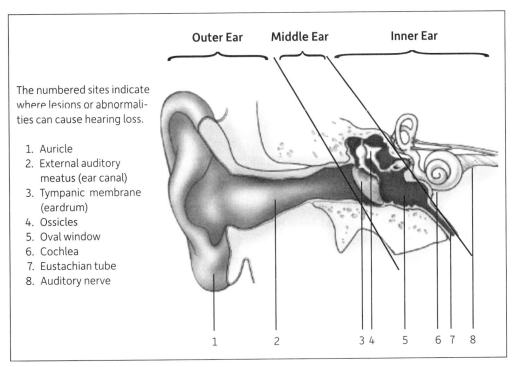

FIGURE 10.4. Anatomy of the ear.

brane to vibrate freely. When you are at a high altitude (e.g., in an airplane or on top of a mountain) and experience pain or a feeling of fullness in an ear, the eustachian tube is not allowing enough air out of the middle ear cavity to equalize the pressure on both sides of the tympanic membrane. Yawning, chewing, or swallowing sometimes relieves this condition because they cause the end of the eustachian tube in the nasopharynx to open, allowing air to pass into or out of the middle ear cavity. The eustachian tube provides the route by which infections travel from the throat to the middle ear cavity, causing earaches.

Inner Ear, Auditory Nerve, and Central Auditory Nervous System

The inner ear contains the **semicircular canals**, the **vestibule**, and the **cochlea** (see Site 6 in Figure 10.4). Each of these structures is filled with fluid. The semicircular canals and vestibule are responsible for balance and equilibrium. The cochlea is responsible for hearing. The cochlea contains many microscopic structures that **transduce** sound-induced vibration into a form of electrochemical energy. Vibrations are conducted from the middle ear to the cochlea by way of the stapes and oval window. The **auditory nerve** (see Site 8 in Figure 10.4) transmits electrochemical energy generated by the cochlea to the CANS.

Summary of Sound Vibration Transmission

The process by which sound-induced vibrations are conducted from the outer ear to the inner ear can be summarized as follows, with the numbers corresponding to the sites in Figure 10.4. The sound waves enter the outer ear at the auricle (1) and are conducted along the external auditory meatus (2) to the tympanic membrane (3). The sound waves cause the tympanic membrane to vibrate, which in turn causes the three little bones in the middle ear (4)—the malleus, incus, and stapes—to vibrate. The vibration of the stapes causes the oval window (5) to vibrate, thereby conducting sound-induced vibrations to the cochlea in the inner ear (6). Electrochemical energy from the cochlea is then transferred to the auditory nerve (8) and then the CANS. The eustachian tube (7) does not function to transmit sound. Rather, its function is to equalize atmospheric pressure in the middle ear and to protect the middle ear from excess pressure and loud sounds.

Types and Causes of Hearing and Auditory Disorders

People who have a hearing disorder have some degree of difficulty understanding speech or hearing environmental sounds (e.g., automobile traffic noise). The severity of the disorder can range from occasional difficulty localizing the sources of sounds to being unable to hear anything (i.e., being totally deaf).

A number of conditions (e.g., diseases, **congenital** abnormalities, types of trauma) can result in children and adults being unable to hear and understand speech as well as their peers. People can have one or more of these conditions, each of which contributes uniquely to a hearing disorder.

Conductive Hearing Loss

People who have **conductive hearing losses** have a bilateral (i.e., both sides) or unilateral (i.e., one side) lesion or abnormality in the outer or middle ear (refer back to Figure 10.4). Those who have a **bilateral conductive hearing loss** experience speech and other sound as being relatively "soft." How soft depends on the severity of the loss. They experience what you experience if you listen to a radio or TV with the volume set very low. You only understand what is being said if you concentrate very hard and the room is relatively quiet. Individuals with a bilateral conductive hearing loss may have lost the ability to equalize air pressure on both sides of the tympanic membrane, which impedes the membrane's ability to vibrate and conduct vibrations to the inner ear.

People with a **unilateral conductive hearing loss** ordinarily experience speech and other sound as being adequately loud unless the sound is soft and on the same side as the impaired ear. Their main problem usually is localizing—that is, finding the source of a sound. The brain needs information about the relative intensity of a sound at both the right and left sides of the head to localize it in space. Consequently, if the ears are not equally sensitive to sound, the brain cannot accurately interpret differences in loudness as reflecting differences in distances between the sound source and the right and left ears. Localization errors occur as a result.

A conductive hearing loss, by itself, cannot cause a person to become deaf. This is true even if the structures of both the outer and middle ear are missing bilaterally, because sound energy can also be conducted to the inner ear through vibration of the bones of the head.

Conductive hearing losses are caused by a lesion or abnormality in the outer or middle ear. This lesion or abnormality prevents sound-induced vibrations from being conducted normally into the inner ear—hence, it's called a conductive loss. Several types of lesions and abnormalities can interfere with the conduction of sound-induced vibrations from the outer ear to the inner ear. I describe some of these in the paragraphs that follow.

Cerumen Impaction

Cerumen impaction occurs when an overabundance of cerumen partially or totally blocks the external auditory canal. This impedes the conduction of sound-induced vibrations. Cerumen is a less efficient medium for conducting vibrations from the auricle to the eardrum than air. When the excess cerumen is removed (preferably by a physician), hearing level should return to normal.

Congenital Atresia of the Outer Ear

A child may be born with a **congenital atresia**. The auricle may also be absent or deformed. This abnormality can occur in one or both ears and is present from birth. The explanation for why congenital atresia causes a conductive hearing loss is similar to that for cerumen impaction—bone or fibrous tissue is a less efficient medium than air for conducting sound-induced vibrations from the auricle to the eardrum. If it is possible for a plastic surgeon to construct an auricle and external auditory canal, the hearing loss should be either reduced in severity or eliminated, provided the structure and function of the ear are otherwise normal.

Otitis Media

Otitis media is an inflammation of the middle ear—the space between the tympanic membrane and the oval window—in one or both ears. It may be the result of a eustachian tube malfunction or a bacterial or viral infection. The space becomes filled with a fluid, which impedes the vibration of the ossicles. As a result, the vibrations that reach the oval window are weaker than normal. Both children and adults can develop otitis media. It can be a chronic, or recurring, condition, and it may lead to a perforation of the tympanic membrane. Fluid in the middle ear can often be eliminated through medical treatment if it is caused by a bacterial infection—for example, administering antibiotics to eliminate the infection producing the fluid.

Once the fluid has been eliminated, the magnitude of the vibration of the ossicles increases and hearing improves.

Medscape (2014) reported that otitis media is the most common condition for which children in the United States under 5 years of age receive medical treatment. Seventy-five percent of children experience at least one episode of otitis media by their third birthday. Otitis media recurs in approximately 20% to 30% of children under 5 (Pichichero, 2000). Health costs for otitis media in the United States are reported to be $2.88 billion per year (Ahmed, Shapiro, & Bhattacharyya, 2014). For a comprehensive overview of otitis media, see the National Institute on Deafness and Other Communication Disorders (NIDCD; 2014b) web pages on ear infections in children.

Cholesteatoma

A **cholesteatoma** is an abnormal accumulation of a fibrous material that can occur in the middle ear behind the typmpanic membrane. It may be **congenital** or acquired, and it can damage the ossicles. The most common are the result of poor eustachian tube function. The effect of a cholesteatoma on the conduction of vibration in the middle ear is somewhat similar to that of otitis media—the fibrous material lessens the magnitude of vibration of the ossicles. The effect on the magnitude of these vibrations (and thereby on hearing) tends to be greater if the ossicles are damaged.

Otosclerosis

Otosclerosis is a disease in which the third little bone in the middle ear, the stapes, becomes immobilized in the oval window. Because the stapes cannot move normally, it cannot conduct noise-induced vibrations normally to the oval window. The fixation of the stapes can sometimes be corrected through surgery. To learn more about otosclerosis, visit the NIDCD (2014c) website.

Ossicular Discontinuity

The three ossicles bridge the space between the eardrum and the oval window. If one of the bones breaks or separates from the other two, vibration can no longer be conducted through them to the oval window. **Ossicular discontinuity** can result from a number of conditions, including severe head trauma. Treatment is usually ossicular-chain reconstruction.

Sensorineural Hearing Loss

People with a lesion or abnormality in the inner ear (refer back to Figure 10.4) have a **sensorineural hearing loss**. Those who have a loss in both ears (i.e., bilateral) experience speech and other sound as distorted and usually as relatively soft. The sound distortion occurs because the ability of the inner ear to transduce sound-induced vibrations into electrochemical energy is not impaired to the same degree for all frequencies. It tends to be more impaired for transducing relatively high frequencies than for transducing relatively low ones. Consequently, the higher the pitch of a sound, the more difficulty a person with a bilateral sensorineural loss is likely to have hearing it.

When people with this type of hearing loss listen to someone speak, they tend to hear certain speech sounds less well than others. They are particularly likely to have difficulty hearing sounds that contain a great deal of high-frequency energy, such as the consonant /s/. Box 10.2 illustrates how a person with a bilateral sensorineural hearing loss may hear certain words. If his or her hearing loss is extremely severe, the person will be unable to hear any sounds (except possibly those that are very low pitched) and will be referred to as deaf.

What is it like listening to distorted sound? You can simulate the experience by listening to your favorite music through the speaker (not your earbuds or earphones) on your phone or on a low-end laptop computer. A loudspeaker is a transducer that converts electrical energy into acoustical energy. Because the small speakers in such phones and laptops are not equally sensitive to all sound frequencies, they will reproduce some frequencies louder than others, thereby distorting the music. You probably will not like what you hear.

If your ability to hear has ever been impaired temporarily after being exposed to loud noise (e .g., at a concert), you have had firsthand experience with a hearing loss of this type. You have experienced what is known as a **temporary threshold shift**.

Some people who have a sensorineural hearing loss experience **tinnitus**. In some cases the noise is described as a diffuse roaring or rushing sound, with its source somewhere in the head. In others the source is localized in one or both ears. The American Tinnitus Association (2014) provides a detailed description of tinnitus. To hear several examples of what tinnitus sounds like, go to the Nottingham Hearing Biomedical Research Unit's (2014) webpage.

Another phenomenon that individuals with a sensorineural hearing loss may experience is **loudness recruitment**. In an ear in which there is recruitment, an in-

---

BOX 10.2   An Illustration of Sensorineural Hearing Loss

Word said	Word heard
sold	old
slate	late
smile	mile
trucks	truck
sink	ink
books	book
house	how
place	play
grocer	grower
since	in

crease in the intensity of a sound will tend to increase in the person's perception of loudness as compared to in the case of a normal ear. Recruitment typically results from damage to the sensory cells in the cochlea and must be considered when fitting a person with a hearing aid. If the person can hear loud sounds normally (or nearly so) without amplification, such sounds can be too loud with amplification and can produce physical discomfort.

Etiology

As I mentioned above, a lesion or abnormality in the inner ear can produce a sensorineural hearing loss. The inner ear converts the vibrations conducted to it by the middle ear into electrical signals that are sent to the brain through the auditory nerve (see Site 8 in Figure 10.4). A transducer changes, or transforms, one form of energy into another form of energy. The inner ear transforms mechanical energy into electrochemical energy. If the inner ear is functioning normally, it will convert the information contained in the vibrations it receives from the middle ear into electrochemical signals without distorting them. However, a lesion or abnormality in the inner ear can cause the information contained in the vibrations to be distorted when they are transduced into an electrochemical signal. The part of the inner ear mechanism responsible for transducing relatively high-frequency mechanical energy into electrochemical signals appears to be more vulnerable to damage than that responsible for transducing relatively low-frequency mechanical energy.

If the mechanism of the inner ear is severely damaged, little (or none) of the information contained in noise-induced vibration will be transduced into electrochemical signals and sent on to the brain. When the mechanisms of both inner ears are severely damaged or destroyed, little or no information is sent on to the brain, and the person is referred to as deaf. Hence, the greater the damage to the inner ear, the greater the distortion of the information in the vibrations conducted to it. A number of conditions can cause the mechanism of the inner ear to function abnormally.

The Aging Process

Sensorineural hearing loss resulting from the effect of the aging process on the inner ear is referred to as **presbycusis**. Aging ordinarily damages rather than destroys the inner ear. Hence, patients with presbycusis usually complain of an inability to understand speech (because they cannot hear certain consonant sounds) rather than an inability to hear. They report that it sounds to them like people are mumbling. The Department of Medicine at NYU Langone Medical Center (2014) provides additional information regarding presbycusis.

Drugs

Ingesting certain drugs can damage the inner ear or cause it to function abnormally. The resulting hearing loss is usually bilateral and of approximately the same magnitude in both ears. One drug that can produce a sensorineural hearing loss when ingested in high doses is aspirin—the hearing loss may disappear when use of the drug is discontinued. There is also some evidence of moderate to profound hearing loss following prolonged use of certain prescription painkillers that combine hydrocodone and acetaminophen. If hearing improves after the use of a drug is discontinued, the effect of the drug on the inner ear probably was to cause it to function abnormally rather than to damage it.

Loud Noise

Brief exposure to extremely intense noise—such as that produced by a loud explosion—can damage the inner ear. Trauma to the ear caused by brief exposure to extremely intense noise usually affects hearing almost instantly. Also, prolonged exposure to loud noise can damage the inner ear or cause it to function abnormally. An immediate hearing loss does not occur from trauma caused by prolonged, or chronic, exposure to loud noise. The effect of such trauma is insidious; a person can work in a noisy environment for many years and be unaware of developing a hearing loss because this type of trauma initially damages a part of the inner ear mechanism that transforms relatively high-frequency information—that at a frequency of approximately 4000 Hz—into electrical signals.

There are several reasons why noise exposure affects the 4000-Hz frequency, including the possibility that the anatomical structures of the inner ear associated with receiving and transducing frequencies near 4000 Hz are more susceptible to acoustic trauma. The loss of acoustic information at this frequency ordinarily does not interfere with understanding speech. However, as the trauma process continues, portions of the inner ear mechanism are affected that transduce information above and below this frequency. Eventually, the damage becomes so widespread that the person experiences difficulty understanding speech. Unfortunately, the person does not become aware of the problem until considerable damage has occurred.

Which types of noise can cause acoustic trauma and result in a noise-induced hearing loss? Almost any loud noise that a person is exposed to repeatedly can do this. Firefighters can develop a loss over time from the noise they are exposed to while riding in a fire engine. Musicians can develop a loss by playing frequently with a heavy-metal rock band. And anyone can develop a loss by frequently attending concerts or by frequently playing very loud music through headphones. Hearing Education and Awareness for Rockers (H.E.A.R.) is a nonprofit organization dedicated to helping musicians and music lovers learn about the dangers of noise exposure that can lead to permanent hearing loss and tinnitus (H.E.A.R., 2014).

Noise loud enough to damage the inner ear sometimes produces a temporary hearing loss before producing a permanent one. Such a loss is referred to as a temporary threshold shift, which means the threshold of hearing has shifted upward. If, after leaving a very noisy environment, your ears felt "stuffy" or you had tinnitus, you experienced a temporary threshold shift.

Viral Infections

Viral infections are thought to be the most common cause of noise-induced hearing loss. Several types of viral infections can damage the inner ear or the auditory nerve.

The measles virus, for example, can produce enough extensive damage to both inner ears to cause a severe sensorineural hearing loss. Measles was one of the main causes of childhood deafness prior to the development of vaccines, which became available in 1963. The mumps virus can also produce a severe sensorineural hearing loss. In addition, upper respiratory infections and influenza can result in sudden hearing loss.

Tumors

Acoustic tumors (neuromas) are almost always benign and slow growing. But as the tumor grows, it can apply pressure to nerve fibers in the inner ear, thereby damaging them. The resulting sensorineural hearing loss is usually unilateral. These tumors can also affect balance and induce tinnitus.

Ménière's Disease

The primary symptom associated with **Ménière's disease** is vertigo, or dizziness. People who have Ménière's disease also experience tinnitus and a feeling of fullness in the affected ear. These disturbances are ordinarily episodic rather than constant, and they can last anywhere from a few minutes to several hours. Individuals can remain symptom free for weeks, months, or even years. The hearing loss associated with this disease is usually unilateral.

Trauma

Injuries to the skull can damage the inner ear. Such injuries can result from accidents, bullet wounds or blows to the head, and surgery (particularly mastoid surgery). The hearing loss associated with trauma is usually unilateral and may last up to a year after trauma. After that time, if a hearing loss still remains, it will most likely be permanent.

Sensorineural Hearing Loss From Auditory Nerve Damage

The right and left VIIIth cranial nerves (vestibulocochlear nerve) are components of the peripheral nervous system. Each has two branches, one of which is the auditory nerve. The other—the vestibular nerve—controls the mechanism for balance and equilibrium, which is located in the inner ear. The auditory nerve transmits nerve impulses from the inner ear on each side to the parts of the brain that make up the CANS. Its function is similar to that of an electrical wire, or cable—that is, to convey electrical energy signals from one point to another. If an auditory nerve is severed or otherwise made inoperable, electrical information will not be sent from the inner ear on that side to the CANS, and the person will be deaf in that ear. If an auditory nerve is damaged (not destroyed), the information sent to the CANS will be incomplete and what the person hears will be abnormally soft, distorted, or both.

Disorders of the auditory nerve, like those of the inner ear, result in hearing losses that are classified as sensorineural. Two common early symptoms of auditory nerve disorders are a hearing loss that is greater for speech sounds containing considerable high-frequency energy (e.g., /s/) and tinnitus. If a sensorineural hearing loss is unilateral, the cause is more likely to be damage to the auditory nerve than to the inner ear.

Etiology

Lesions of the auditory nerve can occur as a result of trauma, disease, irritation, or pressure on the nerve. One of the most common causes is a tumor that impedes the functioning of an auditory nerve by pressing on it. Such tumors (usually referred to as acoustic neuromas) are usually benign and unilateral. Two other conditions that can interfere with the functioning of this nerve are **acoustic neuritis** and **multiple sclerosis**. To learn more about the symptoms and etiology of hearing loss from auditory nerve damage, see Deaf websites (2014).

Mixed Hearing Loss

Individuals with a mixed hearing loss have a lesion or abnormality both in the outer or middle ear and in the inner ear or auditory nerve. They exhibit a combination of the symptoms associated with conductive and sensorineural hearing loss. If conductive components predominate and the loss is bilateral, the deficit will be primarily one of speech being perceived as too soft. If sensorineural components are predominant with such a loss, the deficit will be one of speech being distorted and probably also perceived as too soft. Mixed hearing loss ranges from mild to profound.

Any of the causes for conductive and sensorineural hearing loss that I have already discussed can contribute to the etiology of a mixed hearing loss. Damage to the inner ear may predate that to the outer or middle ear, or the reverse could be true.

Hearing Difficulties From Central Auditory Disturbance

Information conducted to the inner ear and changed by it into electrical signals is sent to the brain via the auditory nerve for integration, organization, and interpretation. The brain cells that perform this function—which are located in the brain stem, medulla, midbrain, thalamus, and cerebral cortex—make up the CANS. Central auditory disturbances do not cause a loss of hearing; rather, they cause difficulties with how sounds are processed.

Damage to the CANS can disturb the ability to localize sound and understand speech in a variety of ways. The characteristic symptoms caused by a CANS lesion are determined by its location. Lesions at specific locations in the CANS tend to produce predictable symptoms regardless of their cause. In the following paragraphs I discuss some disturbances in hearing that can result from lesions in the CANS.

Disturbed Localization Ability

Information from both ears is integrated in the CANS in a way that enables the source of a sound to be located. Someone who has a lesion in the brain cells responsible for mediating this function has difficulty locating the source of sounds, such as a car horn while driving, someone's voice if he or she is not in immediate view, or the sound of an emergency vehicle in traffic.

Disturbed Bilateral Synthesis Ability

The CANS does not usually receive exactly the same information from both ears. (It can only be identical if its source is equidistant from each ear.) The function of some cells in the CANS is to synthesize this information. Consequently, a person whose bilateral synthesis ability was severely disturbed probably would not perceive stereo music or music heard through headphones or earbuds normally.

Disturbed Ability to Separate Figure From Background

People who have difficulty separating the figure from the background, which is sometimes referred to as **auditory agnosia**, have difficulty concentrating auditorily. What they have trouble listening to is the figure (i.e., target sound) rather than all the other sounds present in the environment (i.e., the background). For example, not being able to listen to a teacher or instructor talking because the air conditioner noise is distracting.

If our CANS is functioning properly, we usually have the ability to concentrate on what somebody is saying without being distracted by sounds in the environment. In fact, we may not even be aware of them. Have you ever been in a building, such as a doctor's office, where there is music playing and you are not consciously aware of it until you have been there for a while? People whose CANS is intact only have difficulty concentrating auditorily when the degree of separation between figure and background is quite small. This might occur where there is considerable background noise, for example, at a party. If several conversations are going on near you at such a party, you may have difficulty concentrating on one and ignoring the others because they all compete for your attention at once.

Short Auditory Memory Span

People with a short auditory memory span have difficulty remembering what they hear as well as what other people their age can remember. (The ability to store and recall what one hears increases with age during childhood.) People with a short auditory memory span may answer questions incorrectly (particularly relatively long questions) because they cannot remember them. They also may fail to follow instructions accurately for this reason.

Disturbed Ability to Segment Phonemes

You will remember that conversational speech consists of strings of **phonemes** uttered one after the other. You must be able to segment this string of sounds into words to understand what you are hearing. People with this condition have difficulty understanding speech because they have less than normal ability to segment sequences of phonemes into words. The process involved is analogous to that in segmenting this sequence of letters into words: *disturbedabilitytosegmentphonemes.*

Disturbed Ability to Relate Heard Words to Experience

Words consist of groupings of phonemes arranged in particular sequences. When we listen to words being spoken in a language that we do not understand, we hear groupings of phonemes, but these groupings seem meaningless. We cannot relate them to our own experiences. A lesion in the CANS can disturb the ability to relate heard words to our experience. An example of this is Wernicke's aphasia, which I discussed in Chapter 5.

Abstract–Concrete Imbalance

A lesion in the CANS can disturb the ability to categorize and generalize. Persons who have such a disability tend to be overly concrete; that is, they tend to "lose the forest for the trees." This imbalance can interfere with their ability to understand speech because it prevents them from relating some of the words they hear to a sufficiently broad spectrum of experience. They may visualize only apples when they hear the word *fruit*. Or when they hear the word *chair*, they may think only of an upholstered chair, not also a rocking chair, a beanbag chair, or a metal folding chair. This condition is considered a language disorder rather than a hearing disorder.

Etiology

Central auditory disturbances are caused by damage to the brain—specifically, those parts of the brain that make up the CANS. Any condition that can damage the brain can produce a central auditory disturbance. The following are several such conditions.

Insufficient Blood Flow to the Brain. Brain cells require oxygen to live. Oxygen is carried to brain cells by the blood traveling through arteries. If the flow of blood to any part of the brain is disrupted, the cells in that part will be deprived of oxygen, a condition known as **anoxia**. This is likely to result in injury or destruction if the disruption lasts for more than a few minutes.

A number of conditions can disrupt the flow of blood to the brain. A **thrombus** can form on an arterial wall, cutting off the flow of blood to a part of the brain. An **embolus** can obstruct an artery, thereby restricting the flow of oxygen-rich blood to brain tissue. An artery in the brain could also rupture—the resulting **hemorrhage** can prevent oxygen from reaching brain cells. For more information on emboli, visit Fact Monster's (2014) webpage.

Trauma. Several types of injuries to the skull can damage the brain. A *penetrating wound* involves something (e.g., a bullet) penetrating the skull, producing brain damage in the path of entry. A second type of trauma in which the skull is not penetrated is known as a *cranial blow*. The brain may be lacerated at the point of impact or the blow may cause intercranial hemorrhaging that can damage brain tissue related to hearing.

Tumors. Tumors (i.e., **neoplasms**) are abnormal growths within the brain. They may be malignant (i.e., cancerous) or benign (i.e., not cancerous). These can disturb the functioning of the various structures within the CANS, including the auditory nerve. They can destroy brain tissue directly as they increase in size. They can also destroy brain tissue indirectly by pressing on cranial arteries, thereby decreasing blood flow through them.

Infections. Bacterial and viral microorganisms can cause an inflammation of brain tissue, known as encephalitis. One possible complication of encephalitis is the formation of **brain abscesses**. These cavities can destroy brain tissue as they expand.

Degenerative Changes. Several other conditions can cause the gradual loss (i.e., **degeneration**) of brain cells, one of which is the aging process. With increasing age there is a slow, progressive degeneration of brain tissue that can result from reduced blood flow as a consequence of the thickening of the walls of the cerebral arteries. The thicker the wall of an artery, the smaller the diameter of the opening in it and, hence, the slower the rate of blood flow through it. This thickening of the walls of cerebral arteries is known as **cerebral arteriosclerosis**. Disease, such as **Huntington's disease**, can also result in the gradual degeneration of brain cells.

Functional Hearing Loss

Functional (i.e., nonorganic) hearing losses are so called because they do not appear to have an organic cause. This does not necessarily mean that there is no organic cause—there may well be one that has not yet been discovered. People who do not respond appropriately to speech or other sound and who do not appear to have an abnormality or lesion in their ears, auditory nerves, or CANS tend to be classified as having a functional hearing loss. This type of hearing loss has also been referred to as psychogenic hearing loss, pseudohypacusis, and idiopathic sudden deafness. Males appear to be more commonly affected than females. Of people with pseudo-hypacusis, some are malingerers (i.e., they feign having a hearing loss) and some have emotional disorders. Pseudohypacusis often occurs in populations in which having a hearing loss can result in financial compensation.

Hearing Loss and Cognitive Decline

A recent investigation into the relationship between hearing loss and cognitive decline showed that older individuals who have a hearing loss and normal brain function at age 75 are more likely to develop problems with thinking and memory than their age peers whose hearing is normal (Lin et al., 2013). Lin et al. reported that the cognitive abilities of the individuals with hearing loss declined between 30% and 40% faster than their normally hearing age-peers. Furthermore, the amount of hearing loss was directly related to the level of declining brain function.

Lin and his colleagues suggested that one possible explanation for the cognitive decline is the social isolation that often accompanies hearing loss. Another is that a hearing loss requires the brain to use significant energy to process sound, which leaves less energy for thinking and remembering.

A study by Allen et al. (2003) demonstrated that at least some individuals with a diagnosis of dementia or Alzheimer's disease can successfully use hearing aids with the appropriate training, and another conducted by Palmer, Adams, Bourgeois, Durrant, and Rossi (1999) showed that for at-home individuals with Alzheimer's with hearing loss, hearing aids significantly reduced communication problems for the individuals and their caregivers.

Deafness and Deaf Culture

Until the latter part of the 20th century, deafness was regarded as a disability. In the United States, deaf people were described in terms of not being able to hear and, therefore, not being able to communicate by speaking and hearing—in other words, what they could *not* do. The majority of deaf educators emphasized teaching deaf children to speak and to use speechreading to understand what was being said. However, many children with profound hearing loss were unable to acquire spoken language skills to the same degree as their hearing age-peers and, as a result, had significant difficulties learning to read and write.

More recently, however, as I pointed out earlier in this chapter, research has shown that if typically developing deaf children are exposed to ASL (or, in other **cultures**, their respective sign languages) from birth, they develop language and communication abilities commensurate with those of their typically developing hearing peers who are learning spoken language (Gallaudet University Laurent Clerc National Deaf Education Center, 2014). In other words, the mode of communication is not important as long as the child is exposed from birth to a language she or he can understand.

At the same time, Deaf people in the United States became more vigorous in asserting that they belong to a vibrant culture that differs substantially from the culture of the hearing world. Deaf people prefer interacting with other Deaf individuals who use ASL to communicate and who share a common history, social beliefs, art forms, literature, music, poetry, and social values. Often, hearing family members identify more with Deaf culture than hearing culture.

In contrast to the U.S. hearing culture, which is individualistic and emphasizes privacy and personal space, Deaf culture is highly collective and collaborative. Deaf individuals view themselves as part of a close-knit group in which sharing information is highly valued. Not sharing information is considered rude, and what are considered polite forms in hearing culture are seen as circular and indirect in Deaf culture. Conversely, some communication behaviors that are common among Deaf individuals using ASL are seen as rude by hearing people. An example is staring at one another's face while conversing, which in the Deaf culture is considered necessary for effective communication.

Several national and international organizations exist both to support Deaf people and to educate hearing persons about deafness. One is the National Theatre of the Deaf, which has been a powerful force for removing the stigma from using ASL and legitimizing its use on television, on the stage, and in movies (National Theatre of the Deaf, 2014). Another is Gallaudet University, founded in 1857 and granted university status in 1986. Ninety-five percent of the undergraduate students at Gallaudet are deaf, while hearing students make up 5% of each class. The graduate programs at Gallaudet are open to deaf, hard-of-hearing, and hearing students and offer a wide variety of programs at the master's, doctoral, and specialist levels (Gallaudet University, 2014). For a first-hand look at being Deaf, visit PBS's (2014) feature *Deaf Culture*.

Assessment

Screening

Audiological screening, usually performed by **audiologists**, is used to determine whether a person is likely to have a hearing loss, while audiological assessment involves administering a battery of tests in order to thoroughly evaluate an individual's hearing or auditory processing abilities.

In all states in the United States, newborns are screened by medical personnel employing an **otoacoustic emissions test** (OAE), in which a microphone and a miniature earphone are placed in the baby's ears to pick up the sounds produced by the inner ear when the cochlea responds to a sound. You'll remember that inside the cochlea, hair cells vibrate in response to sound. When they vibrate, they also produce a very faint sound that echoes back into the middle ear. Sounds are played, and in babies who hear normally, the echo that is reflected back into the ear canal is picked up and measured by the microphone. In babies with hearing loss, no echo is measured on this test, and the infant may then be tested using auditory brainstem response. In **auditory brainstem response** (ABR), small electrodes are placed on the baby's head to detect responses, and sounds are played to the baby's ears. The ABR test measures how the acoustic nerve responds to the sounds and identifies babies who have a hearing loss.

Audiological screening is also used in schools and some senior centers to identify individuals who may have a hearing loss and need further evaluation. These screenings are conducted by audiologists or, in some instances, public health nurses or credentialed school nurses using pure-tone audiometers (I'll describe these below) and calibrated earphones. The test involves the individual listening to pure-tone signals of at least three different frequencies and at a loudness level at which people with normal hearing can hear without difficulty. Anyone who fails the screening is then either given a pure-tone threshold test or referred for the test. In a threshold test, again using a pure-tone audiometer, the individual listens to tones of at least four different frequencies and at intensity (loudness) levels that decrease to the point at which the individual can no longer hear them. The idea is to determine the lowest intensity at which the person can hear at each of the four frequencies.

Evaluation

Three basic questions underlie the evaluation of a person's hearing. Before you can be helpful to an individual who has a hearing disorder, you have to identify the reason(s) for it, which I discussed earlier in this chapter. Second, the person's hearing mechanism and function must be assessed to determine the type and degree of disorder. And, third, depending on the nature and type of hearing disorder, you must determine whether assistive or augmentative systems and devices would be beneficial for the individual. To answer these questions, audiologists employ a range of assessment procedures to fully evaluate an individual's hearing ability.

Case History and Otoscopic Examination

One of the first steps is to take a complete case history, which I discussed at length in Chapters 4 and 6. Of course, in taking a case history from a person with a suspected hearing loss, the focus will be on hearing rather than language or speech. Box 10.3 lists some of the most common questions asked during an audiological case history.

After taking the case history, the audiologist will examine the person's ears using an **otoscope** to see whether there is anything untoward in the ear canal and whether the tympanic membrane looks abnormal, either of which usually results in a referral to a physician.

Pure-Tone Audiometry

Pure-tone audiometry helps answer such questions as,

- Is the person's hearing ability within normal limits?
- If the person's hearing ability is not within normal limits, how severely impaired is it?
- What is the cause of the person's hearing impairment?

BOX 10.3   Audiological Case History Questions

The audiologist will ask the following:

- when the person first noticed the loss
- whether the loss was sudden or gradual
- whether one or both ears are affected
- if the person has ringing in the ears
- if the person has a history of ear infections
- if there is a family history of hearing loss
- whether others have noticed any difficulties or symptoms
- whether the person has had exposure to loud noises
- whether there are environments in which the person has difficulty hearing
- whether the person asks conversational partners to repeat

Using pure-tone audiometry, the audiologist assesses the individual's ability to hear tones of specified loudness and pitch. Pure tone audiometry identifies the faintest tones an individual can hear at a variety of pure-tone frequencies, ranging from low to high. The individual wears earphones so that tones can be sent to each ear independently. The procedure involved in pure-tone testing requires that the individuals being tested signal to the examiner whenever they hear a tone.

A pure-tone audiometer is an electronic device for generating sounds. The kinds of sounds it generates are known as pure tones because the acoustical energy in them consists of only one frequency. The pure tones generated are at frequencies within the range of human hearing—approximately 20 to 20,000 **hertz** (**Hz**). The higher the frequency of a pure tone, the higher its pitch; hence, a pure tone of 1,000 Hz would have a higher pitch than one of 500 Hz. The tones can be presented through earphones or loudspeakers at many loudness levels.

Sometimes young children cannot tolerate wearing the earphones. In this situation, the testing is conducted in a sound booth—an insulated booth designed to reduce ambient noise as much as possible. When testing very young children, audiologists use a play-like procedure in which the child is trained to look toward a sound source. Each time the child looks toward the sound source, the audiologist triggers a visual reinforcement, such as a flashing light or a toy that moves. Once the child is consistent in responding, the audiologist systematically lowers the intensity of the tones to discover the lowest intensity at which the child hears tones at each frequency tested. The procedure used with toddlers and preschoolers differs in that, when the child hears the tone, she or he places a toy in a container. Testing without earphones is less accurate than that using earphones because the child listens to the tones with both ears. Further testing is often required in order to discover whether the child has a unilateral hearing loss that was missed.

The results of pure-tone testing are charted on an **audiogram**, which shows the type of hearing loss, its severity, and its configuration. Figure 10.5 shows an example of an audiogram of a person with a moderate conductive hearing loss in the left ear.

When looking at the audiogram in Figure 10.5, you probably noticed another set of markings (< and >). These marks are used to chart the levels at which a person can hear the same pure-tone frequencies as those presented through the headphones or loudspeakers, but they are delivered through an oscillator that is placed on the mastoid bone behind each ear. Called **bone conduction** testing, this procedure is used to determine the degree to which the inner ear is functioning. The audiogram in Figure 10.5 depicts normal inner ear functioning.

Evaluating the Integrity of the Auditory System

Two types of evaluation of the integrity of the auditory system are used: electroacoustic and electrophysiological. The electroacoustic measures used with children and adults are otoacoustic emissions (OAEs, which I described above in the section on testing newborns) and acoustic immittance. During acoustic immittance testing, also called impedance or compliance testing, a probe is placed into the external ca-

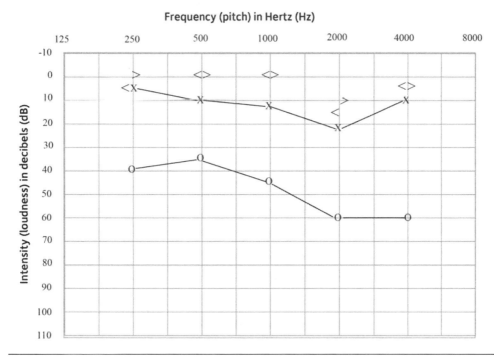

FIGURE 10.5. Audiogram showing a moderate conductive hearing loss in the left ear.

nal. A continuous pure tone is directed into the canal. At the same time, air pressure in the canal is adjusted, which causes the tympanic membrane to respond as the pressure increases and decreases. The action of the tympanic membrane is measured to determine its flexibility.

Certain conditions reduce this flexibility, giving the audiologist valuable information regarding how to proceed with the client. For instance, in children who have otitis media (or scarring from frequent previous ear infections), the tympanic membrane may move very little, which is also the case when the person's ossicles are somehow dislocated or impeded. A perforated eardrum will also not move during impedance testing.

The results of acoustic immittance testing are plotted on a **tympanogram**, which is a graph that shows the response of the tympanic membrane to changes in air pressure between the external canal and the middle ear. The graph shows three different levels of air pressure: neutral room air pressure (the air pressure in the outer canal and the middle ear are the same), positive air pressure, and negative air pressure. In people with normal impedence or flexibility of the tympanic membrane, the membrane shows much less stiffness at neutral air pressure. With both positive and negative air pressure, though, their tympanic membrane responds by becoming much stiffer. Figure 10.6 shows an example of the tympanogram of a person with normal impedence.

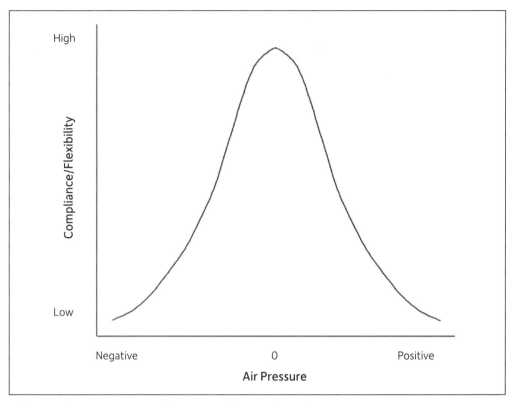

FIGURE 10.6. Tympanogram of a person with normal impedence.

Electrophysiological measures are used to record the responses of nerve cells to sound. Collectively, these measures are called **auditory evoked potentials (AEPs).** The auditory brainstem response (ABR) I described above in the section on newborns is an example of an AEP and is often used with older individuals with developmental delays or impairments in cognitive functioning.

Determining the Severity of the Hearing Loss

Earlier in this chapter I listed the three primary goals of assessment of hearing, the second of which is to determine the type and degree of the hearing loss. In previous sections, I described the assessment process involved in ascertaining the type of hearing loss. One marker of severity can be determined from the results of pure-tone threshold testing. Box 10.4 shows a commonly used classification system relating degree of hearing loss to the thresholds (in dB) the individual displayed during pure-tone testing.

Determining Whether Augmentative or Alternative Systems/Devices Would Benefit the Individual

An alternative or augmentative system or device that works for one individual may be completely inappropriate for another. Even if two people have identical hearing losses, each brings her or his own attitudes, capabilities, and family support. For

BOX 10.4   A Commonly Used Classification System for Determining Severity of Hearing Loss Shown in dB HL (Hearing Level)

Normal hearing	up to 25 dB for adults
	−10 to 15 dB for children
Slight hearing loss	16 to 15 dB for children
Mild hearing loss	26 to 40 dB for adults
Moderate hearing loss	41 to 70 dB
Severe hearing loss	71 to 90 dB
Profound hearing loss (including deafness)	>91 dB

adult clients, the audiologist reviews the evaluation results and discusses with the client the options available given the type and severity of the hearing loss. For children, this discussion takes place with the child's family or caregiver. During these discussions, the audiologist carefully weighs what she or he knows about the client from the case history and from the client's responses throughout the evaluation process. Some may be able to manage hearing aids; others may not. Some may be able to learn speechreading. Again, others may not. The point is to match any augmentative or alternative approach with the client's strengths and abilities. In the following section on treatment, I discuss the various types of alternative or augmentative systems and devices that are most often used with hearing loss.

Evaluating Central Auditory Processing

Central auditory processing disorders (CAPD) often exist alongside attention-deficit/hyperactivity disorder (ADHD), which I described in Chapter 4. Some of the symptoms of each are similar, which means that **speech–language pathologists (SLPs)** and audiologists must take extra care when evaluating CAPD. In both conditions, children exhibit difficulties paying attention and following directions, they are easily distracted and often hyperactive, and they are easily frustrated.

Evaluating CAPD usually involves at least an audiologist, an SLP, and a psychologist. The purposes of assessment are to define and describe the specific aspects of auditory processing the child is experiencing and to recommend appropriate intervention and treatment. Testing by the audiologist includes

- presenting speech and nonspeech sounds that are frequency-distorted, compressed, or presented with a competing signal (usually noise);
- presenting different signals to each ear simultaneously (dichotic listening), which forces the individual to either synthesize the signals or separate them;

- presenting a pattern of signals of different frequencies and asking the individual to indicate the sequence of the pattern (e.g., high, high, low; low, high, low), commonly called *temporal processing*; and
- presenting words and masking most of the information the individual hears (low-redundancy testing), which requires the individual to rely solely on their auditory systems to decipher each word.

In most situations, the SLP will administer a battery of tests to assess the individual's receptive and expressive oral language skills. You can refer back to Chapter 4, where I described the assessment procedure for oral language. The psychologist is responsible for assessing the individual's cognitive function and helping the individual and family interact with academic, work, and social situations.

Treatment

Augmentative and Alternative Communication Systems and Devices

One approach to reducing the severity of hearing disorders is attempting to correct the cause medically or surgically. If a person has a conductive hearing loss because of a middle-ear infection (otitis media), an attempt would be made to clear it up, possibly with an antibiotic. On the other hand, if a person has a conductive hearing loss because the footplate of the stapes is fixed (i.e., unmoving) in the oval window, an attempt might be made to surgically correct it.

It is possible in some cases to restore the auditory system to normal (both anatomically and physiologically) through medical intervention. If this is done, the person will no longer have a hearing disorder, and further intervention will be unnecessary. In other cases, it is not possible to completely restore the system to normal through medical or surgical intervention. An example would be treating profound, bilateral sensorineural hearing loss (deafness) by surgically inserting **cochlear implants** in the patient's inner ears. Cochlear implants can be considered a form of hearing aid since they attempt to make speech audible and understandable. However, cochlear implants use more sophisticated signal processing than **hearing aids**; they use electrical currents to stimulate remaining auditory nerve fibers. Furthermore, cochlear implants are surgically implanted, and their success is less dependent on the degree of hearing loss than conventional hearing aids.

Some patients who have had cochlear implants receive only minimal benefit, with limited improvement in their speechreading ability and environmental sound recognition. Others, however, obtain very high levels of word recognition. They can converse on the telephone and communicate face to face as if they had a mild hearing loss. Even persons with total hearing loss can usually perceive sounds with cochlear implants, though most people require some time to learn how to adjust to them. Although cochlear implants offer significant advantages to people with profound bilateral sensorineural hearing loss, there are also risks that individuals need to consider. The U.S. Food and Drug Administration (2014) lists both the advantages and the most serious risk factors involved. For specific information about cochlear implants, visit the National Institute on Deafness and Other Communication Disorders cochlear implant webpage (NIDCD, 2014a).

In some rare instances, children are born without an auditory nerve, in which case a cochlear implant would not be warranted. A relatively new procedure, auditory brainstem implant (ABI), is being tested on a small number of children in the United States. The ABI delivers electrical stimulation directly to the neurons on the brainstem, which is normally the function of the auditory nerve. The child wears a microphone on the ear to detect sound. The microphone includes a processor to convert the sound waves to electrical signals that it beams to a stimulator under the child's skin. The stimulator then sends the electrical signals to the surgically implanted electrodes on the brainstem.

Although the ABI procedure has been used since 2000 with adults and teenagers whose auditory nerves were destroyed by surgery or a rare type of tumor, researchers are hopeful that the procedure will provide greater benefit to young children, whose brains are more flexible than those of teenagers or adults.

People with severe to profound hearing loss benefit from a range of augmentative systems and devices. Two that are currently used for facilitating telephone communication are instruments known as **text telephones (TTYs)** and **telecommunication relay services (TRS)**. Alerting devices are another type of tool used to help hearing impaired individuals.

The TTY enables deaf people to communicate with others who have a TTY. Users type their messages and responses on a keyboard. TTYs are basic, dedicated microcomputers that have a modem and telecommunication software built in to them. The designation *dedicated* implies that, unlike most microcomputers, they are designed for (i.e., dedicated to) a single task—in this instance, telephone communication. Both iPhones and Android phones are capable of interacting with standard TTY machines through the use of an adapter. In addition, the iPhone uses a setting that allows users to interact with other people using TTYs or smartphone TTY adapters.

Telecommunication relay services enable people who are deaf or severely hard of hearing to communicate on the telephone with persons who do not have a TTY. TRSs also enable persons who cannot speak clearly enough to be understood on the telephone to communicate with others via the telephone. A relay call can be initiated either by the person who has the communication impairment or by someone who wants to communicate with that person. In all U.S. states, the relay call is initiated by calling 711. A person with a hearing impairment would make the call with either a TTY or a standard microcomputer with a modem and appropriate communication software. A person who wants to communicate with the deaf person would use an ordinary telephone.

The operator, known as a communication assistant (CA), will ask for the number the person wants to call. The CA will then dial this number and wait for a person to answer, then ask the caller for the first message. The CA will then relay this message—either by keyboarding it with a TTY or by saying it to the person who answered the phone. The recipient will then be given an opportunity to respond, and the response will be relayed by the CA. The conversation can continue in this manner for as long as the parties desire. The Federal Communications Commission (FCC) has adopted 711 as a dialing code anyone can use to reach TRS services, speech-to-speech (STS) relay services, and voice carry over (VCO) TTYs (FCC, 2014).

The information conveyed cannot be divulged to anyone because it is treated as confidential by law. The call will cost no more than a regular call between the two points. For more information about TRS in general, visit the NIDCD (2004) webpage on the topic.

Alerting devices are designed to do what their name implies: to alert a person with a hearing loss to important sounds, such as a doorbell, a baby crying, a fire alarm, or an emergency. Some of the devices are mechanical and provide visual signals (e.g., flashing lights) or sound in the person's hearing range. Assistive dogs, called hearing dogs, are used by many people with hearing loss to alert them to these sounds and other emergencies, such as fire, an intruder, unexpected water, high heat, or extreme cold.

Hearing Amplification

The goal of nonmedical treatment for people who have a hearing disorder is to both augment their ability to hear and reduce the negative impact the disorder has on their life. One of the most common ways to augment a person's ability to hear is to fit him or her with a hearing aid. For this to be helpful, the individual must have some usable residual hearing.

Hearing aids amplify sounds through small microphones that pick up sounds from the environment. A computer chip then converts the incoming sound into a digital code, which the computer analyzes so it can adjust the sound, factoring in the individual's particular hearing loss, the surrounding sounds, and the person's unique listening needs. These signals are then converted back into sound waves that are delivered to the ears through speakers.

Although most hearing aids consist of parts worn externally, bone-anchored hearing aids use a surgically implanted titanium prosthesis with a small head exposed outside the skin. Sound is transmitted to the titanium implant by means of a sound processor, which sits on the titanium head. The implant vibrates the skull. This vibration stimulates the hair cells in the inner ear, which carry the signal to the auditory nerve.

According to the Mayo Clinic (2014), some of the features of currently available hearing aids include

- directional microphones that focus in one direction to improve hearing ability in noisy environments;
- telephone adapters that make it easier to talk on a compatible telephone

(most that are capable of doing this switch automatically when the phone is held next to the hearing aid);

- bluetooth technology that allows hearing aids to connect with some bluetooth-compatible devices, such as cell phones, music players, or televisions;
- programming capacity that allows preprogrammed settings for a range of listening needs and environments;
- remote controls, so the individual can make adjustments without touching the hearing aid; and
- direct audio input that allows the individual to plug the aid into a television, computer, or music device.

From the list of available features, it is obvious that current hearing aids are digital and include a computer chip that moderates volume and amplifies selective frequencies. This means that people using hearing aids can program them to filter out background noise (e.g., a noisy restaurant, wind, traffic noise). Those that are bluetooth-enabled allow users to control the aid's features using their smart phone and stream music wirelessly directly to the hearing aid. In addition, the digital format has meant that hearing aids are no longer big and bulky. Many fit into the ear canal and are almost invisible.

Speechreading

Another way to augment a person's ability to hear is to teach him or her to do a better job of **speechreading**. We all use visual information to help us "hear" better, particularly in noisy environments. If you don't believe it, the next time someone is speaking to you in a noisy environment, look away from the person and observe the difference in your ability to understand what he or she is saying to you.

For individuals with some residual hearing, whether aided or not, speechreading augments their communication skills to a considerable extent. Speechreading is not easy to learn, nor is it simple. It is often taught to clients in conjunction with other communication strategies, such as learning the most effective ways in which to repair conversations (I discuss this in more detail below) and modifying listening environments.

People who have the most success with speechreading are those who are fluent in the language being spoken and who have some residual hearing. Sometimes, people whose hearing loss occurs gradually over a long time period teach themselves to speechread without knowing that is what they are doing. Box 10.5 lists the factors that increase the difficulty of speechreading.

Modifying Listening Environments

Different environments shape and modify sound in a variety of ways. For instance, a room with soft surfaces, such as carpets, drapes, and cloth furniture, alters sound

> **BOX 10.5** **Situations That Increase the Difficulty of Successful Speechreading**
>
> - noisy environments
> - a conversational partner with a foreign accent or unusual pronunciation
> - unfamiliar vocabulary
> - a person with a speech disorder
> - people who barely move their lips, use few gestures, and keep their facial expressions neutral
> - people who speak rapidly
> - people with bushy mustaches
> - people chewing gum, eating, or smoking

much less than a room with hard surfaces. Sound waves reverberate and reflect against hard surfaces, which interferes with the original sound. Think about how much easier it is to understand speech in a room with soft surfaces than in one with hard surfaces, particularly when many people are talking at the same time.

People with hearing disorders have a more difficult time understanding sound if it reflects and reverberates against surfaces. For this reason, modifying the environment is sometimes used to increase these individuals' ability to hear and understand speech. Most public school classrooms do not offer ideal listening characteristics for children with hearing disorders and need to be altered to offer less interference.

Ideally, the best way to modify such environments is to reduce background noise and eliminate sound reverberation and reflection. However, such a modification is not always possible. Think of a school cafeteria that is also used as an auditorium—installing carpeting on the floor would be disastrous! However, it is possible to increase a student's ability to hear specific voices (e.g., the teacher's) through the use of what is called an **assistive listening system (ALS)**. Some of these devices are used with individual students, and others can be hooked up to several students simultaneously. ALSs are used by people with varying degrees of hearing loss, including individuals who use hearing aids and those with cochlear implants. These products, like hearing aids, use digital technology, but they offer fewer features than custom-fitted hearing aids. However, they are beneficial for amplifying sound with a smart phone and earbuds, or for listening to television or other audio devices with earphones. Some have separate frequency and volume controls, and some personal FM systems are compatible with cochlear implants.

Communication Strategies

There are two major strategies used to develop effective communication systems for individuals with a severe-to-profound hearing loss. The **oral method** of communication focuses on teaching individuals with hearing impairments how to use speech effectively; **manual communication** systems teach individuals to communicate using nonspeech communication systems.

Manual Communication

Children with severe-to-profound hearing loss are at high risk for not developing language unless a functional communication system is developed—as early as possible—for the child and his or her family. Within the Deaf community, children—whether hearing or not—learn sign language in the same way that hearing babies of hearing parents learn spoken language. Sign language, like spoken languages, is passed from generation to generation.

The primary goal is for the child to acquire the linguistic and associated cognitive processes necessary to develop a complete language system. Because the oral approach has not been effective for most deaf children with severe-to-profound hearing loss, several manual communication systems have evolved. Some manual systems use manual gestures associated with spoken English. As I described earlier, **American Sign Language** (ASL) is a manual–visual language based on precise and specific gestures and movements of the head, neck, hands, arms, shoulders, and torso.

Perhaps the most widely used manual communication system based on spoken English is **Signing Exact English** (SEE; Gustason, 1983). SEE uses a system that links a manual sign to each individual English morpheme that is spoken. For example, in the sentence "I am going home," all morphemes (including *-ing*) are signed. The speaker also speaks at a normal rate. One of the disadvantages of SEE is the high number of signs associated with each English word and the necessity for children to understand the concept of morpheme in order to use the system. In addition, most individuals in the Deaf community do not endorse the use of SEE.

American Sign Language does not mirror the English language, or any other spoken language. ASL evolved as a combination of French Sign Language, brought to the United States at the beginning of the 19th century, and a sign language already in use by people who were deaf in the United States. ASL has its own grammar, although its vocabulary overlaps considerably with English. In contrast to SEE, ASL does not follow standard English rules; rather, it is considered a language with its own syntactic rules. People who use ASL consider themselves to be members of a unique culture, who become bilingual and bicultural when they learn to read English and to communicate with hearing people who rely on English.

A component of ASL is the American Fingerspelling Alphabet, shown in Figure 10.7. The American Fingerspelling Alphabet is used to spell words that have no exact sign and to communicate with hearing people who know the alphabet.

Children who grow up seeing and responding to ASL from an early age develop language and cognition just as easily and fluently as hearing children develop spoken language, unless they have other problems in addition to hearing loss. Difficulties arise when children who are deaf grow up in hearing families and are not

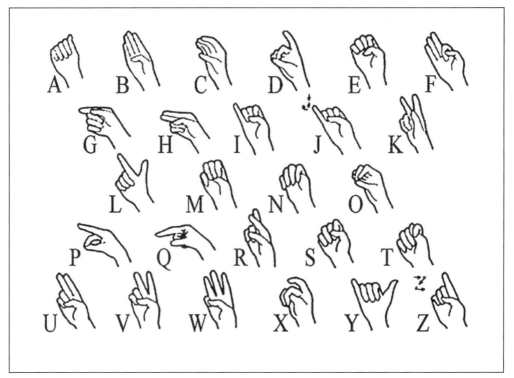

FIGURE 10.7. American Fingerspelling Alphabet.

exposed to ASL. However, hearing children born to deaf parents using ASL develop fluency in ASL and in spoken English, becoming bilingual and bicultural.

Many people who are deaf utilize services provided by professional interpreters for the deaf when it is necessary to communicate with hearing persons who do not know ASL or when they are attending public events. In addition, interpreters are used in classrooms, business meetings, and doctor's appointments, and during court appearances. You can obtain further information about this profession from organizations for the deaf in your state or by visiting the Registry of Interpreters for the Deaf (2005) website.

Oral Communication

Children with some residual hearing are often taught communication through what is called the oral method, in which the focus is on using the child's residual hearing to acquire communication and language. Many families prefer this method because they believe that the world is primarily oral, and their children must be able to communicate in that world. How well the oral method works is directly linked to the amount of residual hearing the child has and to her or his age. Advocates of the oral method do not believe in using sign language because they believe deaf children can catch up to their hearing peers if they are given the appropriate intervention through the oral method. However, many in the Deaf community oppose teaching through the oral method because they believe using ASL is the natural way that deaf children learn to communicate and because using ASL encourages a sense of belonging to the Deaf community.

Aural Rehabilitation

Aural habilitation is the term used to describe efforts to modify or remedy hearing loss that occurs at an early age, while *aural rehabilitation* is the term used to describe the intervention strategies used with individuals who lose hearing after they have acquired spoken language. You will remember that many in the Deaf community do not support aural habilitation in deaf children. However, children whose hearing can be amplified enough for them to hear spoken language are fitted with hearing aids or assisted listening devices.

People who experience hearing loss as adults face significant changes to their lives. These include the emotional stress of frequent communication breakdowns, adjusting to medical or surgical procedures and their results, and increased strain on family relationships. Aural rehabilitation focuses on

- helping people understand how hearing works and how their hearing loss has affected their hearing mechanism;
- teaching people about their medical or surgical procedures and what to expect afterwards;
- teaching people how their hearing aids work and how to maintain them for maximum effectiveness;
- developing effective communication strategies following the hearing loss, including the use of visual clues; and
- investigating assistive devices and their appropriateness.

In addition to focusing on communication abilities, clinicians can help people with impaired hearing through counseling. Audiologists are frequently the professionals who offer support to individuals and their families as they adjust to hearing loss, and, for those who are fitted with hearing aids, adjust to amplification and to hearing again. In addition to offering specific information and support, the audiologist may also recommend that the individual (and family, when appropriate) speak with other people who suffer from hearing loss, perhaps through joining a support group.

Adults who experience a hearing loss later in life are often disoriented and feel as if their identity has suddenly altered in a frightening way. Having developed a personality and identity as a hearing person, individuals who develop a hearing loss may go through several stages of grief (Kubler-Ross, 1997):

- deny the reality of the loss and feel extremely isolated, perhaps refusing amplification;
- express anger about the loss and its effect on their life;

- try to bargain in some way in order to reverse the loss;
- become sad and depressed; and
- accept the loss and its implications for their life.

Whenever an individual or family member shows a severe emotional response to the hearing loss, it is imperative that the audiologist recognize the limits of her or his professional role and refer to an appropriate mental health care professional.

Communication Sciences and Disorders: The Profession

The profession of communication sciences and disorders encompasses a wide range of specialties, all of which aim to understand the normal processes of communication and to assist people whose communication abilities are impaired in some way. Throughout Part 5, I use the term *clinician* to include both speech–language professionals (SLPs) and audiologists.

Chapter 11 introduces the field of communication sciences and disorders, beginning with a brief summary of how the field developed, followed by a description of the roles of SLPs and audiologists, the training required to become one or the other (or both), and typical work settings. The remainder of the chapter is devoted to professional issues: the importance of evidence-based practice, intervention with multicultural populations, ethics, and the impact of the DSM-5 on clinical practice.

Chapter 12 focuses on one of the most important aspects of the profession of communication sciences and disorders—the clinical relationship: what it is, the characteristics of a good therapeutic relationship, and the variables that can influence a clinical relationship.

In Chapter 13, I provide a discussion of clinical assessment, evaluation, diagnosis, and intervention. I describe how assessment and evaluation lead to diagnosis and then to intervention and how intervention includes ongoing assessments that measure the client's progress and guide the clinician in planning further intervention and dismissal from therapy. I describe how to establish goals, design intervention programs, document progress, and terminate therapy.

In Chapter 14, I offer a perspective of the clinician's responsibilities in providing clinical services to clients (and their families), to colleagues, and to the profession. I describe the roles clinicians play in both providing those clinical services and at the same time engaging in the clinical research process.

chapter 11

Professional Roles, Work Settings, and Ethics

Learning Objectives

Describe how an awareness of the history of communication sciences and disorders can help you become a more effective clinician.

Discuss how to avoid jumping on a bandwagon in assuming that a new and fashionable therapy approach is necessarily better than an existing one.

Describe the roles and responsibilities of speech–language pathologists (SLPs).

Describe the roles and responsibilities of audiologists.

List the primary requirements for obtaining a Certificate of Clinical Competence.

Name the work settings of professionals in communication sciences.

Name the professional organizations in the communication sciences.

List the most typical work settings for SLPs and audiologists.

Define evidence-based practice.

List the four Principles of Ethics that guide members of the American Speech-Language-Hearing Association.

Describe the basic principles involved when providing services to multicultural populations.

Describe some of the impacts of the DSM-5 on clinical practice.

Overview

The profession of communication sciences and disorders emerged as a profession in the early 20th century. Although the profession is young compared to some others, attempts to help people with **communication disorders** have been made for thousands of years. Some of those attempts have been more successful than others and have endured, some have disappeared entirely, and some reappear periodically.

Why is it important to be aware of the history of the profession? In other words, why should you spend your time reading about it? I think there are at least five reasons. First, if you aren't aware of the mistakes others have made in their attempts to help people with communication disorders, you are more likely to make them yourself. If you are familiar with what others have attempted and why those attempts failed, you can spend your time more effectively pursuing approaches that have been shown to work.

Second, some approaches have disappeared because they were ineffective. Many of the intervention strategies that were tried in the past were rejected for good reason. Research and clinical experience may have failed to yield evidence that the interventions did what they were intended to do or, for that matter, anything else worthwhile. Or they may have been effective in doing what they were intended to do, but their unpleasant **side effects** discouraged their use.

Conversely, other approaches that were discontinued because they were not effective are periodically rediscovered, only to be discarded once again when they are demonstrated to be ineffective or even harmful. Along the same lines, knowledge of history will help you be less likely to assume that what is claimed to be new is really new. Instead, you will be able to recognize an approach that has been used in the past, regardless of what it may be called or how it may be marketed.

Third, to be maximally effective as a clinician, you will need to be able to distinguish between **intervention strategies** that are simply not effective and those that could be effective if used with a different type of client or for accomplishing a different goal. For example, an intervention strategy that was used for a particular purpose with preschool-age children and found to be ineffective may be effective for accomplishing the same goal with older children or adults. Or, an intervention strategy that wasn't particularly effective for accomplishing its intended goal may have a side effect that makes it usable for accomplishing a different goal.

Fourth, understanding how clinical practice has developed will help you be less likely to reject clinically relevant information that is more than 25 years old. Similarly, you are less likely to assume that just because an approach is new, it is necessarily better than approaches that have been around longer.

The fifth and last reason to study the history of the profession is that you will be aware of how cultural factors impact trends regarding etiology and management of any given impairment at a particular point in time. You will see how cultural influences can alter the way any particular approach is viewed and the degree to which the approach can be successfully utilized.

A Short History

Attitudes about society's responsibility to people with communication disorders (or other physical or mental disorders) have evolved considerably during the past 4,000 years. In early Rome during the seventh century BC, for example, along the **Appian Way** there were cave-like apertures on the rocky outcrop on either side of the thoroughfare. Persons who were mentally handicapped, deformed, and communicatively impaired (particularly ones who stuttered) were caged there to provide entertainment for travelers (Eldridge, 1968). In some ancient **cultures**, many children born with physical deformities, like **cleft palates**, were murdered by their fathers because they were regarded as useless and likely to bring bad luck to their families. Those who were not murdered were often sold and trained to be prostitutes or beggars (Eldridge, 1968). This behavior was condoned by society because such disorders were regarded as an expression of the wrath of a deity.

Eldridge (1968) suggested that the first time a **speech disorder** was referred to in writing was approximately 4,000 years ago (2000 BC) during the Middle Egyptian Dynasty with a hieroglyph translated as meaning **stuttering**. Approximately 700 years later (1300 BC), in the Bible, Exodus 4:10,11 refers to Moses as having a speech disorder, probably stuttering. Jewish folklore includes this explanation of Moses' stuttering: One day when Moses was a young child and sitting on Pharaoh's lap, he grabbed Pharaoh's crown and placed it on his own head. Pharaoh's astrologers were horror-struck. "Let two braziers be brought," they counseled, "one filled with gold, the other with glowing coals, and set them before him. If he grasps the gold, it would be safer for Pharaoh to put the possible usurper to death." When the braziers were brought, the hand of Moses was stretched out toward the gold, but the angel Gabriel guided it toward the coals. Moses plucked out a burning coal and put it to his lips and, as a consequence, for life remained "heavy of speech and heavy of tongue."

In 400 BC, Thucydides, the Greek historian, described a condition that was probably **anomic aphasia**. He reported that many who suffered from the plague in Athens found that upon recovery, they had forgotten not only the names of their friends and relations but also their own names (Klingbeil, 1939a). Around that same time, Herodotus, another Greek historian, recorded the treatment of a young man for a speech disorder that appears to have been stuttering, and Demosthenes, the Greek orator, was treated for a speech disorder by means of **speech** exercises in which some pebbles were placed in his mouth. Demosthenes may have been the first to combat stuttering through the use of speech exercises (Klingbeil, 1939b). Hippocrates, "the father of medicine," appears to have been aware that disorders of speech result from lesions in the left cerebral hemisphere (Benton, 1981).

Aristotle, the Greek philosopher, suffered from a lisp, which may have been what motivated him to study speech disorders. Aristotle felt that stuttering was due to defective movements of the tongue. He stated that stutterers find it difficult to change the position of their tongue when they have to utter a second sound (Eldridge, 1968). He also wrote about disorders associated with deafness. He stated in this regard that there was no possibility of teaching the deaf to speak.

In the seventh century AD, St. John of Beverly is reported by the Venerable Bede to have helped a deaf boy acquire speech, which, according to Eldridge (1968), the saint (then a bishop) accomplished. This account indicates an awareness that deaf persons can be taught to speak and that Aristotle's pessimism may not have been warranted.

In the 11th century AD, Abu Ali Hussain Avicenna, a court physician of Arabia, blamed the tongue for causing stuttering. He also suggested other causes, including lesions of the brain and nerves, and a spasm of the epiglottis, which he advised should be treated by taking a deep inspiration before speaking (Eldridge, 1968). This advice has been given and acted upon periodically since then—even during this century—though it rarely, if ever, produces any lasting benefits.

In the 16th and 17th centuries AD, two Spanish monks, acting independently, developed a systematic approach to educating the deaf, including the first recorded use of using the hands to sign.

Lord Francis Bacon, the English philosopher, wrote a comprehensive treatise on speech disorders and blamed coldness of moisture of the tongue, or occasionally its dryness, on all the disorders (Klingbeil, 1939b).

Dr. Nicholas Tulp, of Amsterdam, published a case study of a young man known as "Johannes the Dumb," who learned to speak following a partial **glossectomy** (Eldridge, 1968).

In the 18th century, Abbé de L'Epée, a French priest, was the first to educate persons with **congenital** deafness, regardless of their social or financial status. He also was the first to found an institute for deaf education. He advocated the teaching of manual sign rather than oral speech (Eldridge, 1968).

An important medical procedure related to the field was developed during this time period. Le Mounier, a French dentist, performed the first successful operation for closing a cleft of the soft palate (Eldridge, 1968).

Several different theories regarding the cause of stuttering were developed during the 1700s. Johann Komad Amman, a Swiss physician, believed that stuttering was due simply to a vicious habit (Klingbeil, 1939b). This belief was a precursor of the theory currently advocated by many authorities that stuttering is a learned behavior.

Johann Gottfried von Hahn, a German physician, laid the blame for stuttering on the hyoid bone (Klingbeil, 1939b). His idea is a forerunner of a contemporary theory that views stuttering as resulting from some type of laryngeal malfunction.

The early 1800s again saw considerable focus on stuttering causes and intervention. Erasmus Darwin, an English physician and naturalist, believed that emotions, such as awe or bashfulness, caused stuttering. He advocated constant practice of the sounds on which stuttering occurs, with as much softening as possible of the initial consonants of words (Klingbeil, 1939b). Some **speech–language pathologists (SLPs)** still advise stutterers to produce the initial consonants of words with a "light contact."

J. M. G. Itard, a French physician, believed that stuttering was caused by a general debility of the nerves that stimulate the movements of the **larynx** and tongue. He recommended that a gold or ivory fork be placed in the cavity of the lower jaw to support the tongue, and that systematic "gymnastics" of the articulators be done against this obstacle. Doing so was supposed to strengthen the tongue (Eldridge, 1968; Klingbeil, 1939b).

Yates, a New York physician, believed that stuttering was caused by a spasm of the glottis, and treated it by advising stutterers to raise the tip of the tongue to the palate and hold it there while speaking (Klingbeil, 1939b). This is another precursor of the theory that stuttering is caused by some type of laryngeal malfunction.

Colombat de L'Isere classified persons who stutter into two groups: (1) those in whom the blockings resulted from spasms of the lips and tongues and (2) those in whom the spasms occurred in the larynx and respiratory muscles. He advocated the use of breathing exercises and vocal rhythms, including the pacing of speech with a metronome device he invented (Eldridge, 1968). There was a revival of interest in training stutterers to pace their speech with miniature metronomes during the 1970s.

Johann Frederick Dieffenbach, a German surgeon, believed that stuttering was caused by a spasm of the glottis and could be cured by surgery. His operation consisted of removing a triangular wedge from the root of the tongue. The operation was performed on hundreds of people, some of whom died following surgery (Eldridge, 1968).

Another important first during the early 1800s was that the first **laryngectomy** was performed. In 1859 the first artificial larynx for laryngectomized persons was produced (Eldridge, 1968).

During the second half of the 19th century, English physician William John Little presented one of the first comprehensive descriptions of **cerebral palsy**. Cerebral palsy then became known as Little's Disease. Unfortunately, he felt it was hopeless to habilitate children with this disorder, a theory now disproved (Eldridge, 1968).

This time period proved much more positive for persons with **hearing** impairments. Alexander Graham Bell moved to the United States from Scotland and contributed significantly to the teaching of speech to individuals with hearing impairments. His contributions are summarized in Box 11.1.

Helen Keller, who was both deaf and blind, was taught by Annie Sullivan to communicate using the manual alphabet. She also learned to produce intelligible speech and to understand speech by touching the lips of speakers (Eldridge, 1968).

Another view on stuttering emerged during this time period. Klencke, a German physician, believed that stuttering reflected stutterers' need for psychological help—for treatment of their whole personality (Eldridge, 1968). Some contemporary authorities view stuttering as a symptom that should be treated by psychotherapy.

In the late 1800s, the profession of communication sciences began to emerge. The Berlin School of Speech and Voice Therapy, founded by the Gutzmans (father and son), began a training center for teachers wishing to specialize in the treatment of speech disorders (Eldridge, 1968). This was one of the first attempts to train non-medical persons to work with those having such disorders. In Hamburg, Germany,

---

BOX 11.1   Alexander Graham Bell (Eldridge, 1968)

The man who probably has had more influence than anyone else in the world on the speech education of the deaf was Alexander Graham Bell (1847–1922). His name and his fame live on, primarily as the inventor of Bell's Improved Telephone, but sometimes we forget that he belonged to the third generation of a family that was professionally and vocationally devoted to speech. His grandfather, Alexander Bell, was a teacher of elocution in Edinburgh; Alexander Melville Bell, of the second generation, also taught elocution in Edinburgh, and evolved a system of symbols, showing the position of the speech organs when making sounds.

In 1870, Graham Bell and his father went to the United States. Here the name of Bell became famous. The invention of the telephone brought fortune as well as fame to Graham Bell, and his wholehearted philanthropy prompted him to use a large part of his fortune to found the Volta Bureau, an organization devoted to promoting and diffusing knowledge of the problems of the deaf, and later to found the Volta-Bell Fund, dedicated to oral teaching of the deaf. His technical skill was of incalculable value in the development of hearing aids. All of his work for the Deaf was directed toward encouraging the use of oral speech.

---

speech therapy for stuttering was provided in elementary schools (Eldridge, 1968); this was one of the first attempts to do so. Also, the first association for teachers specializing in speech–language pathology was formed in Germany. It was called (in translation) The Association of Teachers of Remedial Speech Training (Eldridge, 1968).

During the early 1900s, virtually the only treatment available to people with speech handicaps in the United States was that offered by privately owned commercial schools specializing in the treatment of stuttering. Patients paid large fees (in advance) for "guaranteed cures" (Eldridge, 1968). However, during this time period, many other intervention options were developed.

Centers for treating school-age children with speech disorders were established in school systems in the United States, Germany, Denmark, and England. Speech correction services were offered in the public schools of a number of American cities, including New York, New Haven, and Philadelphia. Treatment centers for people with communication disorders were also established at several U.S. universities, including Columbia, the University of Pennsylvania, and the University of Wisconsin (Eldridge, 1968).

During World War I, hospitals for the treatment of people with brain injuries were established in various parts of the world, particularly Germany. Work done with soldiers with brain injuries resulted in the first large-scale attempt to rehabilitate people with aphasia. Charles K. Mills, a Philadelphia physician, published the first paper in English describing the successful treatment of people with aphasia (Sarno, 1981).

Following World War I, **psychoanalysis** became popular as a way to treat people who stuttered (Eldridge, 1968).

It was also during this time period that the International Association of **Logo-pedics** and **Phoniatrics** held its first convention, in Vienna. This worldwide organization continues today for professionals and scientists in communication, voice, speech–language pathology, audiology, and swallowing (International Association of Logopedics and Phoniatrics, 2014).

The communication science professions grew rapidly during the mid-1900s. The American Speech Correction Association was formed in 1934 and published the first issue of the *Journal of Speech Disorders* in 1936. It was the first journal in English that allowed practitioners to share information on services for people with communication handicaps. Currently known as the **American Speech-Language-Hearing Association (ASHA)**, it is the national professional association for American SLPs; audiologists; speech, **language**, and **hearing** scientists; and professional support personnel.

Also in the middle of the 20th century, Congress authorized the United States Commission of Education to match the amounts spent by cities and states to defray the extra cost of educating "Speech Defectives" and children with other physical handicaps. The availability of this funding motivated many school systems to provide speech therapy services and thereby created a need for more SLPs to provide them. Many colleges and universities began training programs to meet this need. Students training to become SLPs had to learn long lists of Greek and Latin names for communication disorders. As the field evolved away from a strict medical orientation, these names were used less frequently.

Audiology began as a separate profession during these decades—an outgrowth of treatment programs established at Veterans Affairs (VA) hospitals for World War II veterans with hearing impairments. Audiometers were designed to test hearing.

World War II also resulted in increased services for those with brain injuries. Several army hospitals in the United States established special programs for soldiers with aphasia resulting from brain injuries. Following the war, such programs were established in many Veterans Health Administration hospitals. A number of approaches currently used for treating people with aphasia are based on knowledge gained from these programs.

After World War II, the professions of speech–language pathology and audiology grew significantly. The number of training programs and practitioners more than tripled. The minimum level of academic training for ASHA certification was first raised from a bachelor's to a master's degree for both SLPs and **audiologists**, and then to a professional doctorate (AuD) for audiologists. States began to require a **license** to practice both speech–language pathology and audiology. The **scope of practice** (i.e., what a professional is legally and ethically permitted to do) for both SLPs and audiologists expanded considerably. And an information explosion occurred that improved treatment approaches for most types of communication disorders. Similar growth, incidentally, occurred in both professions in most industrialized countries.

Some of the people who had the most impact on speech–language pathology early in this period were Charles Van Riper, Wendell Johnson, Elise Hahn, Mildred

Templin, Helmer Myklebust, Doris Johnson, and Mildred Berry. Influential people later in the period included Laura Lee, Raymond Carhart, Leo Doerfler, James Jerger, Margaret Lahey, and Lois Bloom.

You will have noticed how the field concentrated first on speech, then stuttering and voice. Until late in the middle of the last century, language was thought to consist solely of articulation. In the late 1960s, when language development was first addressed, only preschool language was described. Then, beginning in the 1980s, the study of language development began to cover school-age and adolescent language. For a more complete description visit Duchan's (2011) website, where she describes the history of speech–language pathology in the 20th century.

Social Influences

Culture has had and continues to have an impact on how communication and its disorders are viewed. The management of communication disorders is also affected by cultural perceptions of the cause of what is considered "abnormal" behavior. For instance, in ancient Rome (as well as in a number of other ancient societies) mental and physical impairments were regarded as punishment for sinning or otherwise angering the gods. The appropriate treatment was to seek the gods' forgiveness through prayer or deed. This view influenced how communication disorders were treated in these societies.

One of the main influences on the treatment of abnormal behavior at the end of the 19th century and during the early part of the 20th century was Freudian psychoanalysis. Psychoanalysts considered abnormal behavior to be an overt manifestation (i.e., symptom) of an unconscious, unresolved conflict or repressed need. The appropriate treatment was to help the patient identify and deal with the conflict or need through the process of psychoanalysis, which was used during this period for treating several communication disorders.

During the 1960s, in a dramatic shift, the prevailing view in psychology and psychiatry was that almost all abnormal behavior is learned. Consequently, the appropriate treatment was thought to be helping the client unlearn the behavior through application of what were called laws of learning. This approach was then used to treat almost all communication disorders that were not considered to have an organic etiology.

When pragmatic theory was introduced into the field in the 1970s, attention shifted from the behaviorally based learning model used in the previous decade to one emphasizing the social interactions surrounding and permeating communication. Therapy, particularly for children with language disorders, focused on helping them engage in socially meaningful and relevant communicative interactions.

Most recently, as I pointed out in previous chapters, professional attention has centered on **evidence-based practice**, which is an effort to develop intervention based on practices that are demonstrably effective and that have a proven track record.

We can draw two salient conclusions from reviewing the history of the profession. First, what may be marketed as a "new" or "revolutionary" approach may actually be a reappearance of a technique or approach that was used in a previous time. Second, new is not necessarily better. Because something is touted as new does not mean that it will work better than an approach that has existed for some time. What is important is to determine whether there is evidence to support the use of any given approach for any given client.

Speech–Language and Audiology Professionals

The professionals who have the primary responsibility for helping individuals cope with communication disorders are SLPs, speech–language pathology assistants (SLPAs), audiologists, and audiology assistants. Both SLPAs and audiology assistants are **paraprofessionals**, people who assist professionals in either speech–language pathology or audiology. Audiologists and SLPs are considered **independent professionals**, while SLPAs and audiology assistants work under the direct supervision of an SLP or audiologist.

What Does an SLP Do?

The primary functions of SLPs are to prevent communication disorders when possible and, when a communication disorder exists, to identify it, assess the individual's communication strengths and weaknesses, and provide intervention that helps individuals develop communication skills to their maximal potential. SLPs provide services for spoken, written, manual, and pictorial language and communication systems.

From your reading of previous chapters about the various types of communication disorders, you will have inferred that SLPs work with speech disorders, language disorders, social communication disorders, cognitive–communication disorders, and swallowing disorders (dysphagia). SLPs also provide

- communication services (aural rehabilitation) for people who are deaf or hard of hearing;
- augmentative and alternative communication (AAC) systems for individuals with severe communication disorders (e.g., **autism** spectrum disorder, or ASD; some types of aphasia; progressive neurological disorders); and
- modification services for individuals who want to modify a foreign language accent or enhance their communication skills for social or work purposes.

In the past 20 years, SLPs have undertaken expanded roles, particularly in school settings. Not only do they provide direct service to individuals with communication disorders, but they also offer indirect services through consulting, coaching, collaborating, and educating educators and families. One reason for these expanded roles is that the needs of schoolchildren in the United States are constantly changing (e.g., the number of children with ASD has increased dramatically in recent years). Another is that there is more information available today than ever before about communication disorders: their causes, their physiology, the brain mechanisms underlying some disorders, and genetic factors, to name just a few.

What Does an Audiologist Do?

Audiologists identify, diagnose, treat, and monitor disorders of the auditory and vestibular systems. Their assessment procedures include a variety of hearing tests and assessments of **tinnitus** and balance. Audiologists are qualified to dispense and manage hearing aids. They are also qualified to assess whether a person is a good candidate for a **cochlear implant** and to map cochlear implants. Other services audiologists provide are

- working with industries to design and implement hearing safety,
- designing and implementing newborn hearing-screening programs,
- designing and carrying out school hearing-screening programs,
- counseling families whose infant has a hearing loss, and
- counseling clients and families about compensating for older adults who experience a hearing loss.

Not all speech–language and hearing professionals provide clinical services as their primary function. Some professionals in the field conduct research into the various areas of communication and communication disorders (e.g., synthesized speech, speech recognition, multilingualism) in order to produce information that clinicians can use to better serve their clients. Most of these speech, language, and hearing scientists earn an advanced degree, such as the PhD or EdD. Speech, language, and hearing scientists are usually employed in a wide range of fields, including medicine, academics, advocacy, politics, public policy, and government.

SLPs and audiologists also work in a variety of settings, each requiring a specific set of responsibilities. Very few SLPs or audiologists actually engage simultaneously in every one of the roles described here, but over the course of a career that includes the entire gamut of settings, one could function in a large number of the following roles.

Independent Professionals

What does it mean to be a professional? Professionals have knowledge and expertise usually not possessed by those who seek their services. They are practitioners of occupations that require considerable formal training to perform at the level of competence consumers of their services expect.

As I mentioned above, SLPs and audiologists are independent professionals. Other independent professionals in health-related fields are dentists, **psychiatrists**, and **optometrists**. Most nurses, **physical therapists**, and **occupational therapists** are not independent professionals because they are required by law to only accept referrals from physicians who prescribe what the nurses or therapists are to do.

Independent professionals assume full responsibility for the services they provide for a client or patient. The downside of this is that the professional can be sued for malpractice. Consequently, all independent professionals need professional liability (i.e., malpractice) insurance. SLPs and audiologists in private practice purchase their own professional liability insurance. Those employed by a public school system, hospital, or other institution will almost always have the insurance furnished by their employer.

One of the main responsibilities of SLPs and audiologists as independent professionals is diagnosing and treating communication disorders in order to promote the welfare of people with these disorders. They determine whether people referred to them have a communication disorder, determine the cause of a disorder, and develop and implement an intervention plan for reducing the disorder's severity. If it is not possible to determine the cause, as is the case with many language disorders, the SLP will usually develop an intervention plan that helps the person develop skills to succeed in school or work, compensate for the disorder, or function in everyday life.

Clinician-Investigators

The **Code of Ethics of the American Speech-Language-Hearing Association** states that SLPs and audiologists "shall evaluate services rendered to determine effectiveness" (ASHA, 2010, para. 16). This means that they must do therapy-outcome research in order to function in a manner that is consistent with this code (i.e., they must function as **clinician-investigators** and assess the impact of their therapy programs on their clients). The information gleaned from such assessment enables professionals to improve their effectiveness as clinicians. It can, for example, enable them to identify intervention strategies that are not producing desired outcomes and that, as a consequence, must be modified or discarded.

Clinicians also need to assess the effectiveness of the services they render in order to be accountable. Clinicians are required by their employers and by **third-party payers** (e.g., insurance companies) to document the impact they have on clients. They generate the data needed for **documentation** by doing therapy-outcome research—that is, by being investigators as well as clinicians. You can find ASHA's code of ethics on their website (ASHA, 2010).

Information Counselors

You will recall that in a previous chapter I mentioned that SLPs and audiologists frequently function as information counselors—they provide clients and their families with relevant information about communication disorders and how to cope with them. For example, they provide the families of people with aphasia with the information they need to cope with the behavioral changes that occur with brain damage, or, for an adult who has developed a hearing loss, the audiologist will provide information regarding the best types of hearing aids available for the person's particular loss as well as information about techniques that can maximize the person's understanding of speech in a variety of contexts.

SLPs and audiologists also try to modify attitudes of clients and family members that could impede the rehabilitation process. An example of such an attitude would be the desire to conceal a hearing loss. If this attitude is not modified, it is likely to keep the client from wearing a hearing aid and benefiting from the device.

Furthermore, SLPs and audiologists help clients develop an **objective attitude** toward their disorder. This allows the person to minimize the negative impact of the disorder on his or her life—that is, to make it less handicapping. To learn more about the counseling role of SLPs and audiologists, see Luterman (2008) and ASHA's detailed guidelines for audiologists who provide informational and adjustment counseling to families of infants and young children with hearing loss (ASHA, 2008a).

Educators

All SLPs and audiologists function at times as educators. They provide information to professionals in other fields and speak to professional and lay groups about people who have communication disorders. The majority of SLPs work in schools, so the role of educator is one they engage in daily. Most school-based SLPs work in classrooms, where they teach individuals, small groups, and entire classrooms of students. Many students majoring in audiology or speech–language pathology take a public speaking course to prepare themselves for meeting this responsibility.

Report Writers

SLPs and audiologists are expected to prepare reports on their clients, which become a part of the client's clinical record. On request from the client or the client's family, these reports will be sent to professionals at other institutions or agencies. These reports are expected to include summaries of the findings of evaluations, progress notes, and discharge information.

Reports are one of the ways professionals judge each other's competence. Therefore, it is important that they be well written. Students majoring in speech–language pathology and audiology should develop their writing skills so they can write reports that are clear, informative, and free of grammatical and spelling errors.

Team Members

SLPs and audiologists often function as members of teams on which the professions represented are determined by the client's needs. Team members for a preschool child who is **hypernasal** because of a cleft palate, for example, may include an audiologist, an SLP, a plastic surgeon, a dentist, a psychiatrist, and a **social worker**. They will each evaluate the client and jointly establish goals for the client.

School-based SLPs participate in a variety of teams. The school-based team responsible for writing the student's **Individualized Education Program (IEP)** will include the SLP for students who have communication disorders. In addition, many school-based SLPs provide service through teaching teams that include the classroom teacher, the special educator, an occupational therapist, a physical therapist, and the SLP.

Team members cooperate by each providing services aimed at the client's learning goals, including those related to communication. For example, when working with a child who has cerebral palsy, the SLP will encourage the child to use his or her hands in ways that the occupational therapist has recommended. Similarly, the occupational therapist will encourage the child to communicate in ways the SLP has determined is best for the child's developmental goals. It is important for students majoring in speech–language pathology or audiology to become acquainted with the ways other health-care and education professionals can contribute to the treatment of children and adults who have communication impairments. The Boys Town National Research Hospital website (Boys Town National Research Hospital, 2014) offers a good description of a multidisciplinary team of professionals specializing in deafness and hearing disorders.

Marketing Representatives

People with communication disorders must be aware of services provided by audiologists or SLPs before they can be helped by the services. Raising awareness requires marketing, which most SLPs and audiologists engage in in some form. For example, they give talks to lay and professional groups in which they describe aspects of their clinical service programs. School-based SLPs give presentations to parents, describing their work with students and how it contributes to academic success. To learn more about the marketing activities of SLPs and audiologists, see Matthews (1993).

Lobbyists and Advocates

ASHA's code of ethics states that SLPs and audiologists should hold paramount the welfare of persons served professionally (ASHA, 2010). This refers to all persons who have communication disorders, not just those treated by clinicians.

The welfare of people with communication disorders is affected by both state and federal legislation. Such legislation can influence the availability of funding for needed services. It can influence, for example, whether a child with a severe communication impairment from a low-income family will be able to have the speech-generating communication device or the hearing aid that he or she needs.

One way SLPs and audiologists promote the welfare of people who have communication disorders is by **lobbying** for legislation favorable to client interests and against legislation that could be detrimental to clients. Most lobbying on the federal level is done through ASHA's "Speak Out, Be Heard" program, established in 2011. The purpose of the program is to protect "the current level of services provided by ASHA members" and to "elevate the priorities of communication sciences and disorders professionals before lawmakers" (ASHA, 2014a). In addition to "Speak Out, Be Heard," ASHA encourages grassroots involvement through ASHA members visiting Capitol Hill and by sending email blasts regarding specific legislative items under consideration.

ASHA's "Speak Out, Be Heard" program also includes a political action committee, ASHA-PAC, which represents the professions in the federal political process through contributions to congressional campaigns and attendance at fundraising events related to legislation pertaining to the field. You can learn more about ASHA's advocacy activities on their website (ASHA, 2014a).

SLPs and audiologists also engage in another type of advocacy by promoting the welfare of people with communication disorders. Federal, state, and municipal administrative agencies (e.g., Medicaid, **Medicare**, local school districts), and other **third-party payers**, sometimes deny people services or put them on waiting lists. They may not realize that the client is eligible to receive a service, or their funding may be inadequate to cover all of the services they are supposed to provide. A local school district, for example, may not provide an electronic communication device for a child with a severe communication disorder until the SLP helps provide necessary documentation.

Expert Witnesses

SLPs and audiologists are occasionally asked to testify in trials as **expert witnesses**. They are hired by the attorney for the plaintiff or defendant in a lawsuit to provide evidence-based opinions that will support or refute what has been testified to by the other side. An SLP may, for example, be asked to testify about the competency of a person with aphasia to continue to manage his or her financial affairs, or to testify in a child custody case about which parent would be best able to provide for the child's therapy needs. In a 2007 essay in *The ASHA Leader*, Jill Armour (2007), an audiologist, describes her experience as an expert witness.

Researchers

Many speech, language, and hearing scientists, SLPs, and audiologists spend more than half their time doing either pure or applied research. Their research may be funded by grants from governmental or private agencies. Most of them have a PhD or AuD degree and are on the faculty of a college or university.

Many practitioners in these fields who have master's degrees also do some research, most of which tends to be both clinical and practical. They share their findings with other practitioners in their field by either publishing in professional publications or presenting at professional meetings. ASHA sponsors four major professional journals describing various types of research findings and one online publication that includes news and feature articles for ASHA members:

- *American Journal of Audiology*
- *American Journal of Speech–Language Pathology*
- *Journal of Speech, Language, and Hearing Research*
- *Language, Speech, and Hearing Services in Schools*
- *The ASHA Leader Online*

Supervisors

Many SLPs and audiologists function as supervisors, overseeing the activities of other SLPs, audiologists, or paraprofessionals (e.g., SLPAs or audiology assistants). The facilities in which they supervise include school systems, hospitals, private practice, and rehabilitation centers. They also may supervise student clinicians at a college or university speech and hearing clinic. Any person who has earned a **Certificate of Clinical Competence (CCC)** from ASHA can supervise clinical practicum experiences in his or her area of certification (speech–language pathology or audiology). More specifically, anyone who wishes to supervise must have established competency in the area of practice (e.g., adult aphasia, central auditory processing) in which the supervision is to take place, and some university programs may require additional certification, such as a teaching license or teacher certification in their state.

Administrators

Some SLPs and audiologists function as administrators as well as clinicians in clinical programs. The competencies required for administering a speech, language, and hearing clinical program are the same as those required for other administrative positions. Each graduate education program must be accredited by ASHA, which means that it must have an administrative structure that oversees all aspects of the program. Box 11.2 shows the various aspects involved in such an administrative structure.

Authors

In addition to the writing activities I described in the section on SLPs and audiologists as researchers, many SLPs and audiologists also design computer software, mobile apps, slide presentations, audiotapes, videotapes, diagnostic tests, or therapy kits for use by other clinicians. Also, some invent devices for diagnosing or treating communication disorders. Such activities are not limited to those with PhD or AuD degrees.

BOX 11.2 Components of an Administrative Structure Required of All Graduate Education Programs in Audiology and Speech–Language Pathology

- Regional accreditation from one of six regional accrediting bodies.
- The development and implementation of a long-term strategic plan.
- A faculty that holds authority and responsibility for the program.
- The individual responsible for the graduate education program must hold a graduate degree in speech–language pathology, audiology, or speech, language, and hearing science.
- The individual responsible for the graduate education program must hold a full-time appointment in the institution.
- A nondiscrimination policy that specifies that students, faculty, staff, and clients served are treated in a nondiscriminatory way without regard to race, color, religion, sex, national or ethnic origin, disability, age, sexual orientation, genetic information, citizenship, or status as a veteran of the U.S. armed services.
- The program must provide current, accurate, and available information about the program and the institution.

To review the complete standards for accreditation of graduate education programs, visit ASHA's website (ASHA, 2008b).

Consultants

Most audiologists and SLPs function at times as resource persons, or consultants. They consult with other SLPs about their clients, and they often consult and collaborate with teachers and other professionals to design and implement services. I mentioned earlier that audiologists and SLPs can be called as expert witnesses. In addition, they often provide expertise to business, industry, the courts, attorneys, and public and private agencies.

It is important for SLPs and audiologists to fulfill each of the above roles. However, perhaps one of the most important characteristics of people in the profession is a genuine desire to be helpful to others. A clinician who isn't a people person is unlikely to be successful, regardless of the amount of technical expertise he or she has. You can read about a client's experience with a clinician who was not caring in Box 11.3.

You can read the best description about the human dimension to being an effective clinician, which was written by Charles Van Riper, one of the most influential people in the field during the 20th century, in Van Riper (1979).

Speech–Language Pathology Assistants and Audiology Assistants

Although **paraprofessionals** have been utilized in a number of health-care and education fields (e.g., physical therapy, nursing, teaching) as well as in communication

---

BOX 11.3   **A Client's Experiences With a Clinician**
Who Was Not Caring

This excerpt highlights the importance of a clinician exhibiting a genuine caring attitude. The author, who was a speech–language pathologist, had a stroke at the age of 29 that left her completely unable to communicate for almost one and one-half years.

I feel that the most important trait of a good clinician is a genuine, caring, patient attitude. If one has a lot of "textbook learning" and little empathy for the client, progress will be limited. One speech–language pathologist I had gave me the feeling that when she saw me she thought, "Well, here's Joy again. What shall I have her try today?" Needless to say, I made very little progress with this clinician. She was never really prepared for therapy, and I knew that she was just putting some things together on the spot to keep me "busy." I knew that her knowledge of my condition was severely limited, I think that a client without my background would have recognized this also. I did not get a feeling of professional or personal concern or even professional competency from this clinician. I needed a clinician who cared and was interested in me as a person, a clinician who could make me feel secure in her knowledge of my problem.

Another thing that has a big effect on the attitude of the client is enthusiasm. All speech–language pathologists need to be more enthused about their clients, to greet clients as if they were glad to see them, and to have a positive attitude about the clients. When I was depressed and the clinician was really not interested in me, I became even more depressed. It was wonderful when I would go to therapy and the clinician was cheerful and friendly. Knowing that the clinician cared would bring me out of my depression.

Note. From "I'd Rather Tell a Story Than Be One," by J. G. Post and W. R. Leith, 1983, *ASHA, 25*, p. 27. Copyright 1983 by the American Speech-Language-Hearing Association. Reprinted with permission.

---

sciences and disorders for many years, their widespread utilization in the field of speech–language pathology is relatively recent. ASHA does not register (i.e., grant credentials to) SLPAs. However, it does sponsor an Associates Program, which offers affiliation to individuals working in support positions under the supervision of an ASHA-certified audiologist or SLP.

Speech–Language Pathology Assistants (SLPAs)

ASHA has recommended guidelines for the supervision, use, and training of SLPAs. An SLPA should perform tasks only under the supervision of an ASHA-certified SLP. Box 11.4 lists the tasks SLPAs may engage in.

Not all states allow the use of SLPAs, but in those that do, there are over 25 associate degree programs for SLPAs. The recommended curriculum includes

- general education courses in oral and written communication, mathematics, technology, and social and natural sciences;
- technical courses in the normal processes of communication, communication disorders, anatomy and physiology of the speech and hearing

> **BOX 11.4** **Tasks an SLPA May Perform Under the Supervision of an SLP (ASHA, 2014m)**
>
> The SLPA may assist the SLP in:
>
> - speech, language, and hearing screenings (without any interpretation)
> - assessing students, patients, and clients (again without any interpretation)
> - bilingual translation during screening and assessment activities (without any interpretation)
> - following intervention plans or intervention protocols designed by the supervising SLP
> - engaging in telepractice designed by the supervising SLP
> - documenting client performance
> - programming AAC devices and instructing clients in their use
> - acting as an interpreter for clients/families whose primary language is not English
> - providing services in another language

mechanism, instruction in service delivery as an assistant, workplace behaviors, and cultural and linguistic factors involved in communication;
- on-site observation of an ASHA-certified SLP; and
- fieldwork experiences (100 clock hours).

Audiology Assistants

Like SLPAs, audiology assistants engage only in tasks that are designed and supervised by a certified audiologist, and also like SLPAs, audiology assistants are not permitted in all states. Some of the roles of audiology assistants under the express supervision of a certified audiologist include

- assisting clients with hearing aids or other amplification devices,
- assisting audiologists in treating clients,
- preparing various sorts of materials,
- carrying out analyses of acoustic devices,
- maintaining equipment,
- performing pure-tone audiology reassessments,
- performing hearing testing on newborns, and
- acting as translators or interpreters if fluent in a language in addition to English.

Audiology assistants are *not* qualified to perform the audiological tasks listed in Box 11.5.

Some states require audiology assistants to obtain a license to practice. For instance, Texas's requirements for obtaining a license as an audiology assistant are

- baccalaureate degree with an emphasis in audiology;
- 25 hours of clinical observation;

BOX 11.5 **Some of the Audiologic Tasks**
Audiology Assistants May *Not* Perform

- selecting cases or evaluation procedures for clients
- interpreting any observations or data
- drawing diagnostic conclusions
- designing management procedures
- participating in any team or case conferences unless the supervising audiologist or proxy is present
- deviating from any treatment plan devised by the supervising audiologist
- transmitting any information about any client without the express approval of the supervising audiologist
- discharging any client
- consulting with clients (or family) about a client

- 25 hours of clinical assisting experience; and
- 24 semester hours in speech–language pathology and audiology, with at least 18 in the area in which the applicant is applying.

Becoming an Audiologist or a Speech–Language Pathologist

In large part, the process of becoming an SLP or an audiologist consists of meeting the requirements for the Certificate of Clinical Competence (CCC-SLP or CCC-A). All employers accept the CCC-A as evidence of competency to function as an audiologist, and all employers except the public schools accept the CCC-SLP as evidence of competency to function as an SLP. Although most states require a license to practice as an SLP, the requirements for the license are usually the same as for the ASHA CCC. Each state department of public instruction has its own requirements for certifying SLPs as employable in its schools. Although an SLP who meets the requirements for one state will not necessarily meet those for other states, it is usually not difficult to meet them if you have met those for one state and hold ASHA's CCC-SLP.

In order to earn the Certificate of Clinical Competence (CCC) in Speech–Language Pathology or Audiology, you must earn a graduate degree (master's or doctoral degree for speech–language pathology, doctoral degree for audiology) from an accredited university program, complete the required clinical practicum experiences, and pass a national exam. In addition, you must successfully complete a Clinical Fellowship under the mentorship of a person holding the CCC-SLP or CCC-A during the fellowship. Both audiologists and SLPs must maintain their CCCs through ongoing continuing education.

ASHA's Certificates of Clinical Competence

The formal training program for one of these certificates is usually 6 or 7 years. A student enrolled in the program ordinarily earns both a bachelor's and a master's or AuD degree. The bachelor's portion usually takes 4 years to complete. A master's degree is then completed in 2 years or an AuD in 3 years. Some colleges and universities offer only the undergraduate (preprofessional) portion of the training program. All graduate coursework and graduate clinical practicum experience must have been initiated and completed at a college or university whose program is accredited by the Council for Clinical Certification in Audiology and Speech–Language Pathology (CFCC) of the American Speech-Language-Hearing Association in the area for which certification is sought—speech–language pathology, audiology, or both.

It is possible for a person to earn both certificates. He or she is then qualified to treat anybody with a communication disorder. Meeting the requirements for both certificates usually involves earning two graduate degrees: one in speech–language pathology and one in audiology. The vast majority of members of ASHA are certified in only one of the two areas.

There are five requirements for obtaining one of these certificates: (1) successfully completing academic courses; (2) observing at least 25 hours of diagnostic and therapy sessions; (3) accumulating a minimum of 375 hours of supervised direct clinical practicum experience; (4) successfully completing a clinical fellowship year; and (5) passing a national examination. The following sections describe these five requirements in more detail.

Academic Coursework Requirements

To be employed as an SLP or audiologist, you will need to have certain specific knowledge and skills. Because practitioners in both fields need some of the same information, some of the same courses are required for both ASHA certificates.

Before you can determine whether the speech and language abilities of an individual are within normal limits, you must be familiar with the speech and language skills of typically developing individuals. You have probably already surmised what is necessary by looking at the topics covered in this book. Several sections describe the normal structure and functioning of various mechanisms and processes, one of which, for example, is the normal anatomy and physiology of the speech and hearing mechanisms. To understand how people make sense of speech and how they are able to speak, you have to know how the parts of these mechanisms function. This information can be significant both diagnostically and therapeutically. Diagnostically, it enables clinicians to recognize possible organic causes for their clients' communication disorders. Therapeutically, it can enable them to predict whether it should be possible for a client to improve and, if so, how much.

For example, if an opening in a client's hard palate allows air to flow into the nasal cavity, the clinician would know that the client will continue to be hypernasal until this opening is eliminated by surgery or by fitting a dental appliance into it.

This information is acquired from the required course on the anatomy and physiology of the speech and hearing mechanism, as well as units of other courses that deal with components of this mechanism.

Another thing about normal hearing, speech, and language that you will need to learn pertains to the acoustical signals generated by the speech mechanism and interpreted by the ear. The signals result from the movements of the structures (e.g., the tongue) that make up the speech mechanism. When a person has a speech disorder, there is something abnormal about the acoustic signals being generated by his or her speech mechanism. SLPs attempt to modify these acoustic signals—to make them sound more normal. Information about the acoustics of speech is acquired from courses on speech and hearing science and phonetics.

You must also acquire information about normal language development, which you will need for both diagnosis and therapy. An SLP who does not know the typical development of grammatical rules will not know which ones to teach a 3-year-old client who has a language disorder. Similarly, without information regarding children's development of metalinguistic abilities, the SLP will not be able to design appropriate intervention for children whose metalinguistic skills are not keeping pace with those of their peers. This kind of information is acquired from courses on normal language development.

A third type of information that SLPs and audiologists must acquire pertains to the symptomatology, etiology, prognosis, diagnosis, and treatment of the various communication disorders. Students majoring in speech–language pathology or audiology are introduced to all types of communication disorders—not just to those that are treated by the professionals in their specific field. However, those majoring in audiology acquire information about hearing disorders in much greater depth than those majoring in speech–language pathology, and vice versa.

The clinical relationship is central to what audiologists and SLPs do. It is the structure within which they function clinically. Consequently, you will have to know how to manage the relationship proficiently in order to be maximally effective as a clinician, using the knowledge and skill you acquire in your clinical practicums.

SLPs and audiologists must also know how behaviors are learned and unlearned. Students learn to utilize the various strategies that psychologists have developed for understanding and changing behavior. You will acquire the academic information needed for doing this from psychology courses and the skills for implementing what you learn there in your clinical practicums.

The main responsibilities of most SLPs and audiologists are diagnosis and therapy. You will learn these two skills from both courses that focus directly on these topics (e.g., those dealing with diagnostic methods in speech–language pathology or hearing testing) and those that deal with specific communication disorders (e.g., aphasia, language-learning disabilities). Again, you will also acquire it from your clinical practicums.

Both SLPs and audiologists need information about professional ethics and law as they affect clinical practice. They also need information about establishing and maintaining a clinical practice, record keeping, and marketing clinical services. Many training programs offer a course in which such information is presented (e.g., one on professional aspects of clinical practice in speech–language pathology and audiology).

All SLPs and audiologists function as consumers of research. You will read professional journals in which research is reported, and you will utilize some of the journal information presented in your clinical practice. To know how to evaluate the findings of studies, you must become proficient in reading scientific reports and analyzing this information. You also have to know how to evaluate the impact of your therapy programs on clients—that is, how to produce research. Most training programs offer a course from which you can acquire the information needed for functioning as both a consumer and producer of clinical research.

While most SLPs and audiologists function more often as clinicians than as scientists, they nevertheless have to understand the **scientific method** because they utilize it for clinical decision making. All students majoring in speech–language pathology or audiology are required to take courses in biological/physical sciences and mathematics to facilitate the development of a scientific orientation—understanding how to utilize a systematic and logical approach to discover how things work. A scientific orientation will provide you with the foundation for knowing how to challenge ideas through research and how to rule out alternative explanations until a probable conclusion is reached.

Clinical Observation Requirement

All students majoring in speech–language pathology or audiology are required to observe a minimum of 25 hours of evaluation or therapy before beginning their clinical practicum experiences. This is intended to increase your understanding of the dynamics of the clinical relationship.

Supervised Clinical Experience Requirements

All students majoring in speech–language pathology are required to accumulate a minimum of 375 hours of supervised clinical experience. At least 325 must be accumulated during the graduate study portion of the accredited training program in the professional area in which certification is sought. In addition, these hours must be distributed in certain ways. A specified minimum number must be for evaluation and for treatment, for specific types and severities of disorders, for populations across the lifespan, and for culturally/linguistically diverse populations.

Students majoring in audiology must complete a minimum of 1,820 hours of supervised clinical practicum across six areas of study:

1. foundations of practice in audiology
2. prevention and identification of dysfunction in hearing and communication, balance, and other auditory-related systems
3. assessment, including sensory and motor evoked potentials, electromyography, and other electrodiagnostic tests

4. intervention with individuals with hearing loss, balance disorders, and other auditory dysfunctions
5. advocacy and consultation regarding the communication needs of individuals with hearing loss, other auditory dysfunction, or vestibular disorders
6. education, research, and administration, including analyzing the efficacy and efficiency of practices and programs (evidence-based practice)

Students usually accumulate practicum hours in two types of settings. Almost all practicum hours are likely to be acquired in the clinical facilities of the college or university in which the student is enrolled. The remainder of the hours are accumulated in community facilities that offer speech–language pathology or audiology services, such as public schools, hospitals, private practices, clinics, rehabilitation centers, and nursing homes. All practicum hours must be supervised by a person holding the CCC-SLP or the CCC-A.

SLP Clinical Fellowship Year Requirement

After a student has completed all the academic and practicum requirements for the CCC-SLP and has received a graduate degree, he or she will begin a clinical fellowship year, which is similar to an internship. However, unlike some internships, the person receives a full salary. Any SLP who is certified by ASHA in the student's professional area can serve as his or her clinical fellowship supervisor. This person may or may not be employed by the facility at which the intern is working. The supervisor interacts frequently during this year with the intern and submits a year-end evaluation of the intern's performance to ASHA.

The National Examination Requirement

The final requirement for attaining a Certificate of Clinical Competence is passing a national examination. The examinations are different for those seeking certification in speech–language pathology and in audiology. The tests include discrete multiple choice items. If you fail on the first try, you may take the test again. If that happens, though, you must pass it successfully within the 2-year application period for the CCC.

Work Settings

Audiologists, SLPs, SLPAs, and audiologist assistants provide services in a variety of work settings.

Schools

Public school systems historically have been one of the largest employers of SLPs. The U.S. Department of Labor Bureau of Labor Statistics (2014) reported that in 2012 almost half of SLPs employed work in the schools, partly because schools are required by state and federal special education law to provide speech–language pathology services. Part of the local school district budget for these services comes from state and federal sources.

The clients served in this setting, of course, are school-age children and adolescents. Though the majority are of elementary-school age, federal law requires services to be provided to people from birth to 21 years. Children between the ages of birth and 3 are required by federal law to be offered therapy services if they are at risk for developing a communication disorder.

To qualify a child for special education services, a communication disorder must have a significant impact on a student's educational performance. The majority of children seen by SLPs in public schools have articulation or language disorders. The language services provided by SLPs in the schools address a wide variety of skills, including social language, phonological development, vocabulary development, story comprehension, and organizational skills. SLPs may also help older students with writing, oral presentations, and study skills.

SLPs provide services in school settings for numerous conditions other than language and articulation disorders, including

- autism spectrum disorders,
- childhood apraxia of speech,
- developmental disabilities,
- swallowing (dysphagia),
- learning disabilities,
- augmentative and alternative communication,
- selective mutism,
- traumatic brain injury,
- voice, and
- hearing.

SLPs rather than audiologists do the hearing habilitation in most school districts (except for that involving hearing aids). Some school districts employ audiologists, who spend most of their time testing hearing and assisting children with hearing aids. Far fewer audiologists than SLPs are employed in public schools.

Some private and charter schools have a full- or part-time SLP. If they do not employ one, their students may go to a nearby public school for therapy. ASHA (2007) provides a complete description of the scope of practice of SLPs, including public school settings, on their webpage.

Health-Care Settings

Hospitals, nursing homes, rehabilitation centers, and some HMOs offer speech–language pathology services. The SLP's caseload consists primarily of adults whose communication disorders are caused by brain damage—that is, **aphasia** and **dysar-**

thria. They also work with people who have lost the ability to swallow normally, that is, who have **dysphagia**, which I described in Chapter 7. While assessing patients, SLPs may assist in or perform modified barium videofluoroscopic studies of their swallow.

SLPs who work for HMOs, hospitals, and rehabilitation centers also treat some children. Some SLPs who are employed in hospitals, for example, work with medically fragile infants in neonatal intensive care units. Box 11.6 lists the primary roles played by SLPs providing services to infants—and their families—in neonatal intensive care units (NICUs).

Audiologists employed by HMOs, hospitals, public health departments, and rehabilitation centers have extensive training and skills to perform a wide range of functions, shown in Box 11.7.

BOX 11.6   Primary Roles Played by SLPs When Providing Services to Infants and Their Families in the NICU

- swallowing and feeding evaluation
- communication evaluation
- swallowing and feeding intervention
- communication intervention
- education and counseling for parents or caregivers
- staff education
- collaboration with staff

BOX 11.7   Services Provided by Audiologists in Health-Care Settings

- newborn screening follow-up
- pediatric hearing testing
- pediatric hearing aids
- otoacoustic emissions
- tympanometry
- dizziness and balance testing
- testing for Ménière's Disease
- auditory evoked potential measurement
- adult auditory brainstem response testing (ABR)
- adult hearing testing
- bone-anchored hearing aids
- adult hearing aids
- team member for pediatric and adult cochlear implants

Providing audiological services in health-care settings requires the ability to relate easily with patients/clients and their families/caregivers about the results of testing, the diagnosis of disability, and the plans for rehabilitation. The audiologist must be able to explain to patients the technologies available to assist them with hearing loss or related disorders. Further, the audiologist must be able to consult with other professionals about what it means to have a hearing loss, have a cochlear implant, use an AAC device, or have tinnitus or balance problems. Some audiologists also engage in educational activities for the general public and for policy makers in order to provide them with information about the needs of individuals with hearing disabilities.

Colleges and Universities

Educational institutions offering communication disorders training programs hire both audiologists and SLPs as instructors and as clinic supervisors. Instructors usually have a PhD, and clinic supervisors usually have a master's degree or AuD.

Businesses

Some corporations, particularly those in which employees are exposed to loud noise, employ audiologists. Audiologists who work for industry maintain hearing conservation programs, which involve monitoring environmental noise levels, testing employees' hearing, and fitting employees with ear protectors.

A number of firms that publish books and other materials for SLPs, or manufacture devices for people who have communication disorders, employ SLPs. Some such firms are, in fact, owned by SLPs.

Schools for the Deaf

Among the primary responsibilities of audiologists in schools for the deaf are hearing testing, hearing aid maintenance, and aural habilitation following a cochlear implant. They also may become involved with hearing habilitation, including teaching listening skills and strategies for communication.

SLPs in schools for the deaf typically provide intervention in the areas of voice, articulation, **speechreading**, language comprehension, and language use. SLPs working in schools for the deaf are typically fluent in **American Sign Language (ASL)**, which for many of the school's students is their primary language and, therefore, the language in which the SLP carries out intervention programs. SLPs also provide evaluation and treatment for phonological disorders, velopharyngeal insufficiency, and oral motor and feeding disorders. Some SLPs in schools for the deaf also assist in the maintenance of hearing aids, cochlear implants, and bone-anchored hearing aids. Most SLPs in these settings also offer parent/caregiver counseling.

Residential Facilities for People With Developmental Disabilities

Almost all of these residential facilities offer speech–language pathology services. Intervention focuses on functional communication skills (e.g., vocabulary needed to work at a sheltered workshop or take public transportation) and daily living skills. If a resident has severe developmental disabilities (and, hence, is incapable of acquiring sufficient speech to meet communication needs), services may include teaching gestural communication or use of an augmentative and alternative communication device.

For-Profit Corporations That Sell Services to Other Institutions

These for-profit corporations employ large numbers of SLPs and audiologists whose services are sold to schools, hospitals, nursing homes, rehabilitation facilities, and other institutions. Some of these corporations service institutions in only a single city or a single state; others operate nationally. Many of them also sell the services of other health-care professionals (e.g., physical therapists, occupational therapists, nurses).

Private Practice

The numbers of SLPs and audiologists who enter private practice, either part-time or full-time, have increased dramatically during the past 30 years. A major factor in the increase in the field of audiology is because increasing numbers of audiologists are now licensed as hearing aid dispensers. In addition, as cochlear implants have increased, audiologists in private practice are seeing increasing numbers of people with the implants. Another factor in SLPs' entering into private practice is that in 2008 Congress passed the Medicare Improvements for Patients and Providers Act (MIPPA), which allowed SLPs in private practice to bill Medicare directly.

A number of SLPs in private practice specialize in treating English language learners (ELL). These are usually people who were born in non-English-speaking countries and who are working in the United States. Some corporations will pay for services to improve the intelligibility of their employees' speech.

SLPs and audiologists in private practice usually rent offices in professional office buildings. They function professionally in the same manner as other independent practitioners who are in private practice.

One sign of the increased interest in private practice in audiology and speech–language pathology was the founding in the early 1960s of a professional association for private practitioners—the **American Academy of Private Practice in Speech Language Pathology and Audiology**. The organization acts as a platform for audiologists and SLPs in private practice from which they can share information about the business tools necessary to "establish, maintain, and expand clinical, educational and corporate services in the context of the private practice and to the improvement of the quality of services provided to the public" (American Academy of Private Practice in Speech Pathology and Audiology, 2014, para. 2).

Ethics

Every profession is guided by a set of principles that ensure that its members carry out their professional responsibilities with integrity, according to the highest standards of the profession. For SLPs and audiologists, this set of principles is codified in ASHA's code of ethics (2010). It consists of four basic rules, which I paraphrase below.

1. Individuals must hold paramount the welfare of their clients or people who are participating in research studies. They must treat animals involved in their research in a humane manner. Services must be provided without discrimination and must maintain confidentiality regarding the client.
2. Individuals must achieve and maintain the highest level of professional competence. This includes providing service only in the areas of qualification, and routinely participating in continuing professional development activities.
3. Individuals must promote public understanding of their profession, support the development of services for unmet public needs, and provide accurate information in all their communications regarding the profession. Individuals must not misrepresent their qualifications, credentials, or services.
4. Individuals must respect all professions and maintain harmonious relationships with members of the professions with whom they work. Individuals must not engage in any dishonesty, fraud, deceit, or form of conduct that would reflect adversely on the profession.

ASHA's code of ethics is intended to provide specific standards to cover most situations encountered by SLPs and audiologists. It aims to protect and promote the welfare of the individuals and groups with whom SLPs and audiologists work and to educate members, students, and the public regarding ethical standards of the discipline. Members of ASHA believe that the code of ethics requires a lifelong personal commitment to act ethically; to encourage ethical behavior by colleagues, employees, supervisees, and students; and to consult with colleagues regarding ethical questions and issues.

The Board of Ethics at ASHA periodically reviews the organization's code of ethics to determine whether the code is in need of modification to reflect changes and advances in technology, culture, language use, and population trends. In 2013, the Board issued a statement regarding cultural and linguistic competence (American Speech-Language-Hearing Association, 2014n). In this statement, the Board described the ethnic, cultural, and linguistic changes that have been occurring in the United States and urged audiologists and SLPs not to regard any of the resulting differences as disorders or deficiencies. Furthermore, the statement emphasized that service delivery by SLPs and audiologists must be "respectful of, and responsive to, an individual's values, preferences, and language. Care should not vary in quality based on ethnicity, age, socioeconomic status, or other factors" (para. 6). In other words, audiologists and SLPs are bound by the code of ethics to honor their clients' cultural and linguistic beliefs, values, and conventions regardless of their own personal cultural and linguistic backgrounds.

Multicultural Populations

Cultural perceptions of health, disease, communication, and authority all play significant roles in the intervention process. In planning intervention for multicultural (bilingual and non-standard-English-speaking) populations, clinicians must consider several factors, including the most appropriate language for intervention; any cultural factors that may influence the intervention process; materials that do not offend or upset the client or family; and intervention activities that are culturally appropriate for each client.

Appropriate Language for Children and Adults

Planning any sort of communication intervention with any client involves knowing his or her primary language and any secondary languages. ASHA's code of ethics is clear that clinicians must not discriminate in providing professional services and that if they are not competent to provide services to bilingual clients, they still have professional responsibility for making certain that a client receives appropriate services (American Speech-Language-Hearing Association, 2014f, para. 10).

Choosing which language to use during the intervention process will depend on the nature of the communication disorder and the family's wishes regarding their child's fluency in his or her first or subsequent languages. For instance, parents of one bilingual child with a **language disorder** may wish for intervention in his or her native language, while the parents of another bilingual child with the same disorder may wish the intervention to proceed in the child's second language. In the first case, a clinician who speaks the child's native language would be preferable. In the second case, the clinician must determine whether the child's second language is sufficiently developed for the intervention to proceed in an effective and efficient manner. If not, the clinician will need to counsel the parents about the need to conduct intervention in the child's native language.

Adult clients who cannot speak for themselves because of disease or injury to the brain will most often have family members who will be able to describe to the clinician the client's language abilities prior to intervention. In most cases, it will be obvious which language will be most effective and efficient to use during intervention. In those rare instances when a client has been equally fluent in more than one language, initial diagnostic testing will focus on determining which language faculties, if any, have been retained and are thus available to the intervention process. Ideally, the clinician will be fluent in whichever language seems during diagnostic testing to be most intact.

The political climate regarding bilingual education in the United States often dictates which language may be used in educational settings or how long a child's native language may be used in instruction. Language researcher Judith Johnston (2006) has pointed out that these policies are rarely based on objective research data but rest instead on cultural assumptions and beliefs that often collide with the needs of individuals needing intervention.

Service Delivery With Multicultural Populations

Communication sciences and disorders professionals address the needs of linguistically diverse clients in a number of areas, including accent training for adults who wish to modify their accents for occupational and/or social reasons; diagnosis and intervention for children who have speech, language or hearing disorders; and diagnosis and intervention for adults who have communication disorders following injury or disease.

ASHA (2014p) offers a wide range of resources to assist SLPs and audiologists in developing competence in providing services to clients belonging to cultures other than their own. Box 11.8 lists some of those available.

ASHA has also designed a set of self-assessment checklists for cultural competency that is available online (ASHA, 2014p). The checklists offer an opportunity for you to gauge your beliefs and attitudes toward other cultures, and the degree to

---

BOX 11.8   Some of the Resources Available From ASHA to Assist SLPs and Audiologists in Developing Competence in Providing Services to Clients From Cultures Other Than Their Own

- a cultural competence self-assessment instrument
- international resources to develop cultural competence
- collaborating with interpreters, transliterators, and translators
- bilingual service delivery
- multicultural constituency groups
- multicultural/multilingual issues (MMI) courses in communication sciences and disorders

which an agency or clinic attends to the needs of linguistically and culturally different populations.

The Impact of the DSM-5 on Clinical Practice

In Chapter 4, I introduced you to the *Diagnostic and Statistical Manual, Fifth Edition*, known as the DSM-5, published by the American Psychiatric Association (APA; 2013). This manual serves as the standard used to classify and diagnose what are considered mental disorders, which include several conditions for which audiologists and SLPs provide services and for which they bill insurance companies. The primary conditions from the DSM-5 that affect SLPs are listed in Box 11.9.

One of the major shortcomings of the new classifications in the DSM-5 is that they do not include any mention of oral language, language form, or language content deficits. Therefore, if an individual with autism spectrum disorder (ASD) has difficulties with oral language or with language form or content, clinicians will need to make a dual diagnosis of ASD and Language Disorder in order for individuals to receive the interventions they need and for clinicians to receive insurance reimbursements (ASHA, 2014c).

The APA complicated matters when they added a new category, Social Communication (Pragmatic) Disorder, that is intended to help clinicians identify individuals who have significant problems using verbal and nonverbal communication for social purposes. However, in order to identify an individual as having Social Communication Disorder, clinicians first need to rule out that the individual has ASD, which is characterized by restricted or repetitive patterns of behavior.

**BOX 11.9   Conditions Listed in the DSM-5
Affecting Services Provided by Audiologists and SLPs**

- autism spectrum disorder (ASD)
- language disorder
- speech sound disorder
- childhood-onset fluency disorder (stuttering)
- social (pragmatic) communication disorder
- unspecified communication disorder
- intellectual disability (intellectual developmental disorder)
- major and mild neurocognitive disorders (NCDs); includes dementia and Alzheimer's
- anxiety disorder that includes selective mutism
- specific learning disorder

The APA stated that their intention in creating the Social Communication Disorder category was to "more accurately recognize individuals who have significant problems using verbal and nonverbal communication for social purposes, leading to impairments in their ability to effectively communicate, participate socially, maintain social relationships, or otherwise perform academically or occupationally" (2014, para. 1). The disorder is characterized by problems with pragmatic language (not related to low cognitive ability), including difficulties with acquiring and using spoken and written language and with responding appropriately in conversations.

As a consequence of these changes in the DSM-5, some individuals will be classified as having ASD (but not Social [Pragmatic] Communication Disorder) and possibly Language Disorder (which focuses primarily on vocabulary and grammar), while others may be classified as having ASD and Language Disorder.

If you feel confused at this point, you are not alone! Fortunately, ASHA regularly publishes articles in *The ASHA Leader* to guide clinicians regarding the clinical implications of the new DSM-5 guidelines, the changes clinicians need to make in how they code their insurance claims in order to receive reimbursement, and case studies to illustrate how the changes impact individuals with communication, cognitive, and language disorders. Although the APA follows no prescribed timeline for revising the DSM, the revision process typically takes years; in fact, more than 10 years elapsed between the DSM-IV and the DSM-5. Consequently, clinicians will have ample time to adjust to the latest diagnostic categories and criteria.

chapter 12

The Importance of the Clinical Relationship

Learning Objectives

Identify the interactions that take place within the clinical relationship.

Describe how a therapeutic relationship differs from other relationships.

Identify the characteristics of a good therapeutic relationship.

Discuss how the clinician's beliefs about the cause of a communication disorder affect a client's motivation and progress during intervention.

Describe what clinicians must do to leave their needs outside the therapeutic relationship.

Describe how clinicians can best motivate clients and convey their belief that change is possible.

Overview

The context within which clinical services are dispensed is a relationship involving the clinician, the client, and those close to the client (e.g., parents/caregivers, other family members, friends). This context may be one in which the clinician interacts with a number of members of the client's family or friends. The client is more likely to improve if these interactions are good ones, regardless of the disorder and the intervention strategy being used. Consequently, it is crucial that clinicians be aware of the variables that affect this relationship and, thereby, their ability to be helpful to their clients. In this chapter I discuss some of these variables to give you information that will help you in making your interactions with clients more effective.

The term *client* is used in this chapter and throughout this book to designate the person the clinician is trying to help. Other terms may be used to designate this person, including *patient* or *student*. However, I chose the term *client* both because of its wide utilization in medical and educational settings and because it implies that the person who ultimately is in charge is not the clinician but either the person who sought the clinician's help or a member of his or her family or circle of friends.

What Is the Clinical Relationship?

The **clinical relationship** (i.e., therapeutic relationship) consists of more than the interaction between the clinician and the client. It also includes the relationship between the clinician and each of the client's significant others, and between the client and each of his or her significant others.

Except with young children, the most important of these interactions is usually the one between client and clinician. With young children, the most important interaction is usually between the clinician and the child's parents/caregivers. What these interactions entail is largely determined by the clinician's ability to treat the client as a person rather than as a disorder, or, as Oliver Sacks (1985) so aptly put it, as a biography rather than a disease. The interactions between clinician and client (or significant others) may occur in several settings: in a **therapy room,** in which the client and clinician sit in chairs at a table, or, with young children, on the floor; in the client's natural environment (e.g., home or classroom); digitally (e.g., via e-mail, video conferencing, the use of specialty apps); or on the telephone.

Doing therapy in the client's classroom rather than in a special therapy room is referred to as **collaborative service delivery (integrative treatment model).** Because the Individuals With Disabilities Education Improvement Act of 2004 (Center for Parent Information and Resources, 2014b) requires that children be provided a free, appropriate public education in the least restrictive environment (LRE), **speech–language pathologists (SLPs)** frequently favor providing services in the classroom rather than pulling a child out for individual therapy in a special therapy room. However, because there is very limited evidence-based research regarding the efficacy of doing therapy in the classroom compared with in a therapy room, Cirrin et al. (2010) believed that clinicians "need to select service models carefully, monitor students' progress on a regular and frequent basis, and validate the effectiveness of the intervention program for each student on their caseloads" (para. 47).

Another aspect of the clinical relationship is the relationship between the clinician and the client's significant others. This includes the client's parents/caregivers, spouse, partner, friends, children, classroom teacher, other professionals, and **paraprofessionals,** which I described in Chapter 11. In some instances, this relationship is more important for helping a client than the relationship between the client and the clinician. For instance, when the SLP sees a preschool child whose parents are concerned that he or she is beginning to stutter, the SLP will need to develop a strong relationship with the child's family to provide maximally effective intervention. Some clinicians manage the disorder in such children primarily by counseling the parents.

A third aspect of the clinical relationship is between a client and his or her significant others. This interaction can profoundly influence the likelihood that therapy will be successful. If, for example, those close to a client indicate that they are pleased with how he or she is changing, the client is more likely to continue trying to change than if they indicate dissatisfaction or concern with the client's progress.

This YouTube video describes the clinical relationship from the viewpoint of individuals who have aphasia and from that of several care providers, including SLPs. Sponsored by the National Aphasia Association, it clearly delineates the primary factors care providers need to know in order to communicate most effectively with their clients. Go to the website (http://goo.gl/P8yxI8) or scan the code.

Characteristics of a Good Therapeutic Relationship

In the National Aphasia Association video I mentioned in the previous paragraph, you can see one of the most important characteristics of a good therapeutic relationship: mutual respect. The clinician respects the client and manifests this respect by treating the client as a person, not a "defective mouth" or a "defective ear." Interacting with the client as a person, not as a stereotype, is particularly important for every clinical relationship but especially if the client is from a **culture** different from the clinician's own. Mutual respect also means the clinician refers to the client not as his or her disorder (e.g., "the aphasic," "the LLD kid") but rather as a person who has a particular condition (e.g., "the man with Wernicke's aphasia" or "the student with language-learning disabilities").

While mutual respect is required for a good therapeutic relationship, mutual liking is not. It certainly is desirable for clinician and client to like each other as people, but it isn't essential. We all know people whom we respect a great deal professionally but would not enjoy spending time with socially. Maintaining objectivity and respecting the client as a person allows clinicians to provide services in a professional way whether or not they like the client. When clinicians want to be liked by a client, they can lose their objectivity and become less able to be helpful to the client.

In a good therapeutic relationship, the client can trust the clinician to treat what he or she is told as confidential. Clients must feel free to reveal things about themselves to the clinician that they do not necessarily want revealed to others, even family members.

The participants in a good therapeutic relationship are willing to be honest with each other. They do not tell the other what they want to hear if it is not the truth. Clients, for example, may tell their clinicians that they avoid speaking less often than they do because they want to please them. Or clinicians may not insist that their clients complete assignments regularly because they want to avoid upsetting them and possibly having them discontinue therapy. However, either action could adversely affect progress.

Having **empathy** for one's client helps build a good therapeutic relationship. If the client feels that the clinician does not really understand his or her reactions to the **communication disorder**, the client may not follow through on the clinician's recommendations.

Successful communication between client and clinician is essential for a good therapeutic relationship. Communication is the medium through which the clinician attempts to influence the client and the client attempts to make the clinician aware of his or her needs. Communicating with children whose **language** development is impaired often requires using other modes of interaction (e.g., play) to establish a relationship through which to communicate. In any case, the client is unlikely to be helped by the therapy experience if communication is poor.

In a good therapeutic relationship, the client believes that the clinician values him or her as a person, believes the client's goals are paramount, and wants the client to reach his or her goals. It is crucial that the clinician communicate to the client in every way possible that this is the case.

You are unlikely to be successful with a client you do not value as a person. Every clinician occasionally encounters a client with whom he or she cannot relate well. When such a situation occurs, the client should be referred to another clinician to satisfy the **American Speech-Language-Hearing Association's (ASHA)** ethical requirement to hold paramount the welfare of the client.

Clinicians who continually offer hope that the client can reach the goals they set contribute to a good therapeutic relationship. Although clinicians cannot guarantee improvement, they can offer clients and their significant others hope that they can reach their goals. It is unethical for a clinician to accept a client for therapy or to continue treating a client if there is little likelihood of further improvement. A client who does not really believe that what the clinician is recommending will be effective is less likely to follow recommendations, which would tend to reduce the effectiveness of the therapy program.

In a good therapeutic relationship the clinician gives the client the opportunity to experience success whenever possible. The most successful therapeutic programs are those designed to support clients in moving step-by-step from what they can do to things that are more difficult, eventually culminating in accomplishing things that initially might have seemed beyond the client's capabilities. If clients are asked to do things that are too difficult and that result in failure, they are likely to terminate therapy rather than continue what, to them, is an unpleasant experience. Moreover, when clients set their own goals, they are more likely to want to reach them.

Successful therapeutic relationships are based on a **contract** between client and clinician. The contract (which may actually be written) specifies the obligations each agrees to assume in the relationship. The clinician promises to contribute his or her time and expertise, and the client promises to follow through on the clinician's recommendations for reaching his or her goals, which have been determined through collaboration between client and clinician.

Finally, a good therapeutic relationship is one in which the clinician is willing to share experiences and feelings with the client if the clinician perceives this would benefit the client and encourage the client's reciprocal sharing. The use of life experience stories is one way for the clinician to share experiences and feelings with the client.

Sharing life experiences is one reason why **support groups** (such as that shown in the aforementioned video) for persons who have a particular problem (e.g., Lost Cord clubs, National Aphasia Association, the Learning Disabilities Association of America, the National Stuttering Association) can be very helpful to those with similar experiences and communication needs.

Dr. Carl Rogers (1942), a renowned psychotherapist, described the basic elements of a therapeutic relationship as requiring of the clinician

- warmth and responsiveness,
- openness for the client's expression of feeling, and
- a structure for the therapeutic process.

Variables That Influence a Clinical Relationship

Several variables affect the therapeutic relationship. A clinician's success at being helpful to a client is likely to be determined as much (or possibly even more) by the client as by the clinician's knowledge of therapeutic techniques. The clinician's beliefs, needs, and motivation also play an important role in the relationship. At bottom, though, the model (or combination of models) the clinician uses to provide service will influence the relationship.

The Medical Model

For a long time, the **medical model** was the approach most frequently used by SLPs and audiologists. Using the medical model, the clinician diagnoses the communication disorder and designs and directs the intervention process, which is focused on remediating the disorder. This approach grew out of an effort by the profession of communication disorders to incorporate scientifically supported approaches to the diagnosis and remediation of communication disorders. As Duchan (2001) explained it, the medical model involves "synthesizing what is going on at the biological, psychological and social levels. Such a synthesis is offered by the causal logic of the medical model" (para. 8).

From the perspective of the medical model, the therapeutic relationship is different from other relationships in five ways. First, there is a predetermined time frame during which it can take place. An **evaluation** or therapy session is expected to begin and end at a prearranged time on a prearranged day. The duration of the relationship is likely to be relatively short. In fact, the relationship may exist for only an hour or less (e.g., when an evaluation reveals that a child's **speech** or language development is within normal limits).

Second, the therapeutic relationship exists solely for accomplishing a specific task—eliminating or lessening the severity of the client's communication disorder.

After the task is accomplished, or when further progress seems unlikely, the relationship is usually terminated.

Third, this relationship is not a symmetrical one—the parties play different roles. The client is in the role of the person in need of care, and the clinician is in the role of care provider. For this reason, the client may develop a strong affection for the clinician. This situation can be helpful if handled appropriately by the clinician, because the client is more likely to do what the clinician recommends in order to please the clinician. On the other hand, the situation is less desirable if a clinician becomes overly emotionally attached to a client because the clinician is likely to lose some of the **objectivity** needed to be helpful to the client.

A fourth way the clinical relationship in the medical model differs from others is that one party purchases the services of the other. The client either pays for the clinician's services or arranges for a third party, such as a private or government insurance program (e.g., **Medicare**) or a school district, to make payment.

A final unique aspect of the therapeutic relationship is that only one party is expected to be concerned about the welfare of the other. ASHA's **Code of Ethics** obliges the clinician to hold paramount the welfare of persons served professionally (ASHA, 2010). The client has no such obligation to the clinician.

The Participation Model

As professionals in communication disorders have learned more about the nature of the clinical relationship and expanded the range of settings in which they interact with clients, clinicians (SLPs and audiologists alike) have developed an increasing awareness of other models that offer considerable insight into how we can best assist our clients in their daily lives (Duchan, 2001). One model offered by Duchan is what she calls the **participation model**, in which the focus of the clinical relationship is not the communication disorder but rather on who the client is as a person, how he or she experiences life, and his or her goals (Duchan, 2003). In this model, clients participate fully in the therapeutic process, select their intervention goals, plan the course of therapy, and evaluate their own progress in the context of their life outside the therapy setting.

The therapeutic relationship from the perspective of the participation model has four characteristics that distinguish it from other relationships. Clinicians using the participation model focus on (1) what clients think about themselves, (2) clients' abilities and accomplishments, (3) clients' disabilities, and (4) clients' future (Duchan, 2003). The following are examples of participation models used by clinicians.

1. **Person-centered planning** allows the client to choose from among the many resources and tools offered by the clinician to determine the path he or she wishes to take during the intervention process.
2. **Client and clinician narratives** are used as a means for each to construct an ongoing life experience story that "charts" the therapeutic relationship.

For the client, the story includes narrative regarding progress toward his or her goals. For the clinician, the story includes narrative regarding his or her participation in the client's story (Shields, 1997). Hinckley (2007) proposed the use of autoethnographic narratives, not only as a means of engaging with clients but also as a way for clinicians to reflect on their own growth as clinicians.

3. **Life inclusion intervention** emphasizes the therapeutic relationship as the care and support necessary for the client to be included in his or her community (Calculator & Jorgensen, 1994). Inclusion is considered a core principle in the early intervention systems of most states.

Duchan (2003) suggested that clinicians can best serve their clients by taking the best of both the medical and participation model. She advocates combining them in a creative fashion to suit each client's unique needs and strengths.

The Clinician's Belief About the Cause of the Communication Disorder

The therapy program developed for a client should be based on the clinician's **hypotheses** about the cause(s) of the client's communication disorder, paired with the client's (or family's) perceptions about the goals he or she believes would be best, given his or her life experiences. These hypotheses are developed, in part, from the results of an initial evaluation, which I discuss in more detail in Chapter 13. A therapy program that is based on such hypotheses is more likely to be effective than one that is not.

These hypotheses also help the client and clinician develop realistic goals. The client's potential for improvement is likely to be partially determined by the etiology and severity of his or her communication disorder. If a child is unable to produce the /r/ phoneme correctly, the prognosis for improvement should be better if the reason is faulty learning rather than paralysis of the tongue.

Finally, the clinician's hypotheses can influence whether he or she will develop an intervention plan with the client or will refer the client to another practitioner. An SLP or audiologist is not the appropriate professional to treat some communication disorders. For instance, an adult who exhibits **hypernasality** because of **myasthenia gravis** should be treated by a neurologist because the **dysarthria** responsible for it often can be reduced by medication.

The Clinician's Needs

Clinicians have the same emotional needs as other people, including a need to be liked. However, clinicians must maintain their professional perspective and keep their own emotional needs out of the therapeutic process with their clients. This is not to say that clinicians must refrain from discussing feelings, fears, or perceptions.

Rather, it means that the focus must remain on the clients and their communication needs and strengths.

Failure to act in a professional manner can impact negatively on clinicians' ability to help clients. For instance, they may hesitate to recommend that clients do things that are not "fun," or they may not speak honestly to the client because they don't want to be disliked. Another possible professional pitfall is discussing one's personal problems with clients, which can lead to a role reversal, in which clients function as clinicians and clinicians as clients.

Clinicians must constantly monitor their professional behavior, remembering that one of their primary goals is to promote the welfare of their clients. The therapeutic relationship must have at its center the clients' communication needs and the steps that can be taken to assist them in their efforts to improve their communication abilities.

The Clinician's Ability to Motivate the Client

Clients are unlikely to change unless their **motivation** for change is strong. They will be unwilling to make the necessary investment unless they believe that doing it will be worth the sacrifice—that is, the change will significantly improve the quality of their life. A clinician's ability to motivate a client is an important determiner of the benefit the client is likely to receive from therapy. One way clinicians can motivate clients is through the use of motivational interviewing, which is defined by W. R. Miller and Rollnick (2002) as a "client-centered, directive method for enhancing intrinsic motivation to change by exploring and resolving ambivalence" (p. 25). McFarlane (2012) described motivational interviewing as a combination of

- collaboration—the acknowledgement that the knowledge and perspective of both client and clinician must be considered;
- evocation—the understanding by both client and clinician that the reasons for and decisions to change reside with the client; and
- autonomy—the understanding by both client and clinician that the client is independent and in control of her or his therapeutic process.

A clinician can also motivate clients by making them aware of their progress toward achieving their goals. Clients are more likely to continue investing in their therapy programs if they believe they are making real progress.

Helping the Client Believe Change Is Possible

Clients seeking therapy may not really believe they can change. They may, in fact, believe deep down that they cannot change. Clients who lack confidence in their ability to change are unlikely to do so. In addition, young children and adolescents often see no reason for why they should engage in activities that, from their perspective, lack relevance and meaning. In both these situations, the clinician must be able to communicate with the client in a way that results in the client understanding that the therapy activities lead to desired change.

Why might a client be certain he or she cannot change? One reason may be that previous therapy has been unsuccessful. The more often a client has experienced failure in a therapy experience, the more likely it is that he or she will not believe change is possible. Similarly, children may have experienced therapy that was unpleasant or that took them away from what they perceive as something more interesting. Or, like their adult counterparts, they may perceive previous therapy experiences as unsuccessful and be unwilling to participate further.

Here's an analogy that might help you understand how this situation might arise. Consider a change that you have tried to make at some time in your life (e.g., to lose weight by dieting). If your first diet was recommended by somebody you regarded as an authority on dieting, you probably began with a high degree of optimism. However, if your current diet is your fifth and you regarded the previous four as having been unsuccessful, you probably would not have begun this new diet with as much optimism as you did your first. You may, in fact, have begun it with the expectation (conscious or unconscious) that it would not work, and, consequently, you would be likely to quit at the first indication that it was not working. Of course, going off your diet would result in your not losing weight, which, in turn, would reinforce your certainty that you are unable to lose weight by dieting.

When clients believe they cannot change, their clinician can play a major role in helping them change their mind. The best way is to help them change some aspect of their behavior so they can see they are able to change. While the aspect they change may not be a particularly important one, such a change can cause them to question their certainty that they cannot change—because they have just done it.

If a client enters therapy with the certainty that it will not be effective, he or she is unlikely to change, regardless of the type and severity of the disorder, the skill of the clinician, or the management program used. The clinician may have to engage in activities with which he or she knows the client will be successful, gradually introducing new tasks that are less familiar and more difficult. The key is to provide support throughout the therapeutic process so the client is taking small, successful steps rather than attempting a large one that could result in failure.

A clinician can cause a client to expect a therapy to be ineffective for another reason—by communicating a lack of confidence or competence. If the clinician seems bored, superior, or impatient, the client will surely get the message, regardless of what the clinician says. So, too, will the client if the clinician sincerely believes the client can make little or no progress, despite saying otherwise.

chapter 13

Assessment, Evaluation, Diagnosis, and Intervention

Learning Objectives

Describe the clinical evaluation process.

Differentiate among assessment, evaluation, and diagnosis.

Describe three general approaches for making observations that answer evaluation questions.

Describe how to ensure the validity of the data used to answer evaluation questions.

Describe how to ensure the reliability of the data used to answer evaluation questions.

Describe the process of formulating and testing hypotheses.

List three types of assessment instruments used in the evaluation process.

Describe how the results of the evaluation guide the intervention plan.

Describe how the severity of a communication impairment affects intervention.

Describe the difference between intervention aimed at remediating a disorder and intervention aimed at building compensatory strategies.

Describe the basic steps in the intervention process.

Overview

The clinical evaluation process consists of various assessment procedures the clinician uses in order to diagnose (particularly **differential diagnosis**) an individual's **communication disorder**, which leads to the design of appropriate **intervention** for individuals with communication disorders. Evaluation typically takes place throughout the course of intervention as a way to chart the client's progress. Recall that in Chapter 4 I described the assessment and intervention process as occurring in three phases: (1) assessment, (2) intervention and ongoing data collection, and (3) reassessment. In this chapter, I go into more detail about these three phases.

The Clinical Evaluation Process

The clinical evaluation process begins with the clinician asking specific **questions** and making the observations necessary to answer them. From the answers to these questions, the clinician formulates and tests **hypotheses**. If these hypotheses seem invalid (i.e., not logical or reasonable) or if their validity is uncertain, the clinician reexamines the **observations** on which the hypotheses were based. Next, the clinician may ask and answer some additional questions based on the findings so far. Then, based upon what was learned from the answers to all these questions, the clinician reformulates and retests these hypotheses. The process is repeated until the clinician is satisfied that the hypotheses are sufficiently valid for planning intervention. In the following sections I describe this process in more detail.

Asking Reasonable Questions

The clinical evaluation process is initiated by asking appropriate, answerable questions. Consider the following question: "How well does my client, who has **aphasia**, understand **speech**?" This question is answerable through making certain specific observations. In this example, the necessary observations would be ones that provide information about the client's ability to understand speech.

The following question, on the other hand, does not appear to be reasonable—or answerable: "How well will my client, who has aphasia, understand speech in 2 years?" There is no way to observe this—unless one is a clairvoyant or has the ability to travel in time—which makes it unanswerable. Although the question can be addressed by making a prediction (i.e., prognosis) based on past experience, a prediction is not the same thing as an answer.

The specific questions a clinician will ask during an evaluation are determined by the purpose of the evaluation, which will depend on the type of communication disorder, the age of the client, and the severity of the disorder, among others. Box 13.1 lists examples of specific questions a clinician might ask.

Although some of these questions are not related directly to a client's speech, **hearing**, or **language** functions, the answers to them could directly affect how his or her case is managed and the type, length, and frequency of intervention sessions. If, for example, a client fatigues easily, the clinician might need to keep therapy sessions relatively short.

In addition to questions that are intended to define a client's communication disorder, others are asked after a period of therapy to determine how well a client is progressing. Box 13.2 shows examples of questions that might be asked throughout the intervention process.

BOX 13.1   Examples of Specific Questions a Clinician Might Ask During the Initial Evaluation Process

- Is the client's hearing for pure tones within normal limits?
- Why hasn't the client, who is 4 years old, begun to say words?
- Is the client more likely to understand a spoken or written message?
- Under what circumstances does the client avoid speaking?
- Does the client appear to fatigue easily?
- How concerned does the client appear to be about her syllable and word repetitions?

BOX 13.2   Examples of Questions a Clinician Might Ask Throughout the Intervention Process

- How much reduction (if any) has there been in the severity of the client's stuttering?
- Does the client ask questions in class more frequently than before?
- Has the client learned to produce the /r/ sound correctly at the beginning of words?
- Have the client's parents accepted sign language being taught to their child?
- How well does the client understand speech with the hearing aid he or she is currently using?
- Has the client reached a **plateau**, or is improvement likely to occur with further therapy?

How does a clinician decide which questions are appropriate for a particular evaluation? This decision is based partly on the client's **chief complaint**. However, certain questions are asked routinely, no matter what type of communication disorder the client has (e.g., Is the client's pure-tone hearing within normal limits?).

Answering Questions

After the initial set of questions has been selected, the clinician attempts to answer them. Because the answers are likely to suggest additional questions, the clinician will probably be formulating new questions while answering the original ones. Consequently, two of the tasks in the evaluation process (asking and answering questions) often occur simultaneously.

How do clinicians answer questions? They make observations they hope will yield data that are **valid**, **reliable**, and **representative** of the client's functioning.

The validity of the data used to answer a question is determined by the appropriateness of the observations selected. If a clinician makes observations that are appropriate for answering a question, the data yielded by them are likely to be adequately valid for the purpose. Suppose a clinician wanted to answer the question,

"Does my client have a hearing loss?" Valid data for answering this question would be yielded by a **pure-tone** hearing test. On the other hand, if the clinician clapped her or his hands and observed the client's reaction, the observation would yield an invalid piece of data.

The reliability of the data used to answer a question is determined by the repeatability, or consistency, of the observations selected. If a clinician makes observations in a manner that can be repeated, the resulting data are usually adequately reliable for the purpose. If an **audiologist** tests a client's hearing with a **pure-tone audiometer** that has not been **calibrated**, the reliability of the data yielded by the test will be uncertain. That is, the results might be different at a different time or with a different audiometer.

The representativeness of the data used to answer a question determines if the same answer will be given in other situations (e.g., home, school, work). In other words, are the data generalizable? If a clinician makes observations that are representative, the data yielded by them should possess some generality. Suppose a **speech–language pathologist (SLP)** wanted to answer the following question: "How severe is a child's language disorder?" If the clinician observes the client at home as well as in school, the generality of the answer will be greater because the clinician will have gathered data from more than one context in which the child uses language.

Clinicians use four general approaches for making the observations needed to answer questions: (1) administering tests (**standardized tests**, developmental scales, and criterion-referenced procedures); (2) completing informal observations; (3) interviewing informants; and (4) dynamic assessment.

Administering Tests

One approach that SLPs and audiologists utilize to generate the data they need to answer questions is to administer standardized tests. A wide variety of standardized test instruments is available for evaluating communication disorders, some of which I alluded to in earlier chapters on the various types of communication disorders. Here I describe six basic types of standardized tests.

Audiometric Tests. The two most common audiometric tests are pure-tone audiometric testing and **tympanometry**, both of which I described in Chapter 10. You will remember that pure-tone audiometric tests are used to assess the acuity and sensitivity of a client's ears. They can detect disturbances in the functioning of the outer, middle, or inner portions of an ear as well as the **auditory nerve**. Pure tones of various frequencies are presented at various loudness levels through earphones by an electronic instrument known as a pure-tone audiometer.

One type of pure-tone audiometric test is referred to as an **audiometric screening test**, which is used to determine whether a client's hearing acuity needs further testing. Pure tones of various frequencies are presented to one ear at a time (through earphones) at a loudness level that, though soft, can be heard by most people. Clients are told to raise their hand when they hear a tone. If they consistently respond when tones are presented and refrain from responding when no tones are presented, they pass the test. Otherwise, they fail the test and are usually given a complete audiometric assessment.

Tympanometry, also described in Chapter 10, is the method used to detect disorders of the middle ear. Air pressure in the eustachian tube is varied to test the condition and mobility of the tympanic membrane. Box 13.3 lists the conditions for which tympanometry is most frequently used.

Language Tests for Children and Adolescents. Clinicians use tests to assess children's and adolescents' language functioning across the areas of language development, described in Chapter 4. Recall that in that chapter I explained that most language tests are standardized on a large number of individuals from across the United States who reflect the most current demographic statistics of the U.S. Census Bureau. Scores are collected from all types of individuals, which makes them representative of a wide range of children or adolescents from all areas of the United States. In addition, users can be confident that standardized tests, because they are valid and reliable, measure what they say they measure and will consistently measure the same thing, regardless of who administers the test or when it is administered.

Clinicians use language tests in order to determine whether a child or adolescent has a general **language disorder** that crosses form, content, and use, or whether the child or adolescent has a language disorder in one specific area. The most commonly used language tests assess children's and adolescents' abilities in the following areas:

- Vocabulary (comprehension and production)
- Syntax and morphology (comprehension and production)
- Phonology
- Pragmatics
- Discourse
- Written language

**BOX 13.3   Tympanometry Is Typically Used
to Check for These Conditions:**

- fluid in the middle ear
- otitis media
- perforated (torn) tympanic membrane
- impacted cerumen
- scarring of the tympanic membrane (usually from infection)
- lack of contact between the ossicles
- a tumor in the middle ear
- a problem with the eustachian tube

If a child or adolescent scores below average on a battery of language tests, one of the primary questions the clinician must ask is whether the scores reflect an actual language disorder or a language difference arising from English as the child's non-native language. Children whose language abilities are different purely as a result of not knowing English well enough to score well do not have a communication disorder. Most children in this situation are well able to learn language skills given appropriate support and instruction, while children with language disorders usually require intensive and specific intervention aimed at remediating their deficient language skills.

Language Tests for Adults. Adult language disorders usually stem from brain damage related to stroke, tumor, trauma, or **degenerative** disease. The language tests used with adults differ from those used with children and adolescents in that adult instruments focus on how intact the person's language abilities are following the brain damage, while the tests used with children and, to some extent, adolescents assess primarily developmental language abilities. Most standardized tests for adults with brain damage assess the following:

- Articulation
- Fluency
- Word finding
- Repetition
- Grammar
- Auditory comprehension
- Reading
- Writing
- Visual-motor ability
- Spelling

In addition to **standardized assessments**, many SLPs use functional communication assessment tools, which are often less biased than standardized tests in evaluating clients from linguistically or culturally diverse backgrounds. Functional assessments usually assess the following:

- Telling time
- Using verbal and nonverbal contexts in communicating
- Role playing
- Observing social conventions (i.e., pragmatics)
- Understanding and using humor, metaphors, and absurdities
- Understanding and using number concepts

Articulation Tests. Articulation tests enable clinicians to both identify and inventory a client's articulation errors (i.e., sound omissions, substitutions, and distortions) at the beginning, middle, and end of words. (Refer to Chapter 8 for information about articulation disorders.) One type of articulation test is the picture articulation test, which is used mostly with young children. The child is shown a series of drawings or photographs, as shown in Figure 13.1, and asked to name the objects depicted in them. Their names contain each English phoneme at least once at the beginning of a word (initial position), at the end of a word (final position), and in the middle of a word (medial position). The clinician indicates on a form whether the **target phoneme** was produced correctly and, if it was not, the type of error made. The resulting error inventory is used both for setting therapy goals and as a **baseline** for evaluating therapy effectiveness.

Tests of Motor Functioning. Motor functioning tests are used for assessing the functioning of the muscles used for respiration, phonation, and articulation. These tests provide the data necessary for determining whether the musculature is adequate to support the production of normal speech. A client who fails any of these tests may have a neuromuscular disorder.

One motor functioning test that is used with both children and adults is the determination of **diadochokinetic rates** for certain consonant–vowel syllables (e.g., the initial consonant and vowel in the word *tub*). The number of times the client is able to repeat the syllable in 5 seconds is compared to that of persons his or her age who are not neurologically impaired. Relatively low diadochokinetic rates (e.g., less than one repetition per second) suggest that the functioning of at least one articulator is not adequate to support the production of normal speech.

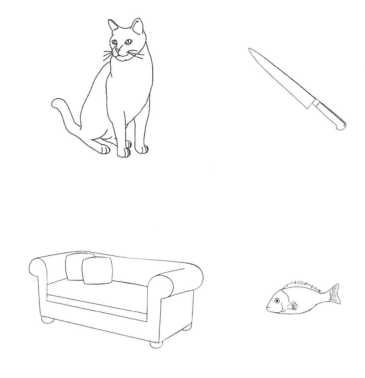

FIGURE 13.1. Figures with the /f/ phoneme in initial, medial, and final position, and one figure with no /f/ phonemes.

Tests of Attitude. Attitude tests can provide some insight into the nature of a client's attitude toward his or her communication disorder. This sort of test contains statements similar to the following:

- A student with a communication disorder should not ask questions in class.

  Strongly Agree, Moderately Agree, Undecided, Moderately Disagree, Strongly Disagree

- A person should be embarrassed if he has a communication disorder.

  Strongly Agree, Moderately Agree, Undecided, Moderately Disagree, Strongly Disagree

The client responds to each statement by circling the words that best describe his or her reaction to it. If the responses are honest, they can provide considerable insight into the degree to which the client is handicapped by having the communication disorder.

Informal Observations

Gathering informal observations entails collecting the data needed to answer questions by observing relevant behaviors in natural contexts rather than by eliciting them in a testing context. For example, to identify and inventory a client's articulation errors, you could tape-record a conversation with the client and later listen to the recording to abstract relevant information from it. Another example would be videotaping a child playing with his or her parent in order to determine mean length of utterance, different types of pragmatic intentions used, and types of words used in expressive language.

As I pointed out in Chapter 4, informal observations have both advantages and disadvantages compared with administering standardized tests. Perhaps the main advantage of utilizing data samples that were gathered by informal observation is that they are more likely to reflect how a client typically communicates in his or her environment than when data samples are elicited by a test. Perhaps the main disadvantage of utilizing data samples that were generated by indirect observation rather than by testing is that this approach may be considerably more time-consuming. This would, for example, tend to be the case for identifying and inventorying articulation errors.

On the other hand, for some questions, informal observation may actually be less time-consuming than testing may be. For instance, if a clinician wants to know if a person with aphasia has a deficit in his ability to understand speech, having an informal conversation with the person would be likely to yield an answer as accurate as administering an **aphasia test**. However, the following question would probably be best answered through the use of a standardized test: "How impaired is the client's ability to understand speech?" Test data collected from a standardized instrument would be more likely than informal observation to yield an accurate estimate.

Keep in mind that informal observations may not be as valid or as reliable as standardized instruments, but what the clinician learns from these observations often leads to a fine-tuning of the assessment process.

Interviewing Family, Teachers, and Other Professionals

Clinicians interview family members, teachers, or other professionals to obtain relevant information about the client. The type of data that can be collected from interviews ranges from the developmental history and background of the communication disorder to current communication functioning in everyday life. Interviews can be performed live between clinician and interviewee, via teleconferencing or videoconferencing, or through interview checklists that are completed by the interviewee(s). Chapters 4 and 6 include detailed descriptions of case histories.

Dynamic Assessment

Dynamic assessment involves a test–teach–retest approach that turns intervention into an ongoing assessment process leading directly to treatment. It is important to note that assessment in this context does *not* equal testing. Rather, the assessment, because it is dynamic, focuses on using the individual's responses to the clinician's supportive probes as guidance for what to do next. It involves finding out what the individual knows (testing), supporting the individual to learn something beyond what she or he already knows (teaching), and reassessing to see what happened (retesting).

Many clinicians utilize dynamic assessment because it is an interactive procedure in which the clinician is an active partner in the individual's learning and rehabilitation process. In addition, because each step involves testing, teaching, and retesting, the clinician knows exactly what the individual is learning. In other words, through the process of dynamic assessment, the clinician is able to collect the data necessary to guide intervention in the most effective and efficient manner.

All four of the above approaches (i.e., tests, observations, interviews, and dynamic assessment) may be utilized for making the observations needed to answer a question. Suppose an audiologist wanted to answer the question, "How well does a child's hearing aid compensate for his or her hearing loss?" To answer this question, the audiologist is likely to administer one or more hearing tests, informally observe how well the child seems to understand what is said while wearing the hearing aid, and question the child's parent about how well the child seems to understand what is said at home while wearing it.

All data yielded by such observations are unlikely to be given equal weight for answering questions. For instance, in the example in the previous paragraph, the audiologist would be unlikely to need to use dynamic assessment as part of the process of determining how well the child's hearing aid compensates for her or his hearing loss. In addition, some of these approaches are regarded as having greater validity, reliability, and generality for the purpose than are others. The more valid and reliable the data used for answering a question, the more confidence a clinician can have in the accuracy of the answer.

Formulating, Testing, and Reexamining Hypotheses

After the clinician's questions have been answered, the next task during an initial evaluation is to use the information obtained to formulate hypotheses about the etiology and severity of the client's communication disorder. If it is an ongoing evaluation, the next task would be to assess the impact the therapy program had on the disorder. An example of such a hypothesis follows: "Based upon the information I currently have available, the most likely explanation for the problem that the client is having with understanding speech is a **conductive hearing loss**."

The phrase "based upon the information I currently have available" suggests an important characteristic of such hypotheses: they always are viewed as tentative and subject to change as new information becomes available. New information may make it necessary to revise or abandon a hypothesis. Of course, it can also support a hypothesis.

An example of a hypothesis about the impact of a therapy program on a client follows: "Based upon the information I currently have available, the program has decreased the severity of the client's **stuttering**."

After the hypothesis has been formulated, it is tested. The approach clinicians use depends on whether the hypothesis deals with etiology or therapy outcome.

Hypotheses Regarding Etiology

Testing hypotheses about the etiology of a client's disorder involves determining whether the hypotheses allow the clinician to make accurate predictions about the disorder's symptoms and characteristics. That is, if a hypothesis about the etiology of a client's communication disorder is accurate, it should predict how the client's symptoms will vary under certain conditions. If, for example, an audiologist hypothesized that a client doesn't comprehend speech normally because of a conductive hearing loss caused by a bacterial infection, he or she would predict that antibiotics would improve the client's comprehension. If the client's comprehension improved under this condition (i.e., using antibiotics), the clinician's hypothesis would be supported. The clinician could also make other predictions about how the client's hearing would vary if the cause was a conductive hearing loss resulting from **otitis media** and check to see if the hearing varied in the way(s) predicted by the hypothesis.

Hypotheses About Therapy Outcome

A second type of prediction deals with the impact of intervention. If the hypothesis about the etiology of the disorder is accurate, it should allow the effect of intervention on the disorder to be predicted (assuming both that the disorder is treatable and other variables, such as a lack of motivation, are not impeding improvement).

The intervention program a clinician develops for a client should be based on the clinician's assumptions about the cause of the client's communication disorder.

The alternative—using the same intervention for all people who have a particular disorder, regardless of its cause—is not acceptable because it is unlikely to be effective.

Testing hypotheses about therapy outcome involves determining what the available data indicate about differences (if any) between a client's current status and status during the earlier evaluation period that serves as a baseline. Conclusions about program effectiveness are, in fact, hypotheses of this type, comparisons between baseline and periodic assessments of current status. Dynamic assessment is a good example of this type of hypothesis testing.

A clinician can reach one of three conclusions about the validity of a hypothesis. If the available data clearly supported it, the hypothesis would tentatively be regarded as valid. If the available data clearly appeared to refute it, the hypothesis would tentatively be regarded as invalid. And if the available data neither unequivocally supported nor refuted it, its validity would tentatively be regarded as uncertain.

Even when the clinician concludes that a hypothesis seems to be valid, the evaluation process does not stop. It is always possible that something may be learned in the future that is not consistent with the hypothesis. If this happens, the clinician will need to reconsider the conclusion that the hypothesis is valid.

If the clinician concludes that a hypothesis is invalid or that its validity is uncertain, the evaluation process continues in the manner shown in the decision tree in Figure 13.2 and described in the next paragraph.

When a clinician judges a hypothesis to be invalid or of uncertain validity, the next step is to reexamine the data on which it is based and decide whether the hypothesis is the only possible one that could be consistent with the data. The clinician then also decides whether additional data are needed to make this decision. If so, the clinician may formulate new questions or collect additional data relevant to ones that were already asked. This process of the clinician reexamining answers, asking and answering questions, and formulating and revising hypotheses will be repeated until the clinician has arrived at a hypothesis that is valid, given the available data.

Questions Clinicians Ask During an Initial Evaluation

The clinical evaluation process for an initial evaluation, which I summarized in the preceding paragraphs, begins with the asking of one or more answerable questions. In this section, I clarify what I mean by an answerable question by examining some of the more common questions SLPs and audiologists ask and attempt to answer during an evaluation.

Are the Client's Speech, Language, and Hearing Within Normal Limits?

This is the first question SLPs and audiologists seek to answer during an evaluation. They do not necessarily assume that people referred to them for an evaluation have

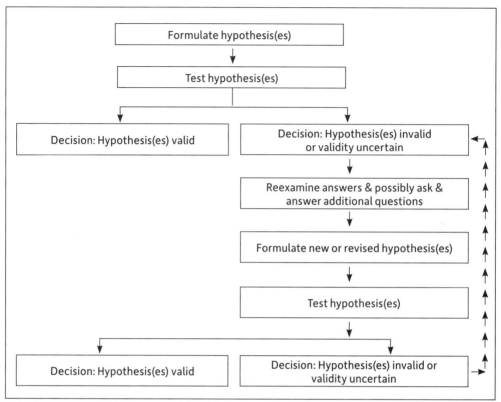

FIGURE 13.2. Testing hypotheses in the clinical evaluation process.

a speech, language, or hearing disorder. Some of them will have speech, language, and hearing that are within **normal limits**. For example, a 3-year-old whose parents are concerned that she isn't saying speech sounds correctly may simply be having difficulty producing the voiced and voiceless "th" sounds. Because many 3-year-olds do not produce these sounds correctly, her ability to produce speech sounds (i.e., articulation) can be judged to be within normal limits.

To determine whether a client's speech, language, and hearing are within normal limits, the clinician compares the person's abilities in these areas to accepted norms. For children, these would be **developmental norms**. Such norms specify the maximum age by which a child can exhibit a particular error (e.g., producing the /r/ sound incorrectly) and not be regarded as having a disorder.

Determining whether a particular aspect of communication behavior is within normal limits is somewhat arbitrary because it is determined by the percentage of the population labeled "atypical" or "abnormal." For instance, different states define "normal limits" differently, which affects the total number of children who qualify for special education services. Some states define "abnormal" more strictly than others, which means they have fewer special education students than states that define "abnormal" less strictly. Even though a clinician may determine that a child has a language disorder, whether the child qualifies for services through the school system depends on how the state defines "abnormal."

Unfortunately, there is no accepted standard for the percentage of children that it is appropriate to label "abnormal." Most clinicians use standardized assessments and procedures to help them make this decision. These instruments and procedures have been carefully standardized on a large population of people with similar speech, language, and hearing characteristics.

Is the Client at Risk for Developing a Disorder?

Although a client may not be judged to have a speech, language, or hearing disorder at the time of the evaluation, he or she may appear to be at greater than ordinary risk for developing one. The clinician arriving at this conclusion has an ethical responsibility to do whatever possible to minimize the risk. If, for example, a client who works in a very noisy environment is given a hearing test and found to have hearing within normal limits, that client would, nevertheless, be at greater than ordinary risk for developing a noise-induced hearing loss. Consequently, the audiologist would be warranted in making some recommendations for hearing conservation.

What Are the Characteristics of Disability and Impairment?

The **World Health Organization (WHO;** 2014b) has suggested that *disabilities* "is an umbrella term, covering impairments, activity limitations, and participation restrictions" (para, 1). The organization further defines an impairment as "a problem in body function or structure" (para. 1) and a disability as "a complex phenomenon, reflecting the interaction between features of a person's body and features of the society in which he or she lives" (para. 2).

Using these definitions for example, if a client has a moderately severe **sensorineural hearing loss**, the hearing loss would be an impairment. If the hearing loss is severe enough to prevent the person from using a telephone or causes the person to avoid parties and other social situations because of embarrassment about being hard of hearing, the inability to communicate in this way would be a disability.

If a client's communication behavior was judged not to be within normal limits, the clinician would attempt to describe the ways it deviated from normal, as well as any ways that it disabled the client. The clinician would do this by making appropriate observations (i.e., by administering tests, observing the client informally, or interviewing informants). The resulting inventory of the client's communication impairments and disabilities would then be used to select goals for therapy.

Preventing or minimizing the development of disabilities and impairments is usually easier than eliminating them or reducing their severity after they occur. Consequently, if an inventory of a client's communication impairments indicates that the disorder is accompanied by disabilities, a management goal should be to minimize the extent. More important, perhaps, than waiting to determine whether the impairment has progressed to a disability or impairment would be for the clinician to provide proactive therapeutic intervention designed to prevent such a progression.

What Is the Cause of the Communication Disorder?

Once a client's communication impairments or disabilities have been identified, the next step is to formulate a tentative hypothesis for the cause in order to design appropriate and effective therapy. If, for example, a clinician assumed that a client is having difficulty understanding speech because of a hearing loss, intervention would be different from that designed for a client whose communication disorder was caused by receptive **aphasia**.

A clinician may have to perform a differential diagnosis before formulating a tentative hypothesis that describes the reason(s) communication deviates from what is considered normal. Making a differential diagnosis is a two-stage process. First, the clinician identifies all the possible reasons for why the communication behavior deviates from normal in the ways it does. Second, the clinician systematically rules out as many of these reasons as possible. Ideally, this process will result in the elimination of all but one, which would be tentatively regarded as being the explanation for the deviation from normal.

For a differential diagnosis to yield the "real" reason for a disorder, all possible reasons for it must be considered. If even one possibility is not considered, the diagnosis yielded by the process could be inaccurate.

To illustrate the differential diagnostic process, suppose that an adult client was reported to be having difficulty understanding speech. The following are some possible reasons that would have to be considered:

- Conductive hearing loss
- Sensorineural hearing loss
- Auditory nerve dysfunction
- **Auditory agnosia**
- Receptive aphasia
- Receptive language disorder
- Reduced auditory memory span
- Slow processing of auditory information
- Difficulty processing abstract information
- Feigning or malingering
- Severe depression
- Frequent petit mal seizures
- Frequent severe fatigue
- Schizophrenia

The information needed to rule some of these reasons in or out could be gleaned from testing, either current or previous; for others, it could be gathered from informal observation; and for still others it could be obtained from interviews with family or caregivers, friends, and other professionals. There may, of course, be other reasons for a client not responding normally to speech sounds.

Is There Any Reason Why the Clinician Cannot or Should Not Provide Therapy?

Just because a client has a communication disorder does not necessarily mean that he or she is eligible to receive therapy. Eligibility is particularly likely to be a problem if someone other than the client or the client's family (i.e., a third party, such as a school system or an insurance company) will be paying for it. To be eligible to receive therapy, the client may have to meet certain criteria, and the clinician will have to gather the data needed to document that the client meets those criteria. In public schools, for example, children are eligible for speech–language services if their communication disorder has an adverse effect on their educational performance. Individual states offer guidelines for assessing eligibility for SLP services, documenting the adverse effect on educational performance that is a result of a speech and/or language impairment, and determining how and when to discontinue SLP services. The Colorado Department of Education provides a good example of these guidelines (2010).

Client motivation is another reason a clinician may decide not to provide therapy services. Almost all of the benefits that can be derived from therapy require a significant investment by the client and/or family. A prerequisite for clients making such an investment is motivation. Although a clinician should be able to generate the necessary motivation in a young child, in an older child or adult a clinician can usually do no more than reinforce the motivation the client already possesses. Consequently, an older child or adult must be intrinsically motivated to make the necessary investments of time, energy, and resources before beginning therapy. Otherwise, the client is unlikely to improve, and he or she may begin to develop uncertainty regarding progress.

Questions Clinicians Ask During a Reevaluation

Clinicians reevaluate their clients periodically for a number of reasons, including the following:

- to meet **third-party payers'** (e.g., **Medicare**) and employers' requirements for accountability and **documentation**

- to check their tentative hypotheses about the communication disorder they are attempting to modify and modifying those hypotheses as necessary
- to assess their clients' progress toward meeting therapy goals
- to decide whether to recommend further therapy
- to fill requests for progress reports from other professionals and agencies (e.g., vocational rehabilitation, mental health services, educational systems)

Regardless of the setting in which SLPs or audiologists are employed, they will be required to document the outcome of intervention with clients. If clinicians are employed by a public school, they will be expected to document how well the goals and objectives specified in **Individualized Education Programs (IEPs)** have been met. If clinicians are employed in a medical setting, they will have to document client progress to receive funding from insurance programs for additional sessions.

To be maximally helpful to clients, clinicians use intervention strategies to modify communication behaviors based on what is hypothesized to have caused them. If clients change in the ways that would be expected if the hypotheses are valid, the change(s) would provide at least partial support for their validity. Unfortunately, if clients do not change in these ways, the reason could be either that the hypotheses are invalid or that some other factor (e.g., a lack of motivation to change) is impeding the clients' ability to change. Regardless, their lack of improvement would trigger a need for further evaluation.

Obviously, without periodic reevaluations it is not possible to gauge clients' progress toward achieving therapy goals. Neither would it be possible to make informed decisions about the likelihood that further therapy would be helpful. As I mentioned above, utilizing a dynamic assessment approach is one way to conduct ongoing assessments throughout the intervention process. In the following paragraphs I address the main questions that are usually asked during a reevaluation.

Has There Been Any Change in the Severity of the Communication Disorder?

This is a routine question to ask throughout the intervention process as well as at the end of therapy, particularly if there were more than a few sessions. If the answer is "yes," the clinician would then ask, "In what way(s) has the client changed?" Answering these two questions involves comparing specific aspects of the client's communication to what they were when therapy began.

Has the Communication Disorder Been Remediated, or Have Compensatory Strategies Been Successfully Established?

This question is a logical extension of the previous one. If there has been change in the severity of the communication disorder—and assuming the change is a positive one—the clinician will want to know whether the change is significant enough that the client would no longer be considered to have a communication disorder. If not, then the clinician will ask whether the client has developed compensatory strategies that are sufficiently robust for use if the client is dismissed from therapy.

How Likely Is the Client to Continue Improving If He or She Receives More Therapy?

This question is asked periodically throughout the intervention process. The answer determines whether additional therapy will be recommended. Data necessary for answering it include information pertaining to the amount of improvement during the previous few sessions. If there has been a significant amount of improvement during this period, the prognosis for continued improvement tends to be better than if there has not been significant improvement. The **Code of Ethics of the American Speech-Language-Hearing Association** prohibits keeping clients in therapy beyond the point they are likely to benefit from it.

Has the Individual or Family Member Chosen Not to Participate Further in Therapy/Relocated/Sought Another Provider?

Sometimes a clinician will meet a client (or family member) who is plainly unwilling to participate in therapy or who becomes unwilling over a period of time. Most clinicians will attempt to further motivate the client (or family member), but if those efforts fail, they will choose to terminate therapy because no further progress is likely to occur. Another factor that can result in a clinician dismissing a client from therapy is poor or inconsistent attendance. Again, most clinicians will attempt to help the client (or family member) attend more consistently, but if that does not happen, they will terminate therapy. Finally, a clinician will, obviously, dismiss clients who relocate or seek help from another provider—not necessarily an SLP but perhaps a debate coach or singing teacher.

The Intervention Process

Throughout this book I have talked about intervention but until now haven't specified exactly what it entails. In its most general sense, intervention is anything that is done with the intention of improving a person's function in some area of his or her life, which in this context means communication. Specifically, intervention for a communication disorder involves applying therapeutic techniques in order to modify an individual's performance in a specific area (e.g., vocabulary, hearing, balance, social language, fluency). The intervention process consists of several components, which I discuss in the following sections.

Defining an Individual's Communication Disorder

The first step in intervention is really one of the last steps in the initial clinical evaluation process: defining the communication disorder as specifically as possible. This process allows the clinician to formulate the hypotheses I described in the earlier section on assessment, one of which will address the cause of the communication disorder, thereby influencing the choice of intervention strategies. If, for example, the reason for a client's difficulty understanding speech is hypothesized to be a sensorineural hearing loss, the client will probably be fitted with a hearing aid. On the other hand, if it is hypothesized to be receptive aphasia, the clinician will design a program of appropriate language stimulation.

Defining the individual's communication disorder provides the baseline against which the clinician can document therapy outcome(s). In other words, to document changes in the severity of a client's disorder after a period of therapy, the clinician compares the individual's communication to what it was at the beginning of therapy—to the baseline.

The behaviors that characterize a client's communication disorder may not consist solely of impairments in speech, hearing, or language. They may also include psychological difficulties that affect the client's life. An example would be avoiding certain situations because of a poor self-concept. It is important to identify these behaviors as well, especially if they are severe enough for a referral to a mental health professional.

Deciding on Individual or Group Therapy

For SLPs who provide both individual and group therapy, part of the intervention process is determining whether a particular client would benefit more from one or the other. In some work settings, such as health-care facilities, individual therapy may be preferred because of the severity of a client's communication disorder or because there are no other clients with the same type of disorder. On the other hand, SLPs working in the schools often provide therapy in group or classroom settings.

Many audiologists and SLPs organize and facilitate support groups for clients with similar communication disorders, such as aphasia, **laryngectomy**, hearing loss, stuttering, or **Ménière's disease**. These groups may meet in person, on social media, or online through an organization. An example is the National Stuttering Association (2014a), which provides links to local support groups and sponsors online social networking groups for parents and groups for teens.

Establishing Intervention Goals

The next step in the intervention process is establishing **long-term** and **short-term goals**. These goals are derived in part from answering the question, "What is the purpose of intervention for this person's communication disorder?" Recall that in Chapter 4, I discussed three purposes for intervention: changing the problem causing the disorder, changing the disorder, and teaching compensatory strategies. To set appropriate long-term goals and short-term objectives, the clinician must first identify which of these purposes is most likely to be achieved given the nature and severity of the disorder, the client's age, previous intervention successes or failures, and the client's communication needs in everyday life.

Both long-term and short-term goals are usually documented in written form. Box 13.4 shows the required components for IEPs in schools. The success of any intervention program is determined largely by the appropriateness of the goals and objectives to the client's specific disorder and communication needs.

Selecting goals affects therapy in at least two ways. First, it determines what is to be done to help the client. Second, it influences the client's level of motivation to invest in therapy. A client is likely to work harder to achieve some goals than to achieve others. Children, in particular, need to see how therapy goals are related directly to their everyday life.

The distinction between long-term goals and short-term goals is not absolute. A goal that is a first step or means to an end for one client may be the ultimate goal for another. For instance, the long-term goal for one client might be to become aware of the communication disorder. For another client, the first short-term objective might be to become aware of the voice disorder while the long-term goal might be to significantly change the use of voice at home and in school in order to eliminate vocal stress.

Long-Term Goals

Long-term goals specify the outcomes the clinician is attempting to accomplish through the intervention process. Attaining long-term goals should result in a meaningful reduction in the severity of the client's disorder. Some common long-term goals used by SLPs follow:

1. *The client will produce speech that is at least 80% intelligible to most people.* This is the type of long-term goal a clinician establishes when it is not feasible for a client to completely eliminate a communication impairment but it is feasible for him or her to develop speech that can be understood by most people. A clinician might set such a goal for a client whose speech musculature is not functioning normally because of a neuromuscular disorder (i.e., someone who has dysarthria) or for someone who is deaf or has had a glossectomy.

2. *The client will produce the / ʃ / phoneme correctly in all positions in words during nonstructured conversational speech at least 95% of the time.* This is the type of long-term goal clinicians establish when they believe it is feasible for a client to eliminate a speech disorder. A 100% success level is not expected because it might take years to achieve. In addition, it is reasonable to assume that if a client has learned to produce the / ʃ / correctly 95% of the time, he or she should be able to learn to produce it correctly

BOX 13.4   What Is an IEP, and What Does It Include?

An IEP is an educational program, specifically tailored to each individual child, taking into account his or her capabilities and limitations, and setting forth specific goals for the child's learning and personal growth.

The IEP is mandated by the federal law, most recently IDEA 2004 (Individuals with Disabilities Education Improvement Act of 2004), governing special education. The IEP states the educational needs of the student, the goals and objectives directing the student's educational program, the student's educational programming and placement, and the evaluation and measurement criteria that were developed during the creation of the IEP.

Speech–language pathologists and audiologists who work in the schools use the IEP as a way to describe the goals and objectives that drive intervention for students with communication disorders. The following must be included in the IEP:

Present levels of performance. The IEP must provide a statement of the child's present levels of academic achievement and functional performance in all areas of concern, including academics, physical functioning, social and behavioral skills, communication, and life skills.

Annual goals. The IEP must include a statement of measurable annual goals, including academic and functional goals. The IEPs of children who take alternate assessments must include a description of benchmarks or short-term objectives.

Educational progress. This is a description of how the child's progress toward meeting the annual goals will be measured and when periodic reports on the progress the child is making toward meeting the annual goals will be provided (e .g., through the use of quarterly or other periodic reports, report cards, or other). This description must also describe how it will be conveyed to parents/caregivers.

Special education and related services. The child's IEP must include a statement of the special education and related services, and supplementary aids and services to be provided to help the child toward meeting educational goals. Services must be based on peer-reviewed research to the extent practicable. IEPs also include a statement of the program modifications or supports to be provided by school personnel.

Statement of participation in regular education program. Because the law requires that children be educated in the least restrictive environment, the IEP must specify how the child will participate in the general education program with typically developing children. It must also specify the amount of time the child will participate in general education programs.

Testing adaptations and modifications. The child's IEP must include a statement of any individual appropriate accommodations that are necessary to measure the academic achievement and functional performance of the child on state and districtwide assessments. The IEP must state why these adaptations and modifications are necessary for this child.

Length and duration of services. The IEP must include a statement regarding when services will begin and end, the frequency of the services, where they will be delivered, and how long they will be provided.

Transition. The first IEP after the child is 16 (and updated annually) must include appropriate and measurable goals that address postsecondary training, education, employment, and independent living skills (when appropriate) and the transition services necessary to assist the child in reaching these goals.

The complete final regulations are available from the U.S. Department of Education (2006).

100% of the time without the need for further therapy. Consequently, it would almost always be safe to discharge a client who had achieved this level of success.

3. *The client will communicate functional, everyday needs.* This is the type of long-term goal clinicians establish for clients who have a severe communication impairment—people whose speech is inadequate (temporarily or permanently) for meeting at least some of their communication needs. In Chapter 5, I described some of the various strategies and devices that are used with such clients to augment their ability to communicate.

4. *The client will use figurative language correctly in a written story.* This long-term goal is typical of the type school-based SLPs establish for students with language-learning disabilities. These students frequently have difficulty with the **metalinguistic** aspects of language, especially in writing.

A number of factors can influence a clinician's selection of long-term goals for a client. A few are listed here.

The Severity of the Communication Disorder. Generally, the more severe the communication disorder, the more likely it is that long-term goals will focus on helping the client develop communication that is adequate for everyday functional needs. The less severe the communication disorder, the more likely it is that long-term goals will focus on speech, language, or hearing improvements that bring the client as close as possible to normal communication.

People with severe communication impairments either have no **intelligibility** or lack sufficient intelligible speech to meet their **functional communication needs**. Some of the conditions that result in severe communication impairments are **cognitive disabilities**, **autism**, **cerebral palsy**, aphasia, deafness, glossectomy, and laryngeal pathology (including laryngectomy).

Clinicians who work with people with severe communication impairments have as their ultimate goal helping their clients develop the ability to communicate at a level adequate for meeting their daily, functional needs. To achieve this goal, clinicians will typically help their clients develop more intelligible speech (assuming this is possible) as well as provide them with communication strategies (which may include devices) to augment their ability to communicate. These strategies provided might include **American Sign Language (ASL)**, **American Indian Sign Language** (sometimes referred to as *Hand Talk*—more information about American Indian Sign Language is available from Plains Indian Sign Language, 2014), **Gestural Morse Code**, **communication boards**, and electronic communication devices. Augmenting a client's speech and other natural communication abilities by one or more of these strategies or devices can enable clients with sufficient cognitive abilities to meet their communication needs—or come closer to meeting them.

The Client's Communication Needs. Perhaps the greatest factor involved in designing long-term goals is the client's communication needs. The clinician first identifies these needs and then determines what the client has to develop, eliminate, or modify in order to meet their needs. Intervention consists of the clinician helping the client make the necessary changes.

To illustrate this point, suppose a clinician must develop long-term goals for an elementary-school-age girl who has normal intelligence, hearing, and vision, but who is unable to speak, write, or walk because of cerebral palsy. What are this child's communication needs? First, she should be able to converse with people face-to-face. A communication board as shown in Figure 13.3, or a laptop computer to synthesize speech, might enable her to meet this communication need. The clinician might also decide to use a communication board app, many of which are now available for mobile phones, tablets, and computers. Friendship Circle (2011) has descriptions of several iPad apps on their website.

Second, she must be able to do written work in the classroom. A laptop computer and printer can enable her to do this if she has sufficient motor control to use the keyboard. Third, it would be desirable if she could communicate by telephone. The clinician can contact their state's **telecommunication relay service (TRS)** to arrange for telephone services that are functionally equivalent to those available to other telephone users. And, to communicate more informally, the clinician can assist the girl in learning to use the computer (and/or smartphone) for e-mailing and social networking.

The Client's Prognosis for Improvement. When establishing long-term goals for a client, the clinician will need to consider the client's potential for change. Obviously, the clinician will design goals she or he believes the client is capable of achieving, because to do otherwise is to act unethically. If the client has difficulty achieving the

I CAN HEAR PERFECTLY			PLEASE REPEAT AS I TALK THIS IS HOW I TALK BY SPELLING OUT THE WORDS							WOULD YOU PLEASE CALL	
A	AN	HE	AM	ARE	ASK	BE	BEEN	BRING	CAN	ABOUT	ALL
HER	I IT	ME	COME	COULD	DID	DO	DOES	DON'T		AND	ALWAYS
MY	HIM	SHE	DRINK	GET	GIVE	GO	HAD	HAS	HAVE	ALMOST	AS
THAT	THE	THESE	IS	KEEP	KNOW	LET	LIKE	MAKE	MAY	AT	BECAUSE
THEY	THIS	WHOSE	PUT	SAY	SAID	SEE	SEEN	SEND	SHOULD	BUT FOR	FROM
WHAT	WHEN	WHERE	TAKE	TELL	THINK	THOUGHT	WANT			HOW IF	IN
WHICH	WHO	WHY	WAS	WERE	WILL	WISH	WON'T	WOULD	ED	OF	ON OR
YOU	WE	YOUR	-ER	-EST	-ING	-LY	-N'T	-'S	-TION	TO UP	WITH
A	B		C	D	E	F		G		AFTER	AGAIN
H		I		K	L	M				ANY	EVEN
N	O		P	Qu	R	S	T			EVERY	HERE
U	V		W	X	Y	Z				JUST	MORE
1	2		3	4	5	6	7			ONLY	SO
8	9		10	11	12	30				SOME	SOON
										THERE	VERY
SUN. MON. TUES WED. THURS. FRI. SAT. BATHROOM			PLEASE THANK YOU GOING OUT MR. MRS. MISS. START OVER MOTHER DAD DOCTOR END OF WORD							$ ¢ ½ (SHHH!)? *Lynda Miller*	

FIGURE 13.3. Example of a communication board.

goals, the clinician will reevaluate the goals to determine whether they are too difficult and need to be reformulated.

Available Resources. The resources available for treating a client can influence the long-term goals a clinician develops. Such resources include available funding, administrative support, adequate physical facilities, access to appropriate materials, and continuing education opportunities.

Short-Term Goals (Objectives)

Short-term goals specify the abilities clients must develop in order to achieve long-term goals. These abilities often have to be developed in a specific sequence, as illustrated in Figure 13.4. The tasks specified in this figure almost always have to be carried out in the sequence indicated. A client, for example, would almost always have to be able to produce /s/ correctly in single words before doing so in sentences.

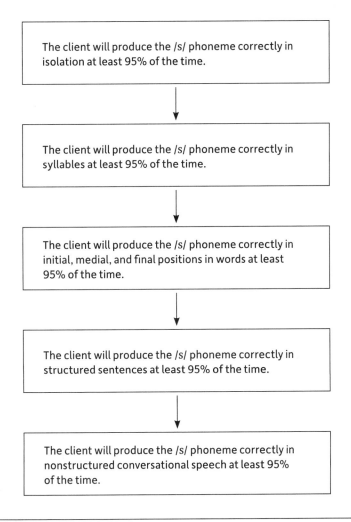

FIGURE 13.4. Some short-term goals (objectives) a client must achieve before being able to produce /s/ correctly during nonstructured conversational speech at least 95% of the time.

Developing Intervention Strategies

The development of intervention strategies arises directly from the long-term goals and short-term objectives the clinician establishes for the client. Several factors, including the following, affect clinicians' choices of which intervention strategies to use:

1. *The number of strategies that are appropriate for achieving a particular goal with which a clinician is familiar.* Clinicians can select only from among the strategies they know. If a clinician is familiar with only a single strategy for achieving a goal, the selection process will be easy. However, clinicians are more likely to be successful in achieving a particular goal if they know more than one strategy, because there are few (if any) that will work with all clients!

2. *The clinician's hypothesis about the primary cause(s) of the behavior to be changed.* The intervention strategies clinicians choose are influenced by the assumptions they make about the reason(s) the client continues to exhibit the target behavior. The client may continue this particular behavior for physiological or psychological reasons, or a combination of the two. If the clinician's hypothesis is accurate, intervention is more likely to be successful than it would be if the hypothesis turns out to be inaccurate.

3. *The time and financial investments required.* Some intervention strategies require more time or greater financial investment than others. The more time a clinician must invest to implement an intervention strategy, the greater the cost to the client (or whoever is paying for the therapy). It may be possible, for example, for a clinician to reduce the time investment that is required to attain a particular goal and, consequently, the cost, by conducting some sessions through videoconferencing, texting, custom apps, or e-mailing. For instance, clinicians who work with preschool children can teach parents several techniques for talking with their preschooler, and then text parents daily reminders to use one or more of the strategies. Or, clinicians with experience developing apps for mobile devices can design a custom app for a school-age child who can use it to practice specific speech sounds in between therapy sessions.

4. *The client's treatment history.* If a client has had previous therapy and believes that the approach used was effective, the clinician is likely to continue using it. On the other hand, if the client does not believe it was effective, the clinician will want to use a different approach. A client's beliefs about the effectiveness of an intervention can reduce or enhance its effect. Clients tend to invest more time and energy in therapy when they anticipate success than when they anticipate failure.

5. *The client's intellectual level.* A client's level of cognitive functioning can influence the choice of an intervention strategy. It probably wouldn't be possible, for example, to use a communication board containing the al-

phabet and commonly used words, as in Figure 13.3, with people with significant cognitive deficits.

6. *Evidence-based practices.* You will recall from Chapter 11 that **evidence-based practice (EBP)** means integrating the clinician's individual clinical expertise with the best available external clinical evidence obtained from systematic research. The **American Speech-Language-Hearing Association** defines EBP as using current best research results to make clinical decisions about client care. Based on the evidence from a comprehensive literature search and review of published research studies, the clinician develops interventions appropriate for each client.

Implementing Intervention Strategies

SLPs and audiologists implement a wide range of intervention strategies. Much of learning to be an SLP or audiologist focuses on acquiring an understanding of these strategies. Table 13.1 provides an illustration of the link between intervention strategies and the goals they are intended to help a client attain; in the example, the client has an articulation disorder.

Documenting Progress

A clinician cannot ethically continue providing intervention if the client does not demonstrate measurable progress toward the long-term goal established at the beginning of therapy. The clinician can modify the intervention strategies being used, refer the client to another professional, or terminate therapy. In any case, the clinician must be able to show whether the client's communication behavior changed, and, if it did, how. The easiest way to show these changes is to document the client's communication behaviors during each therapy session. One way to document progress is to keep a running tally of the client's attempts to produce a target communication behavior, for example, the number of correct productions of the /s/ phoneme in initial position in words from a specified word list.

Another approach to documenting progress is to track the number of targeted communication behaviors used from session to session. For instance, a clinician working with a school-age child on developing the ability to tell a spontaneous story could track the story components the child included at the beginning of therapy, after four sessions, and again after eight sessions. If the intervention strategies used are appropriate, the number of story components the child includes will increase measurably.

Dismissing the Client From Therapy

The final step in the intervention process is dismissing the client from therapy and writing a summary report. Ideally, all the client's initial goals have been achieved

TABLE 13.1. Example Goals and Intervention Strategies for an Articulation Disorder

Goal	Intervention strategy
The client will produce the /s/ phoneme correctly at the beginnings of single words at least 95% of the time.	The client will read aloud lists of words that begin with the /s/ phoneme. After the client says each word, the clinician will signal whether it was said correctly. The client will repeat the task until she is producing /s/ correctly at least 95% of the time in this context.
The client (who has a sensorineural hearing loss) will be fitted with a hearing aid that will enable him to understand at least 90% of words spoken in a quiet environment.	The client will be fitted with a hearing aid, and the percentage of the words on one or more special lists that he identifies correctly will be determined. The words will be presented over a loudspeaker in a sound-treated room. If the client doesn't appear to understand at least 90% of them, the process will be repeated with other hearing aids.
The client (who has a flaccid paralysis of the soft palate and is extremely hypernasal) will produce speech that is at least 90% intelligible.	The client will be fitted with a palatal lift prosthesis to reduce hypernasality and thus increase the intelligibility of his speech. First, a sample of the client's speech will be recorded with the prosthesis in place. Then, several listeners will transcribe the sample to determine whether it is at least 90% intelligible. This is an example of intervention for a communication disorder that requires the involvement of a clinician who is not an SLP or audiologist. In this case, the clinician involved probably would be a dentist who specializes in prostheses (i.e., a prosthodontist).

and there doesn't appear to be a need for new ones. However, several factors can result in terminating therapy before the client has reached his or her goals. Probably the most common is that the clinician determines that the client is unlikely to make further progress toward the goals. Unless the client is likely to benefit from further therapy, the clinician is ethically bound to terminate the intervention process. This does not mean, however, that the clinician concludes that the client will never benefit from further intervention. To the contrary, often the clinician will arrange for periodic reevaluations to determine whether further therapy at that time would be beneficial to the client.

Another reason clients may be discharged before achieving their goals is that they want to change clinicians. Changing clinicians may result from the client moving away from the area or from the client having decided to enter the intervention process with a different clinician. A third factor influencing discharging clients before they have achieved their goals is that they can no longer afford the clinic's fee. For instance, their insurance benefits for this type of therapy may have been exhausted, or their budget does not allow payment of further fees. In this situation, clients may seek therapy at a less expensive facility, such as a university speech, language, and hearing clinic.

Finally, clients may be discharged before their goals are achieved simply because they want to be. They may no longer have time for therapy or be motivated to continue it, or they may feel capable of functioning as their own clinician. In fact, for some clients—particularly those whose communication impairments cannot be completely eliminated—assuming the responsibility for continued improvement may be one of the goals established when they began the therapeutic process. For these clients, terminating therapy with a clinician signals the achievement of their goal.

chapter 14

The Clinician's Responsibility

Learning Objectives

Describe how evidence-based practice (EBP) benefits SLPs and audiologists in designing and providing services to clients.

Describe why SLPs and audiologists need to gather and disseminate information about the effectiveness of the clinical tools and techniques they use.

Describe the clinician-investigator role and the benefits that SLPs and audiologists derive from undertaking this role.

List the six steps in the clinical research process.

Describe why it is necessary to establish scientific justification for answering clinical questions through research.

Demonstrate how the same data can be presented to imply greater or lesser improvement.

Define 25 statistical terms that are used in clinical research in professional journals.

Overview

Like most other health-care professionals, **speech–language pathologists** (SLPs) and **audiologists** rely considerably on the experience of others in their work. Most clinicians create few, if any, of the evaluation procedures and intervention strategies that they use. Instead, they acquire them by talking with colleagues, taking courses, reading books and professional journals, surfing the Internet, participating in continuing education activities, and attending professional meetings.

For clinical services to be maximally effective, clinicians need to share information about what works and what does not, which I described in Chapter 2 as **evidence-based practice (EBP)**. Because a publisher claims that a particular diagnostic test yields data that are **valid**, **reliable**, and **representative** does not necessarily mean that it actually does. However, publishers of **standardized assessments** almost always publish the statistical information necessary to determine whether their tests do possess adequate statistical power to be considered valid, reliable, and representative. Clinicians typically evaluate this information as part of deciding whether or not to use the test.

Similarly, because a particular **intervention strategy** is claimed by its creator to have been proven effective does not necessarily indicate that it really has. The amount of confidence a clinician can have in both these conclusions depends on who generated and interpreted the data. Unlike test instruments, which undergo rigorous statistical design and analysis, intervention programs are only recently being evaluated with the same rigor. Unfortunately, the desire of someone who creates an intervention process or program to have his or her creation be regarded as valid, reliable, and effective can bias both how he or she gathers data to evaluate it and how the data are interpreted. This phenomenon is referred to as **experimenter bias**.

Consider this illustration of how experimenter bias can affect the gathering of data to both evaluate and interpret an intervention program. A hypothetical language program for school-age children has 23 participants enrolled in a summer program. The goal of the 8-week program is to increase the children's expressive language skills. At the beginning and end of the program, each child is interviewed by a clinician who records the conversation and then calculates the number of different sentence types used by each child. The results indicate that at the beginning of the program the children used mostly simple, active, declarative sentences. At the end of the program, the children's conversations contained several examples of compound sentences, **interrogatives**, and embedded phrases. From this information, the program director, who designed the program, concludes that the program is effective because the children's expressive language skills changed over the course of the intervention sessions.

If you look more closely at the data, however, you will see that there is no way to compare the children's sentences at the start of the program with their sentences at the program's conclusion. To measure and document actual change the director would have needed to document changes through some sort of rigorous comparison of the children's expressive language skills at the beginning and end of the program. One way to do this would be to administer a well-documented test of expressive language skills to all the children at the beginning and again at the end of the intervention program. Then the director could compare the pre- and postprogram scores to see whether the changes, if any, reflect statistically significant differences.

Unfortunately, for most therapies for speech, language, and hearing disorders, most (sometimes all) of the outcome data available were generated either by their creators or by people who are closely associated with them (e.g., their graduate students). Consequently, questions can legitimately be raised about the validity, reliability, and generality of data used to support statements about their effectiveness. How can the accuracy of such statements be assessed? Perhaps the best way is to encourage clinicians with no investment in the effectiveness of any given therapy to assess it.

My primary purpose in this chapter is to acquaint you with how clinicians gather and disseminate information about the effectiveness of clinical tools and techniques. I begin with a review of evidence-based practice and follow with a discussion of clinicians functioning as **clinician-investigators**. Then, I describe the clinical research process, emphasizing seven questions clinicians address when judging the effectiveness of any particular therapy.

Evidence-Based Practice (a Review)

You will recall that in Chapter 2 I described evidence-based practice as the attempt to provide the best possible intervention for each client through utilizing a combination of evidence from scientific studies, clinical experience and judgment, and the unique needs of each client. I listed the four-step process ASHA recommends that clinicians use to employ evidence-based practice (see Box 14.1).

To support clinicians in engaging in EBP, **the American Speech-Language-Hearing Association (ASHA)** offers the following variety of easily accessible tools (2014s):

- Evidence maps for a variety of disorders and procedures used by audiologists and SLPs. These evidence maps contain the most current research findings and how they relate to specific practices. For instance, the evidence map for spoken language disorders contains information on findings regarding such practices as early intervention, narrative interventions, pragmatics/social skills/discourse, and behavioral approaches.
- Client and patient handouts that provide information to help consumers understand how SLPs and audiologists assist individuals with speech, language, or hearing disorders.

BOX 14.1   The Four-Step Process of Engaging in Evidence-Based Practice, Recommended by ASHA

- *Frame the clinical question:* Analyze the specific communication disorder presented by your client; compare possible intervention approaches to determine which would offer the best outcome for your client; formulate the desired outcome for this client.
- *Find the evidence you need in order to plan intervention:* Analyze existing practices that are considered highly efficacious; systematically review the scientific evidence regarding your particular clinical question; analyze the individual studies that relate to the clinical question regarding this client.
- *Assess the evidence:* Determine its relevance to the specific clinical question you're asking; consider who wrote and published the evidence you're analyzing.
- *Make the clinical decision:* Combine your clinical experience and expertise with the evidence you've gathered; determine which intervention approach would be best for your client.

- Templates and tools such as **documentation** templates (e.g., clinical swallowing evaluation, pain assessment); EBP web-based tutorials; a compendium of EBP guidelines and systematic reviews; and the National Outcomes Measurement System (NOMS), a tool that guides clinicians in collecting data, setting goals, and making claims for services provided to **Medicare**.
- Information on clinical topics and issues that help clinicians translate evidence and expert opinion into practice.

Practicing clinicians can also utilize ASHA's evidence-based systematic reviews (ASHA, 2014d), which are conducted annually and form the basis for EBP guidelines. Each year, the review assesses the body of scientific evidence related to specific clinical questions and provides the extent to which a particular diagnostic or intervention approach is supported by the evidence. For instance, a review (McCreery, Venediktov, Coleman, & Leech, 2012) examined 26 databases regarding the effects of digital noise reduction hearing aids or directional microphones in school-age children with hearing loss. Their conclusion was that digital noise reduction neither improved nor degraded speech understanding. Directional microphones were found to improve speech recognition only in controlled settings, but their effectiveness in actual everyday listening environments was unclear.

Two clinical conclusions can be drawn from this systematic review. One, until further evidence is generated to suggest otherwise, digital noise reduction does not seem to affect speech understanding in school-age settings. Two, directional microphones can positively affect a student's speech recognition in controlled optimal settings, but the evidence does not address whether directional microphones are effective in a student's everyday listening contexts.

The Clinician as Clinician-Investigator

SLPs and audiologists need to systematically evaluate and document their therapy in order to prevent experimenter bias and to determine whether the techniques and strategies they are using are effective. One way to systematically evaluate and document one's therapy is by functioning as a clinician-investigator. The research clinicians do, usually **single-subject research**, results in the documentation necessary to show the effectiveness of particular therapy strategies and methodologies. It also serves an important function related to the ASHA code of ethics, which states that clinicians must evaluate the services they provide in order to determine their effectiveness. Further, this type of research contributes to the evidence surrounding the use of particular techniques and strategies.

Although there is considerable variation in the amount and type of therapy outcome research that individual SLPs and audiologists perform, they are all required to do some, regardless of whether they are employed in an educational, medical, or other setting. If you are employed in the public schools, you will be required by your employer (usually the school district) to conduct research to document effectiveness because your employer needs the documentation to be eligible for reimbursement from the federal or state government for at least a part of your salary. If you are employed in a medical setting, you will be required by your employer to document your practices because your employer needs the documentation to be paid for your services by private and governmental insurance entities (e.g., Medicare).

Another way people with communication impairments benefit from SLPs and audiologists functioning as clinician-investigators is that they receive the highest-quality services. Therapy service improves when SLPs and audiologists share information with their colleagues. An SLP, for example, may find that an intervention approach that is effective with one clinical population is also effective with another. An example is the recognition by Weiss (2004) that many children who stutter—especially school-age children and adolescents, whose language is more complex than that of younger children—can be helped by providing therapy for pragmatic language skills. Box 14.2 describes how one SLP used specific pragmatic language strategies to increase fluency in a 10-year-old boy.

Clients also benefit when their clinicians routinely assess therapy outcomes because these clinicians are more likely to monitor more carefully the services they

---

BOX 14.2   **An Example of Using Pragmatic Language Therapy to Increase Fluency in a 10-Year-Old Boy Who Stutters (Weiss, 2004)**

Weiss proposed that, because children who stutter often exhibit increased disfluency in conversational contexts, clinicians can successfully incorporate pragmatics therapy into intervention for stuttering. She described an example of conversation-based therapy for a 10-year-old boy who was particularly anxious about going to school because he stuttered when his teacher called on him in class and when he attempted to talk to classmates during free time.

The SLP designed an intervention plan for him that began with having the boy select the topic of conversation in which he could use his fluency strategies. Initially, the SLP had the boy tell a monologue or story rather than engage in turn taking. Once the boy became comfortable and fluent in this context, the SLP increased the challenge by selecting a random topic.

The boy practiced using his fluency strategies while initiating a topic, maintaining the topic, and changing the topic in conversation with the SLP. When his fluency remained constant during these contexts, the SLP first added conversational partners, then changed the setting of the conversations from the therapy room to the boy's classroom, all the while monitoring the boy's fluency. Eventually, the SLP and the boy collaborated on activities and conversational situations in which he could practice his fluency strategies in his life outside of the therapy room and his classroom.

provide. Through this monitoring, clinicians are likely to identify and correct problems sooner, thereby increasing the likelihood that clients will benefit.

Finally, functioning as clinician-investigators makes it possible for clinicians to improve their effectiveness. By systematically evaluating the services they provide, they obtain information needed to identify both strategies that work for their clients and themselves and those that do not. In addition, one strategy may be more compatible with a clinician's personality and belief system than another, which affects that clinician's expectation that one particular strategy is more likely to help a client than another.

The Clinical Research Process

The clinical research process involves assessing and documenting therapy. This process is similar in many ways to the clinical evaluation process I described in Chapter 13. Like the clinical evaluation process, the clinical research process involves asking **answerable questions** and making the observations needed to answer them. The clinical research process is diagrammed in Figure 14.1.

Asking Relevant and Answerable Questions

The clinical research process starts with the clinician asking one or more answerable questions that are relevant for improving clinical effectiveness—that is, they answer the "so what" and "who cares" questions regarding therapy. Questions regarding therapy outcome are examples of clinically relevant questions and carry the greatest **scientific justification**. Clinicians assessing the impact of a particular approach ask questions such as the following.

> *What is the impact of the approach on the communication behavior(s) that it is intended to modify?*

By "behavior" I also mean the client's attitudes and feelings. We become aware of clients' attitudes and feelings by observing their behavior. We look at behaviors as indicators of attitudes and feelings.

In most cases, if the answer to this question is that an approach has no meaningful impact on the behavior it is intended to modify, then answers would not be sought to any of the other questions listed below. However, occasionally one encounters a therapy approach that does not appear to do what it is intended to do but, nevertheless, has a very desirable side effect. Because such an approach might be considered worthy of further evaluation because of this **side effect**, answers would be sought to the following questions.

> *What is the impact of the approach on other aspects of a client's communication?*

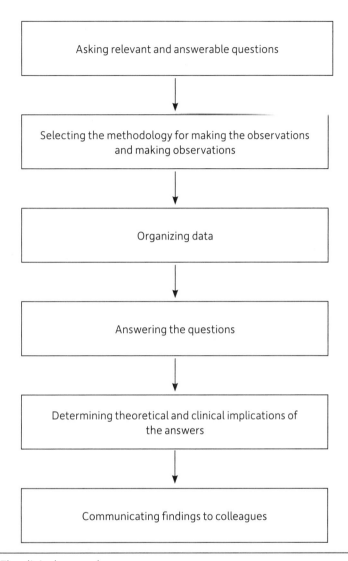

FIGURE 14.1. The clinical research process.

An approach that has a desirable impact on behaviors that contribute to a client's communication disorder may have an undesirable impact on other aspects of the client's communication, including speaking rate, auditory acuity, speech rhythm and articulation, voice intensity and quality, language formulation, verbal output, spontaneity, or credibility as a communicator. If, for example, a person with a fluency disorder is taught to monitor speech for moments of stuttering and to voluntarily reduce their severity, this may result in a reduction in the stuttering severity but also reduce speaking rate, spontaneity, and inflection. If a client's communication behavior following intervention attracts more adverse attention than it did prior to intervention, the value of the approach would be questionable.

What other effects is the approach having on the client?

In other words, are there any side effects that are not directly related to communication? If so, are they desirable or not? Children with **autism**, for example, may often exhibit self-stimulating hand movements, which can lead to poor self-concept, reduced peer acceptance, disturbed biological rhythms, and increased anxiety. However, some children with autism exhibit fewer of these side effects after they have been taught a gestural communication system such as **American Sign Language**, or when they are engaged in particular physical activities, such as a therapeutic horsemanship program.

What is the client's attitude toward the approach and its effects on his or her communication and other aspects of life?

A client's attitude toward an approach and its effects can reduce or enhance its effectiveness. If, for example, a client who has a hearing aid refuses to wear it, having the aid will not improve his or her ability to hear (unless, of course, the client's attitude can be changed through counseling). On the other hand, a client who has a strong belief that a particular therapy program will be of benefit is likely to invest the necessary time and energy in the program, which, in turn, will probably enhance its effectiveness.

What are the attitudes of a client's significant others toward the approach and its impact on the client's behavior?

Therapy is more likely to be successful if the clinician and the client's significant others believe it will be beneficial. For example, if a family member lacks confidence in the effectiveness of an approach, this reduces the odds that it will be effective. On the other hand, if the client's family and friends have a positive attitude toward the therapy, the client will be more likely to respond positively.

What investment is required of the client and clinician?

Each type of therapy requires various types of investment, including financial, time and energy, and willingness to be uncomfortable. An approach may be effective but too expensive to be practical for many clients. For example, a highly sophisticated speech-generating communication device may cost enough that many persons with severe communication impairments cannot afford it. Or an approach may be effective but cause clients to be so uncomfortable that few would be willing to make the necessary investment. One such approach is voluntary stuttering—fake stuttering—outside the therapy room. Many individuals who stutter find this activity extremely noxious and refuse to do it.

What is the probability of relapse following termination of therapy?

People who have a **communication disorder**, particularly individuals who stutter, often relapse to some degree after therapy is terminated. Although any client can suffer a relapse, the likelihood of relapse occurring when some approaches are used is unacceptably high. If the benefits yielded by a therapy are highly likely to wear off after a client is discharged, most clinicians would consider the therapy to be of questionable value. Consequently, it is important when evaluating a therapy to take the probability of relapse into consideration.

Selecting a Methodology and Making Observations

Once a research question has been formulated, the next task is to select a methodology for collecting the data needed and to make observations. If the question is answerable, it will indicate (either directly or indirectly) both what and whom to observe. For example, consider the question, "Do 3 months of daily sessions of a particular **aphasia** therapy improve the speech comprehension of people with **Wernicke's aphasia?**"

For this question, the *what* (which aspect of communication behavior to observe) is speech comprehension and the *who* (persons on whom observations are to be made) is clients with Wernicke's aphasia. The speech-comprehension levels of people with receptive aphasia after 3 months of the therapy would be compared to what they were at the beginning of the period (i.e., **baseline**). The method used to generate the data needed to answer the question would be to administer pre- and posttherapy tests of speech comprehension and then compare the scores. If the posttherapy scores were sufficiently high to suggest there had been a meaningful improvement in speech comprehension, the investigator probably would conclude that the program had been effective. To draw this conclusion, however, the clinician must be certain that no other events occurred during the 3-month period to account for the change in the clients' speech comprehension. For instance, if the clients with aphasia had received the therapy program within 6 months post-trauma, an alternative explanation for their improvement would be **spontaneous recovery**.

The data used to answer a question can be quantitative, qualitative, or a combination of the two. **Quantitative data** consist of numerical information, and **qualitative data** consist of observation, interviewing, and document review. Some questions can be answered more accurately by using quantitative data, others by using qualitative data, and still others by some combination of these two.

Organizing Data

After the observations have been converted into data, the next task is to organize or summarize them in a way that makes it possible for them to be used for answering the question. The organizational structure used may be a table (see Table 14.1) or graphs (see Figure 14.2). Tables are appropriate for both qualitative data and quantitative data.

Note that Figure 14.2 suggests a greater degree of improvement than do the scores in Table 14.1 even though both show the same data. The impression of improvement in the graph on the left in Figure 14.2 was enhanced by having the test score scale begin with 30 rather than 0. When the scale is begun with 0, as in the

TABLE 14.1. Example of Organizing Data Into a Table in Order to Compare Pre- and Posttherapy Scores

Test subject	Pretherapy score	Posttherapy score
1	25	50
2	35	60
3	20	70
4	30	31
5	60	65
6	50	45
7	15	18
8	20	20
9	35	40
10	65	70
	35.5 = Mean	46.9 = Mean

Note: Hypothetical pre- and posttherapy scores of 10 people with aphasia

graph on the right, the amount of improvement appears to be less. These examples illustrate the importance of carefully examining the scales on graphs before interpreting them.

Quantitative data can also be summarized by performing various **statistical analyses** on them. For descriptions of those that are used most frequently in speech–language pathology and audiology research, and the terminology associated with them, see Box 14.3, Statistical Terms.

Answering the Questions

Once the data have been organized or summarized in a way that enables the questions to be answered, the questions are relatively easy to answer. Using the hypothetical example shown in Table 14.1, one statistical analysis that could be used to show whether the differences between the pre- and posttherapy scores reflect real change is the *t* test (you'll find a definition of the *t* test in Box 14.3, Statistical Terms). In our example, performing the *t* test would show that the posttherapy scores are significantly higher than the pretherapy scores. As a result, the clinician can conclude with confidence that the therapeutic intervention program used was effective for improving the speech comprehension of clients with Wernicke's aphasia.

Determining Theoretical and Clinical Implications of the Answer

Answering the research question naturally leads to two further considerations. First, what does the answer imply regarding the theoretical basis underlying the inter-

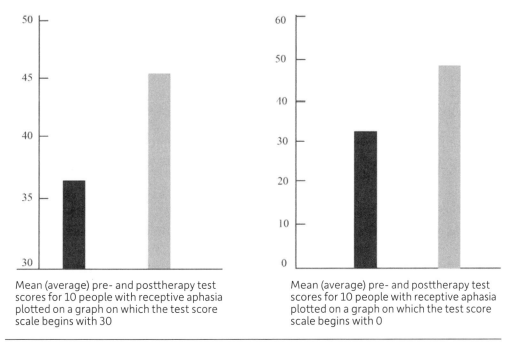

Mean (average) pre- and posttherapy test scores for 10 people with receptive aphasia plotted on a graph on which the test score scale begins with 30

Mean (average) pre- and posttherapy test scores for 10 people with receptive aphasia plotted on a graph on which the test score scale begins with 0

FIGURE 14.2. Two examples of graphs showing data comparing pre- and posttherapy test scores.

vention program? Second, what does the answer imply about possible clinical implications for these clients (or others who may benefit from the same therapeutic approach)?

Using the example from Table 14.1, once the clinician has determined that the intervention was effective in improving the speech comprehension of clients with Wernicke's aphasia, he or she considers what that information contributes to the theory underlying the theoretical approach. For instance, if the therapy involved pairing spoken sentences with the same sentences in print, the clinician could hypothesize that the therapy stimulated the brain with paired sensory stimuli, the theory being that stimulating the client's impaired language abilities increases the chances for improvement in speech comprehension.

One clinical implication that could be derived from the example is that this particular therapeutic approach might also work with children who have impaired speech comprehension. To test this idea, the clinician would use this implication as a beginning hypothesis for another clinical research study that would follow the same steps described here, only this time applying the steps to children with impaired speech comprehension.

Communicating Findings to Colleagues

Clinician-researchers communicate their findings with colleagues in a variety of ways. They can be reported in clinical journals, such as, for audiologists, the *American Journal of Audiology*; *Perspectives*; *Audiology Connections*; *Access Audiology*;

Journal of the American Academy of Audiology; for SLPs, *American Journal of Speech–Language Pathology*; and *Perspectives*; and for both audiologists and SLPs, *Journal of Speech, Language, and Hearing Research*; *International Journal of Speech–Language Pathology*; and *Language, Speech, and Hearing Services in Schools*. In addition, SLPs often submit their findings to journals published in related fields, such as learning disabilities, exceptional children, and autism. Another means of reporting on the results of one's clinical research is to present a platform presentation or poster presentation at a professional meeting, such as the annual convention of ASHA or that of a state speech, language, and hearing association.

BOX 14.3   Statistical Terms

These statistical terms are the most commonly used in speech–language and audiology publications. For a complete list and definitions of statistical terms, see the list compiled by the Department of Statistics at the University of California, Berkeley (2014).

Analysis of variance—A statistical technique used mostly to assess the likelihood that observed differences between more than two means, medians, or other statistics are real ones (i.e., not merely the result of random sampling error). The scientific method requires such observed differences to be shown to be highly unlikely to result from random sampling error (i.e., chance) before they can be interpreted.

Confidence interval—An estimate of the value of a population statistic based on a sample of persons from the population (e.g., the percentage of persons in the United States who approve of the president's job performance estimated from the responses of a sample of 1,000 persons). The estimate is expressed as an interval within which it is 95% or 99% certain that the value falls (e.g., it is 95% certain the president's job approval rating is between 56% and 58%).

Correlation coefficient—A statistic that usually provides information about both the strength and direction of the relationship between two variables (e.g., height and weight). Correlation coefficients range in value from −1.0 to +1.0. The closer the value of the coefficient is to zero, the weaker the strength of the relationship. And the closer it is to either −1.0 or +1.0, the greater the strength of the relationship.

The minus or plus sign in front of a correlation coefficient indicates whether the relationship is a positive or negative one. If the relationship is a positive one, as the value of one variable increases, that of the other does also (e.g., height and weight are positively related). And if the relationship is a negative one, as the value of one variable increases, that of the other decreases (e.g., chronological age and number of articulation errors are negatively related for preschoolers).

Level of confidence—When you're doing a significance test, it is the level at which you want to be confident that an observed difference is real (i.e., not due to random sampling error) before concluding that it is real. The two levels of confidence that are used most often are 95% (0.05) and 99% (0.01). If you declare an observed difference between means to be a real one at the 0.05 (95%) level of confidence, there is a 5% chance that you will be wrong (i.e., that the observed difference really was due to random sampling error).

Box 14.3 (*continued*)

Linear relationship—Either a positive relationship in which both variables increase or decrease in value proportionally or a negative relationship in which the value of one variable increases as the value of the other decreases proportionally. If points for the two variables are plotted on a line graph (that is referred to as a *scattergram*—see A through C), the line of best fit to the points (i.e., the line from which they deviate the least) will be a straight line (rather than a curved line).

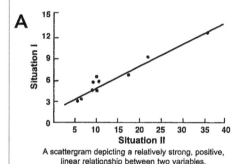

A scattergram depicting a relatively strong, positive, linear relationship between two variables.

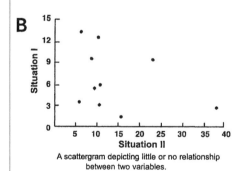

A scattergram depicting little or no relationship between two variables.

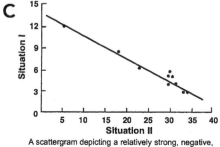

A scattergram depicting a relatively strong, negative, linear relationship between two variables.

Mean—A measure of "central tendency" that is the average of the numbers in a column or row. You add the numbers and then divide the total by how many numbers you added. The mean of the following numbers is 5: 1, 10, 4.

Median—A measure of "central tendency" that is the number at the midpoint of a set of numbers when the numbers in the set are ordered from lowest to highest (or from highest to lowest). The median of the following set of five numbers is 4: 1, 2, 4, 6, 30.

Mode—A measure of "central tendency" that is the most frequently occurring number in a set of numbers. The mode in the following set of 10 numbers is 5: 2, 3, 4, 4, 5, 5, 5, 5, 6, 8.

N—The abbreviation for the number of subjects or other entities (e.g., $N = 10$ subjects).

Negative relationship—If a relationship between two variables is a negative one, as the value of one increases, that of the other decreases (e.g., as children grow older, the number of articulation errors that they exhibit decreases).

Normal distribution—A symmetrical, bell-shaped curve in which certain relationships hold regarding its height at specified distances from its center (see the following example).

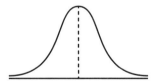

Percentile—The percentage of persons in a population who have a test score, or other numerical designation (e.g., height), that is less than a specified one. For example, having a test score at the 50th percentile means that half of the people who took the test had lower scores. The median, incidentally, is the 50th percentile.

(*continues*)

Box 14.3 (*continued*)

Population—The group of persons to whom an investigator wants to be able to generalize. An example of such a population could be persons who have receptive aphasia and are more than 1 year posttrauma.

Positive relationship—If the relationship between two variables is a positive one, as the value of one increases, so does that of the other (e .g., increases in height tend to be accompanied by increases in weight).

Random error—A form of error present to some degree in all sampling and measurement processes. While such an error can make it difficult to detect relatively small differences and relatively weak relationships, it does not bias the data (i.e., cause incorrect conclusions to be reached about differences and relationships).

Random sample—A sample selected from a population by a random process (e.g., by using a table of random numbers). If a sample was not selected by a random process, the accuracy of conclusions about the population from which it came will be uncertain.

Range—A measure of "variability" that is the difference between the smallest number and the largest number (e .g., the subjects ranged in age from 5 years to 8 years). The larger the difference between the two numbers, the greater the variability.

Sample—A group of people or other entities that were selected from a population of such people or entities either randomly or by some other process.

Scattergram—A two-dimensional graphical display for visualizing the strength, nature (linear or curvilinear), and direction (positive or negative) of the relationship between two variables. It provides almost the same information about the strength and direction of a relationship as does a correlation coefficient.

Significance tests—Statistical techniques for assessing the likelihood that observed differences between means, medians, or other statistics are real ones (i.e., not merely the result of random sampling error). Two examples are analysis of variance and the *t* test.

Standard deviation—A measure of the "variability" of the numbers in a row or column. The larger the standard deviation, the greater the variability. The standard deviation is less likely than the range to overestimate variability (because it isn't affected as much as is the range by a few extreme scores or other measures).

Statistically significant difference—A possible outcome of a significance test. Its usual interpretation is that it is 95% or more certain that the difference between means, medians, or other measures on which the test was performed was not due to chance. However, the difference in the population may not be as large as that observed, nor does it necessarily have any theoretical or practical implications. A difference between pre- and posttherapy measures may be statistically significant, but the amount of change it reflects may not be enough to yield any meaningful reduction in the severity of a client's impairments, disabilities, or handicaps.

Systematic error—A type of error present in a measurement process that biases the data (i.e., causes incorrect conclusions to be reached). For example, if a pure-tone audiometer is not calibrated properly, it may indicate hearing thresholds at one or more frequencies that are higher or lower than they should be.

***T* test**—A statistical technique for assessing the likelihood that the observed difference between two means, medians, or other statistics is a real one (i.e., not merely the result of random sampling error).

Variable—An entity than can assume more than one value. Two examples are chronological age and weight.

glossary

Abduct To move apart.

Ablative surgery Surgical removal of all or part of a structure (e.g., the lips or mandible).

Acoustic neuritis Inflammation of the auditory nerve.

Addition In a speech sound disorder, a sound added to a syllable or word (e.g., "upa" for "up"); the least common articulation error.

Adduct To move together.

Alveolar ridge A ridged shelf in the upper jaw (i.e., maxilla) behind the upper teeth.

Alzheimer's disease A chronic, degenerative disease of the brain that usually worsens over time.

American Academy of Private Practice in Speech Pathology and Audiology (AAPPSPA) An organization devoted to SLPs and audiologists in private practice offering professional support, resources, and interactions among members.

American Indian Hand Talk (Amer-Ind) A manual communication system adapted from one developed by Native Americans hundreds of years ago.

American Sign Language (ASL) A sign language used in Deaf communities in the United States and the English-speaking parts of Canada.

American Speech-Language-Hearing Association (ASHA) A national professional association for audiologists; SLPs; speech, language, and hearing scientists; audiology and SLP support personnel; and students. ASHA acts as the accrediting and credentialing organization for its members and member affiliates.

Amyotrophic lateral sclerosis (ALS) A progressive, fatal neuromuscular disorder, also known as *Lou Gehrig's disease*. Causes damage to nerve cells in the brain and spinal cord.

Anomaly An irregularity; deviation from what is expected.

Anomic aphasia The inability to name things or recognize spoken or written names of things (i.e., severe difficulty with word retrieval).

Anosognosia A condition in which an individual is not aware he or she has a difficulty or condition.

Anoxia Absence of oxygen supply to an organ's tissues.

Answerable question A question that can be answered by making observations and that indicates (directly or indirectly) the observations that have to be made to answer it.

Anterior open bite A type of dental malocclusion in which there is a relatively large space between the upper and lower incisors when the jaws are together.

Antonyms Words with opposite meanings.

Aphasia Partial or total loss of the ability to communicate orally or in writing; caused by damage in the brain.

Aphasia test A test used to identify language deficits that can result from damage to the cerebral cortex, particularly the left hemisphere.

Aphonia Without voice; the inability to produce voice.

Appian Way A road in ancient Rome that had cave-like apertures in the rocky outcrop on both sides, in which people who had mental handicaps, deformities, and communication impairments were caged to provide entertainment for travelers.

Arbitrary As it pertains to language, the absence of any necessary connection between what a word means, how it sounds, or its form.

Articulators The organs that produce speech: tongue, teeth, lips, mandible, hard palate, and velum.

Artificial larynx Two types of artificial larynges are available: (1) a handheld, battery-operated device that produces sound through the cheek, neck, or chin, and (2) an intraoral device that utilizes a sound-producing tube placed toward the back of the mouth.

Aspiration Food or liquid entering the airway.

Assistive listening system (ALS) Any of a number of devices that amplify sound directly into the ear and separate the sounds the individual wants to hear (e.g., speech) from background noise.

Audiogram Graphic record of an individual's hearing ability for a variety of standard frequencies.

Audiologist Audiologists evaluate, diagnose, treat, and manage hearing loss and balance disorders in children and adults.

Audiometer An instrument used to measure hearing acuity through measuring the individual's responses to sounds of different frequencies and intensities.

Audiometric screening test Presenting pure tones in each ear at a set intensity level (usually 20 dB) at three frequency levels (1000, 2000, and 4000 Hz). To pass, individuals must signal that they heard all three tones in each ear.

Auditory agnosia A disorder of the central auditory nervous system in which the person has difficulty separating figure from background noise.

Auditory brainstem response (ABR) A procedure in which small electrodes on an individual's head detect how the acoustic nerve responds to sounds.

Auditory evoked potentials (AEPs) The collective term for electrophysiological tests that measure the neuroelectric responses of the auditory system to sound.

Auditory nerve A branch of the VIIIth cranial nerve that transmits electrochemical energy generated by the inner ear to the central auditory nervous system (CANS).

Autism A group of complex disorders related to brain development, typically manifested by difficulties in social interactions, particularly in pragmatics, and by the presence of repetitive behaviors.

Babbling The vocalizations of infants after approximately 6 weeks of age, characterized by the production of meaningless, though usually articulate, vocal sounds.

Basal ganglia Multiple cell nuclei located at the base of the forebrain; part of the extrapyramidal system.

Baseline The results of an assessment prior to any intervention; an individual's communication skills or abilities before intervention begins.

Basic episode An early developmental story that contains an initiating event or "problem," an attempt to address or solve the "problem," and a consequence.

Bilabial sound Sound produced with closure of the lips.

Bilateral conductive hearing loss A conductive hearing loss in both ears.

Bilingualism The habitual use of two languages, sometimes with equal ability in both, but more commonly with one language being dominant.

Biofeedback The use of various types of instrumentation to provide feedback about particular muscles, sounds, or movements.

Bolus The rounded mass of food formed through chewing and saliva prior to swallowing.

Bone conduction testing Sending a pure tone through a vibrator placed behind the ear or on the forehead, which bypasses the middle ear and stimulates the cochlea.

Bound morpheme A morpheme that is attached to a larger word, such as -s to mark the plural *dogs*.

Brain abscesses Walled-off cavities containing dead or dying white blood cells.

Broca's aphasia A nonfluent aphasia characterized by difficulty forming and understanding complete sentences, retrieving word meanings, and forming speech sounds.

Calibrated An instrument that is calibrated provides systematic increments or gradations of degree, quantity, or volume, as in frequency or intensity. A common example is a thermometer.

Central auditory nervous system (CANS) The auditory nerve pathways from the brainstem to the cerebral cortex.

Central nervous system (CNS) The brain and spinal cord, which are responsible for processing information received from and sent to all parts of the body.

Cerebellum Area of the hindbrain that controls motor coordination, balance, equilibrium, and muscle tone.

Cerebral arteriosclerosis A thickening of the walls of cerebral arteries, resulting in a slower rate of blood flow through them.

Cerebral cortex The outermost surface of the cerebral hemispheres of the brain.

Cerebral palsy (CP) A group of disorders causing physical disability, specifically in movement, balance, and posture.

Cerebrovascular accident (CVA) Sudden death of brain cells because of lack of oxygen as a result of reduced blood flow to the brain. Caused by blockage or rupture of one of the arteries to the brain. Also called *stroke*.

Certificate of Clinical Competence (CCC) The certification awarded by ASHA to those professionals who have met the rigorous academic and professional standards specified by ASHA.

Cerumen Ear wax.

Cerumen impaction An overabundance of ear wax.

Ceruminous glands The glands that secrete cerumen.

Chief complaint The reason given by the client (or the person who requested the evaluation) indicating why the evaluation was requested.

Cholesteatoma A type of tumor that can occur in the middle ear and cause a conductive hearing loss.

Cilia Small hairs on the inner surface of the external auditory meatus.

Classroom discourse The specific language patterns and structures used by teachers and students within the classroom setting.

Cleft palate A congenital disorder in which there is an opening in the hard palate, soft palate (i.e., velum), or both.

Clinical relationship The context within which clinical services are dispensed, involving the clinician, the client, and those close to the client. Also referred to as *therapeutic relationship*.

Clinician-investigator A clinician who does therapy-outcome research, which forms the basis for evidence-based practice. All SLPs and audiologists are required to collect some data on outcomes for purposes of accountability.

Closed head injury An injury resulting from a blow to the head.

Cochlea The sensory organ in the inner ear that is responsible for transmitting sound to the central nervous system.

Cochlear implant The surgical insertion of a small, complex electronic device consisting of an array of electrodes placed in the inner ear, a receiver/transmitter that is placed under the skin just above and behind the ear, and an external microphone and speech processor that sit behind the ear.

Code of Ethics of the American Speech-Language-Hearing Association The document governing the obligations and responsibilities of SLPs; audiologists; and speech, language, and hearing scientists in order to preserve the highest standards of integrity and ethical principles.

Code switching Alternating between two languages in the context of a single conversation.

Cognitive disability Significantly below average intellectual functioning and concurrent deficits in adaptive behaviors.

Collaborative service delivery (integrative treatment model) Providing services to a school-age child (or children) in a general education or special education classroom rather than in a separate therapy room.

Communication Any exchange of information between people using a common code, or symbol system, that is understood by those involved.

Communication board A sheet of cardboard or other material on which the alphabet, commonly used words and phrases, or pictographic symbols are printed. The user communicates by pointing to or otherwise indicating the symbols needed to transmit messages.

Communication disorder An impairment in receiving, sending, processing, or comprehending concepts or verbal, nonverbal, or graphic symbol systems.

Communicative intent An individual's intention to communicate with others.

Conductive aphasia A type of aphasia characterized by *paraphasia*.

Conductive hearing loss Hearing loss caused by pathology in the outer or middle ear.

Congenital Any nonhereditary condition, particularly an abnormal one, that exists at birth.

Congenital atresia A partial or complete absence or blockage of the external auditory meatus.

Conjunct A word or phrase connecting a sentence with previous sentences.

Consistency effect The greater-than-chance tendency for stutterers to stutter on words that they stuttered on previously.

Contract A written or oral agreement that the parties agree to abide by voluntarily. The relationship between the client and clinician is a contractual one.

Conversational repair A speaker's recognition that the listener has not understood something, followed by the speaker's attempt to clarify what she or he meant.

Copula A verb that links the subject and predicate of a proposition (e.g., all the forms of "to be").

Corpus callosum The bundle of neural fibers connecting the left and right hemispheres of the brain.

Cricoid cartilage A ring-like structure at the base of the *larynx* that surrounds the *trachea*.

Cultural context The language-specific situation and setting within which any communicative interchange takes place.

Culture The beliefs, values, customs, practices, and social behavior characteristic of a particular group of people.

Decibel (dB) The unit of measurement for the loudness of sounds. The louder the sound, the larger the number.

Decontextualized language Language that is removed from the immediate situation or context so that meaning is conveyed in a more abstract way.

Degenerative The structure and/or function of affected body parts deteriorate over time.

Dementia A decline in mental ability severe enough to limit or interfere with daily activities.

Developmental norms Ages by which specific percentages of children in a given population have acquired particular abilities.

Diadochokinetic rate The rate at which an individual can accurately and rapidly repeat a series of alternating phonetic sounds, such as /pʌ tʌ kʌ pʌ tʌ kʌ pʌ tʌ kʌ /.

Diaphragm The primary muscle of inspiration and inhalation; dome-shaped muscle separating the thoracic cavity from the abdomen.

Differential diagnosis A process for distinguishing between two or more conditions with similar characteristics by systematically comparing and contrasting their characteristics with clinical findings.

Discourse Various types of verbal communication, including casual conversation, lectures, sermons, stories, and arguments.

Disfluency Hesitations, repetitions, mispronunciations, and interjections in one's speech.

Disjunct A word or phrase that conveys a speaker's attitude toward the content of the sentence it appears in.

Documentation Regarding intervention, describing its impact on clients, using data that possess adequate levels of validity, reliability, and generality.

Dysarthria A neuromuscular disorder that prevents structures within the vocal tract, particularly the oral cavity, from moving properly to produce speech sounds.

Dyslexia A language-based learning disability characterized by difficulty in learning to read fluently and in accurate reading comprehension.

Dysphonia An impairment in the ability to produce voice sounds using the vocal folds and related structures.

Dysrhythmic phonations Disturbances in the normal rhythms of words.

Dystonia A voice disorder characterized by involuntary movements of one or both vocal folds.

Efficacy Degree to which a method or approach results in a specific, beneficial result; effectiveness.

Embolus A blockage (clot) originating somewhere else that travels to a blood vessel (e.g., blood clot).

Empathy The ability to truly understand how another person feels about an event, experience, process, or idea.

Endoscopic assessment A very small, flexible tube with a camera and light on the end is inserted through the nose and into the back of the mouth. The scope is connected to a computer and video monitor with which the SLP can see the person's swallowing function.

Endotracheal intubation Placement of a plastic tube into the trachea to allow an individual to breathe.

Epiglottis The flap of cartilage in front of the larynx that prevents food or liquid from passing into the trachea.

Esophageal speech Speech produced by injecting air into the upper esophagus, causing the esophagus to vibrate, thus creating sound used to produce speech.

Esophagus The tube that carries food and liquid from the mouth to the stomach.

Eustachian tube A hollow structure that connects the middle ear to the back wall of the throat.

Evaluation The first step in the intervention process. The purpose of evaluation is to determine if the client has a communication disorder and, if so, to identify and describe the impairments and handicaps that it has caused or placed the client at risk for developing.

Evidence-based practice (EBP) Basing decisions about the care of individual clients on the best evidence available about what works. In EBP, clinicians integrate their clinical expertise and judgment with the best available external clinical evidence derived from systematic research.

Expectancy phenomenon The ability of stutterers to predict moments of stuttering with greater-than-chance accuracy.

Experimenter bias An experimenter's bias (sometimes very subtle) that the outcome of an experiment will match her or his expectations.

Expert witness A professional whose education, training, skill, or experience provides expertise and specific knowledge about communication disorders. An expert witness may be called upon by either the prosecution or the defense.

Expiration Exhalation; breathing out.

Expository discourse Discourse that describes, explains, argues/persuades, or compares and contrasts.

External auditory meatus The part of the outer ear that is also referred to as the ear canal.

External intercostal muscles Muscles between the ribs that aid in inhalation by moving the ribs upward.

Extrapyramidal system The part of the motor system that controls involuntary movements and reflexes as well as muscle tone and posture.

Figurative language Language that bypasses literal meaning to convey a special meaning on a more abstract level (e.g., metaphor, simile, idiom).

First temporal convolution A longitudinal gyrus (convolution) on the lateral surface of the temporal lobe.

Flaccidity Paralysis or weakness of muscle contraction resulting from damage to muscle fibers, myoneural junctions, or lower motor neurons.

Fluency Smooth and effortless production of connected speech.

Fluent aphasia Aphasia in which an individual's speech production is relatively fluent and connected.

Free morpheme The smallest grammatical unit in any given language; a morpheme that can stand alone as a word (e.g., *dog*).

Frontal lobe The front part of the brain that regulates and mediates decision making, problem solving, emotions, and judgment.

Functional communication needs The basic communication abilities a person needs to function in everyday life (e.g., face-to-face or telephone conversations and writing).

Generative Speakers can create an infinite number of utterances using a limited number of grammatical rules.

Gestural Morse Code A communication system used by persons who have severe communication impairments in which words are spelled out letter-by-letter using gestures (e.g., blinking the eyes) for Morse Code dots and dashes.

Global aphasia The most severe form of aphasia that usually occurs immediately following a stroke.

Glossectomy Surgical removal of a portion of the tongue. Such surgery is usually done to remove a malignant tumor from the tongue tissue.

Glottal sound Sound made with an open glottis.

Glottis The open space between the vocal folds when they are in the abducted position.

Graphophonemic awareness Recognition of the sound–symbol relationships between phonemes and print letters.

Hard palate The anterior portion of the roof of the mouth.

Hearing The perception of sound.

Hearing aid An electronic device worn by an individual in or behind the ear to improve hearing.

Hematoma A pooling of blood, for example, between the skull and the brain, that causes swelling.

Hemianopia Loss of vision in either the left or right half of an individual's visual field.

Hemiplegia Paralysis of the muscles on one side of the body.

Hemorrhage Rapid and uncontrolled loss of blood.

Hemorrhagic stroke A stroke caused by blood hemorrhaging out of a cerebral artery.

Hertz (Hz) The unit of measurement for the pitch of sounds. The higher the pitch, the larger the number.

Homonyms (also known as *homophones*) Words that sound the same but carry different meanings.

Human papillomavirus (HPV) The most commonly sexually transmitted infection in the United States. It is preventable with vaccines.

Huntington's disease A genetic disease resulting in gradual loss of brain cells. Both neurological functioning and intelligence are affected. Also referred to as *Huntington's chorea*.

Hypernasality The voice quality resulting from an excess amount of air passing through the nasal passageways.

Hyponasality The voice quality resulting from too little air passing through the nasal passageways.

Hypotheses In this context, preliminary explanations for clients' impairments, disabilities, and handicaps.

Ideographic A set of graphic characters that symbolize ideas without indicating the pronunciation of the words represented.

Idiom A phrase or sentence that means something different from its literal meaning.

Idiosyncratic Language features that are unique to a particular individual and thus unpredictable.

Incisors The four front teeth in each jaw (i.e., the two central and two lateral incisors).

Incus The second of the three tiny bones in the middle ear.

Independent professional A professional who is not required by law to have his or her activities regulated (i.e., controlled) by a member of another profession. Speech–language pathologists and audiologists (like physicians and dentists) are independent professionals. Speech–language pathology assistants (like nurses and physical therapists) are not.

Individualized education program (IEP) The unique program designed by a team of professionals and family for an individual student who receives special education or related services. The IEP serves as the guide for the provision of special education supports and services.

Inspiration Inhalation; breathing in.

Intelligibility How understandable a speaker is to a listener.

Interjections Sounds, syllables, words, or phrases added between words.

Internal intercostal muscles Muscles between the ribs that help in forced exhalation by depressing the ribs and moving them inward.

Interrogative forms Phrases, sentences, or intonation patterns that serve to ask questions.

Intervention strategy The approach used to try to achieve an intervention goal (i.e., to be helpful to the client).

Ischemic stroke A stroke caused by blockage that disrupts or stops blood flow to a region of the brain.

Labio-dental sound Sound produced with the upper teeth placed on the lower lip.

Language The code used for communicating ideas with others.

Language content The substance of a language, or the meaning of what we are trying to say; also called *semantics*.

Language disorder Disruptions in an individual's understanding and expression of language content, form, or use.

Language use How people use language to negotiate relationships; also called *social communication*, or *pragmatics*.

Laryngeal tone The sound produced by the vocal folds.

Laryngectomy Removal of the larynx and separation of the trachea from the mouth.

Laryngopharyngeal The area where the larynx and the pharynx meet.

Laryngoscopic view The view of the vocal folds possible when using a head mirror and laryngeal mirror.

Larynx The structure that contains the vocal folds (i.e., the mechanism that produces voice), located at the top of the trachea. The larynx also functions as a valve that prevents food and liquids from getting into the lungs.

Learning style The process(es) through which an individual (or cultural group) learns most efficiently.

Left cerebral hemisphere The hemisphere of the brain that controls movement of the right side of the body as well as most functions of language, logic, reasoning, and similar abilities.

License A permit issued by a governmental entity (usually a state) to practice a profession.

Lingua-alveolar sound Sound produced with the tongue against the alveolar ridge.

Lingua-dental sound Sound produced with the tongue between the upper and lower teeth.

Lipreading An older term for speechreading. Using visual facial information to augment hearing for understanding speech.

Lobbying Attempting to encourage the passage of state or federal legislation that is likely to be helpful to persons who have communication disorders and to discourage the passage of legislation that is likely to be harmful to them.

Localization of function The theory that certain functions, such as language, are located in very specific areas of the brain.

Logopedics The study of speech disorders.

Long-term goals Statements that specify the measurable outcomes the clinician is attempting to achieve through the intervention process.

Loudness recruitment An abnormally rapid growth of loudness with an increase in intensity.

Lower motor neurons Neurons (nerve cells) that receive impulses from upper motor neurons and connect the spinal cord and brain stem to muscle fibers; all voluntary movement relies on spinal lower motor neurons.

Lungs The organs in the chest responsible for breathing.

Malleus The first of the three tiny bones in the middle ear.

Mandible Lower jaw; largest and strongest bone in the face.

Manual communication An approach used to teach individuals with hearing impairments how to communicate using their hands in combination with body postures and facial expressions to communicate; signing.

Maxilla The upper jaw.

Medical model An approach to assessment and intervention in which the focus is on the communication disorder. The clinician diagnoses the communication disorder and is solely responsible for designing and directing intervention, which focuses on remediating the disorder.

Medicare A national health-care insurance program in the United States for people age 65 or older and some younger individuals who have serious disabilities.

Ménière's disease A disease of the vestibular system (part of the inner ear) that has a sensorineural hearing loss as one of its components.

Metacognitive ability The various processes used to reflect on one's own thinking and learning.

Metalinguistic skills The processes one uses to reflect on and talk about language and linguistic features.

Metaphor A figure of speech indirectly comparing two dissimilar things.

Metapragmatic ability The ability to talk about how language is used.

Metapragmatics The ability to reflect on how language is used.

Modified barium swallow The individual swallows small amounts of food and liquid mixed with barium while an x-ray captures moving images of the food as it travels from the mouth, through the pharynx, and into the esophagus.

Morphemes The smallest meaningful elements of language.

Morphology and morphological disorder *Morphology* is the study of the way words and parts of words (morphemes) combine to make meaning. A *morphological disorder* is a disruption in the ability to understand or express oneself by using the morphemes characteristic of one's language.

Motivation In this context, the willingness of the client to make the investments necessary to achieve therapy goals.

Motor system The parts of the peripheral and central nervous system that regulate the contraction of muscle fibers.

Multiple sclerosis (MS) A neurological disorder that can affect the functioning of the auditory nerves and other structures within the brain that support motor and sensory abilities. Typical symptoms are weakness, incoordination, paresthesias, speech disturbances, and visual complaints.

Muscular dystrophy Any of a group of diseases causing progressive muscle weakness and loss of muscle mass.

Myasthenia gravis A chronic condition that causes fatigue and weakness in the skeletal muscles.

Myofunctional therapy Therapy intended to eliminate tongue thrusting.

Myoneural junctions The junction between a nerve fiber and the muscle it innervates.

Narrative discourse The forms of language used in storytelling.

Nasal Speech sounds produced with the velum lowered, which allows air to pass through the nose.

Nasal cavity Large air-filled space above and behind the nose.

Nasality The nasalization of speech sounds, as in /m/, /n/, and /ŋ/.

Nasogastric tube (NG tube) A plastic tube inserted through the nose and down into the stomach in order to supply food and medications.

Negation Denial, refusal, or disagreement.

Neoplasm Tumor.

Neurodevelopmental Having to do with how the brain and central nervous system grow and develop.

Neurofibrillary tangles Insoluble, twisted protein fibers that clog the brain from the inside out.

Nonfluent aphasia Aphasia in which an individual's speech production is halting, effortful, and disconnected.

Nonstandardized assessments Non-norm-referenced instruments or procedures used to evaluate the various types of communication disorders.

Normal limits Statistically expected range within which a person's speech, hearing, or language abilities fall.

Norms The statistical grouping of scores collected from a representative sample of individuals.

Objectivity Perceiving, documenting, and managing clients' impairments, disabilities, and handicaps without becoming emotionally involved or losing focus on the client's welfare.

Observations The data used to answer the questions that an evaluation is intended to answer.

Occipital lobes The lobes at the back of the cerebral cortex responsible for visual processing.

Occlude To block or obstruct.

Omission In a speech sound disorder, the deletion of a sound from a word (e.g., "ba" for "ball").

Oncologist A medical professional specializing in cancerous tumors.

Oral cavity The hollow part of the mouth.

Orality Speech sounds produced without undue nasal resonance.

Oral method An approach used to teach individuals with hearing impairments how to use speech effectively.

Oral peripheral exam An assessment of the structures involved in producing voice and speech: lips, teeth, tongue, facial muscles, and larynx.

Orofacial myofunctional disorder Disorder of the muscles and functions of the face, mouth, lips, or jaw.

Oropharynx The top of the throat where the mouth and the pharynx meet.

Ossicles The three tiny bones (malleus, incus, stapes) in the middle ear (also known as *ossicular chain*).

Ossicular discontinuity An abnormal separation of the ossicles.

Otitis media An inflammation in the middle ear that can cause a conductive hearing loss.

Otoacoustic emissions test (OAE) A procedure in which the vibration produced in the inner ear when it is stimulated by a sound is picked up and measured by a probe inside an individual's ear.

Otolaryngologist A medical professional specializing in ear, nose, and throat conditions.

Otosclerosis A disease in which the stapes (the third bone in the ossicular chain) becomes fixated in the *oval window*, thereby causing a conductive hearing loss.

Otoscope An instrument used to examine the ears. It consists of a light source and a magnifying lens.

Oval window The membrane that separates the middle ear from the inner ear.

Palatal sound Sound produced with the tongue against the hard palate.

Paralinguistic signals Vocal or nonvocal signals accompanying speech (e.g., pitch, loudness, rate, fluency, gestures, postures).

Paraphasia A characteristic of anomic aphasia in which the individual transposes sounds in a word or adds syllables or sounds to words.

Paraprofessionals The people who assist professionals in either speech–language pathology (SLPAs) or audiology.

Parentese The modifications in speech and language adults use when talking to babies: raised pitch, slowed rate, singsong pattern, elongated vowels.

Parietal lobe Located behind the frontal lobe and above the temporal lobe, the parietal lobe is responsible for integrating sensory input.

Parkinson's disease A progressive motor system disorder resulting from the loss of dopamine-producing brain cells.

Part-word repetitions Repetitions of sounds and syllables in words.

Participation model A clinical relationship characterized by client and clinician focusing on "what clients think about themselves, their abilities and accomplishments, their disabilities, and their future" (Duchan, 2003, para. 1).

Penetrating injury An injury resulting from a foreign object that enters the brain and causes damage.

Perinatal Something that occurs during the birth process.

Perseveration Continued repetition of a response (e.g., a word or phrase) when it no longer contributes to meaning but instead interferes with communication.

Pharyngeal cavity Links the nasal cavity to the larynx and the mouth to the esophagus.

Pharynx The part of the throat immediately behind the nasal cavity and mouth, and above the esophagus and larynx.

Phonation The production of voice made by the vibration of the vocal folds.

Phoneme collapse The child produces one sound for several different adult target sounds, or deletes several adult target sounds in a given position (e.g., /t/ substituted for /f, p, h, θ, n/).

Phonemes The smallest units of speech sound that carry meaning.

Phoniatrics The study of voice disorders.

Phonics A method for teaching children how to decode new words by sounding them out.

Phonological awareness An individual's awareness of the phonological structures of language.

Phonological disorder A disruption in the ability to learn the rules governing the sound system of a given language.

Phonological processes The phonological patterns young children use to simplify adult articulation until they have the ability to use adult phonological forms.

Phonology The study of the speech sound (phoneme) system in any given language.

Phrase repetitions Repetitions of units of two or more words.

Pictographic A set of graphic pictorial symbols used to convey information.

Plateau A period during which the client makes no measurable progress toward achieving a therapy goal.

Polio A viral disease that damages lower motor neurons and causes flaccidity. The functioning of the velum is frequently affected.

Postlingual deafness Hearing loss that occurs after a child has begun learning language.

Postnatal Something occurring after birth.

Pragmatics and pragmatics disorder Pragmatics is the study of how people use language to negotiate relationships and meet their needs (see language use). A pragmatics disorder is a disruption in the ability to use language effectively, to express oneself appropriately in changing contexts, and to negotiate relationships.

Prelingual deafness Hearing loss that occurs before a child begins learning language.

Prenatal Something occurring prior to birth.

Prepositional phrases Phrases that begin with prepositions—words used before nouns and pronouns.

Presbycusis Sensorineural hearing loss resulting—directly or indirectly (e.g., long-term exposure to noise)—from the effect of the aging process on the inner ear.

Presuppositions Assumptions speakers make about what their listeners already know and don't need to be told specifically.

Prosody The rhythm, tempo, rate, stress, and intonation patterns of language.

Prosopagnosia The inability to recognize faces.

Prosthesis An artificial device to replace or augment a missing body part.

Prosthodontist A person who specializes in the part of dentistry pertaining to replacement of missing teeth and tissues with artificial substitutes.

Proverbs, adages, maxims Short and well-known sayings that offer advice or a cultural "truth."

Proxemics The study of how people in a given culture negotiate personal space during social interactions.

Psychiatrist A medical professional specializing in preventing and treating mental illness.

Psychoanalysis A system of psychotherapy developed in the late 1800s by Sigmund Freud.

Psychologist A professional who provides counseling or psychotherapy.

Pure tone A sound in which particles of air vibrate at a single frequency.

Pyramidal system Motor fibers extending down each side of the spinal column; functions to control voluntary movements.

Qualitative data Information that is difficult to measure, count, or express in numerical terms (e.g., the nature of relationships among various groups).

Quantitative data Data that consist of numerical descriptions of various sorts of attributes.

Referents What a word or symbol stands for or refers to.

Reliable Consistency and stability of measurement over time; research findings that can be replicated. Data that are consistent over time.

Representative Data that are consistent across situations (e.g., home, school, work).

Resonance The modulation of voice as it passes through the various cavities on its way from the vocal folds and out the mouth and nose.

Resonate To exhibit resonance.

Respiratory system The organs and tissues involved in breathing (which delivers oxygen to all parts of the body) and vibrating the vocal folds to produce voice.

Respiratory therapist A trained professional who treats people with disorders that affect the cardiopulmonary system.

Revision-incomplete phrases Disfluencies in which the speaker begins an utterance but does not complete it.

Right hemiplegia Weakness on the right side of the body, usually caused by damage to the left side of the brain.

Right-hemisphere deficits Impairments related to damage to the right cerebral hemisphere.

Scientific justification Providing answers to the "so what?" and "who cares?" questions for why it is important to carry out a particular clinical research project.

Scientific method A process for proposing a hypothesis and conducting methodical observations in order to accept or reject it.

Scope of practice What a communication sciences and disorders professional is legally and ethically permitted to do.

Secondary behaviors Behaviors that accompany moments of stuttering, particularly those of adults (e.g., using interjections or eye blinking). Also referred to as secondaries.

Semantics and semantic disorder Semantics is the study of meaning in any given language and how meaning is constructed through words (vocabulary), parts of words, phrases, sentences, and larger units of discourse. A semantic disorder is a disruption in the ability to understand or express meaning appropriately.

Semicircular canals The structures in the inner ear responsible for the detection of rotation.

Senile plaques Protein that collects outside of cells and forms a mass between neurons.

Sensorineural hearing loss Hearing loss that results from damage to the sensory cells of the cochlea or to the nerve pathways from the inner ear to the brain.

Short-term goals   These are "stepping stones" to achieving long-term goals. They often have to be accomplished in a specific order. Also referred to as *short-term objectives*.

Side effect   Something an intervention strategy changes other than what it's intended to change. A side effect can be physiological, psychological, desirable, or undesirable.

Signing Exact English (SEE)   A system linking a manual sign to each spoken individual English morpheme.

Simile   A figure of speech directly comparing two dissimilar things.

Sine wave   The waveform for a pure tone.

Single-subject research   A research design in which questions are answered by data from individual subjects rather than by data that are derived from the performances of groups of subjects.

Social worker   A mental health professional who helps people improve their lives in a variety of areas, including psychological issues, financial problems, health problems, relationship issues, and substance abuse.

Sound distortion   A sound that is produced inaccurately but sounds similar to the intended sound. The most common type of sound distortion is the lisp.

Sound substitution   Using another sound instead of the intended sound, as in "thun" for "sun."

Spasmodic dysphonia   A form of dystonia resulting from either hyperadducted or hypoadducted vocal folds.

Spasticity   A condition in which certain muscles are continuously contracted. It is the result of a lesion in the pyramidal and extrapyramidal systems.

Speech   The production of phonemes by the vocal tract.

Speech disorder   Any of several impairments that affect the production of normal speech.

Speech–language pathologist (SLP)   Speech–language pathologists (sometimes called speech–language clinicians or speech therapists) assess, diagnose, treat, and aid in preventing communication and swallowing disorders (U.S. Census Bureau, 2014).

Speechreading   Understanding what a person is saying through watching the movements of the mouth; observing facial expressions, gestures, and body postures; and analyzing the context and situation (Gallaudet Laurent Clerc National Education Center, 2008).

Spontaneous recovery   The tendency for aphasia impairments to decrease in severity during the first 6 months posttrauma.

Standard English   The language considered the norm for any given nation.

Standardized assessments/tests   Instruments that use norms gathered from a representative sample of individuals and that are administered in a consistent ("standard") way.

Stapes   The third of three tiny bones in the middle ear.

Starters   A device that individuals who stutter use to avoid stuttering. They inject sounds, syllables, words, or phrases they believe they can say without stuttering before words on which they expect to stutter.

Statistical analyses Numerical analyses for summarizing and otherwise treating quantitative data (e.g., to assess their validity and reliability) in order to answer research questions.

Sternocleidomastoid muscle A large muscle of the neck that is attached to the head, breastbone, and clavicle. Helps to bend, flex, rotate, and extend the head.

Stuttering A speech disorder in which speech sounds, syllables, or words are prolonged, repeated, or blocked, resulting in a disruption in the flow of speech.

Support group A group of people having a particular disability who support each other's attempts to cope with it. Members of such a group may communicate mainly face-to-face or online.

Supramarginal gyrus A portion of the parietal lobe involved in phonological and articulatory processing.

Syllabary A set of written symbols that represent syllables.

Symbolic The representation of one thing by something else (e.g., a word used to represent a thing, as in *chair*).

Synonyms Different words with the same meaning.

Syntax and syntactic disorder Syntax is the study of the structural components (grammar) of a language. A syntactic disorder is a disruption in the ability to understand or use the grammar of one's language to create an infinite number of utterances.

Target phoneme The phoneme that a drawing or word in an articulation test is intended to elicit.

Telecommunication relay service (TRS) A telephone service making it possible for people with hearing or speech–language disabilities to make and receive telephone calls.

Temporal lobe Located beneath the frontal and parietal lobes; responsible for many language functions and long-term memory.

Temporary threshold shift A temporary hearing loss after being exposed to loud noise that affects the functioning of the inner ear.

Tense pauses Pauses filled with barely audible heavy breathing or muscle tightening. Also referred to as blocks.

Therapy room A room, usually quiet, in which a clinician provides assessment and intervention services for a client or a group of clients.

Third frontal convolution A region of the brain in the frontal part of the left hemisphere of the brain, just in front of the face area of the motor cortex.

Third-party payers Private insurance companies and governmental organizations (e.g., Medicare) that pay for client services.

Thromboembolic stroke A stroke caused by an embolus that originates in an artery outside the brain.

Thrombus A blood clot that forms and stays in a vessel.

Thyroarytenoid muscle The muscle tissue forming the body of each vocal fold. It functions to relax the vocal folds.

Tinnitus The perception of sound (ringing, roaring, buzzing, hissing, tinkling) when no external sound is present.

Tongue thrust Thrusting the tongue against the incisors (i.e., front teeth) while speaking and swallowing.

Trachea The rings of mucuous-covered cartilage connecting the pharynx and larynx to the lungs; the windpipe.

Tracheostomy A surgical opening for a tube that is inserted into the trachea to allow an individual to breathe.

Transcortical aphasia In the sensory type, conversation and spontaneous speech are relatively fluent, but speech usually includes jargon. The motor type is characterized by expressive language difficulties.

Transduce Convert energy from one form into another. The inner ear transduces sound-induced vibration into a form of electrochemical energy.

Trauma Damage that is usually accidental to the nervous system or other bodily structures.

Traumatic brain injury (TBI) Injury to the brain caused by a violent blow or jolt to the head.

TTY The most common designator for a text telephone (derived from TeleTYpewriter). Also known as TDD (telecommunication device for the Deaf).

Tympanic membrane The membrane separating the outer ear from the middle ear; the eardrum.

Tympanogram The graph showing the results of tympanometry (the response of the ear to both sound and air pressure).

Tympanometer An instrument that measures the function of the middle ear by varying the pressure within the external ear canal and measuring the movement of the eardrum (tympanic membrane).

Tympanometry The procedure used to assess the mobility of the tympanic membrane and the presence or absence of fluid in the middle ear.

Unfilled pauses Long pauses between words, without tension.

Unilateral conductive hearing loss A conductive hearing loss in only one ear.

Unintelligible Speech that is not understood by listeners because of the speaker's inability to clearly form speech sounds.

Upper motor neurons Neurons in the motor region of the cerebral cortex or brain stem that carry information to the lower motor neurons.

Valid An instrument that measures what it claims to measure. Data that are well grounded on available evidence.

Velar sound Sound produced with the tongue against the velum.

Velopharyngeal closure Elevation of the velum to contact the posterior and lateral walls of the pharynx, thereby closing off the opening between the oral and the nasal cavities.

Velopharyngeal port The space between the soft palate (velum) and the pharyngeal wall. When the soft palate elevates up and back against the pharynx, the port closes.

Velum The soft palate.

Ventilator dependence An individual who must use a ventilator in order to survive, either temporarily, intermittently, or permanently.

Ventricular (vestibular) folds Located just above the true vocal folds, the false vocal folds help keep food and drink out of the airway.

Vestibule The organ of equilibrium located in the inner ear.

Vocabulary The words of a language; also used to describe the words an individual knows.

Vocal folds Two folds of mucus membrane at the base of the larynx that vibrate to produce voice when air passes over them.

Vocal tract The mechanism that molds the "buzz" generated by the vocal folds into speech sounds. It consists of the pharyngeal, oral, and nasal cavities.

Voiced Consonants produced with vocalization.

Voiceless Consonants produced without vocalization.

Waveform the graphic representation of the shape of a wave defined by its frequency and amplitude.

Wernicke's aphasia A fluent aphasia characterized by serious comprehension difficulties and rapid-fire speech that may make little or no sense.

WHO The World Health Organization. A special agency of the United Nations, it was created in 1948 to direct and coordinate international health.

Word-finding problem Difficulty retrieving words from one's lexicon.

Word repetitions Repetitions of entire words. In most cases they are single-syllable.

references

AAC Institute. (2014). *Welcome to the AAC Institute.* Retrieved http://www.aacinstitute.org

Ahmed, S., Shapiro, N. L., & Bhattacharyya, N. (2014, January). Incremental health care utilization and costs for acute otitis media in children. *Laryngoscope, 124*(1), 301–305. doi:10:1002/lary24190

Aitchison, D. (2013, December 24). *Esophageal speech* [Online video]. Retrieved from https://www.youtube.com/watch?v=kyN_NFoBfiw

Allen, N. H., Burns, A., Newton, V., Hickson, F., Ramsden, R., Rogers, J., . . . Morris, J. (2003). The effects of improving hearing in dementia. *Age and Ageing, 32*(2), 189–193.

Ambrose, N. G. (2004). Theoretical perspectives on the cause of stuttering. *Contemporary Issues in Communication Science and Disorders, 31,* 80–91.

Academy of Doctors of Audiology. (2015). *What is an audiologist.* Retrieved from http://www.audiologist.org/what-is-an-audiologist

American Academy of Private Practice in Speech Pathology and Audiology. (2014). *AAPPSPA's purpose.* Retrieved from http://www.aappspa.org/slp-aud.item.9/purpose.html

American Board of Swallowing and Swallowing Disorders. (2014). *Common questions.* Retrieved from http://swallowingdisorders.site-ym.com/?page=commonquestions

American Psychiatric Association. (2013). *Diagnostic and statistical manual of mental disorders* (5th ed.). Arlington, VA: American Psychiatric.

American Psychiatric Association. (2014). *Social (pragmatic) communication disorder.* Retrieved from http://www.dsm5.org/Documents/Social%20Communication%20Disorder%20Fact%20Sheet.pdf

American Speech-Language-Hearing Association. (1985). *Clinical management of communicatively handicapped minority language populations* [Position statement]. Retrieved from http://www.asha.org/policy/PS1985-00219/

American Speech-Language-Hearing Association. (1993). *Definitions of communication disorders and variations.* Retrieved from http://www.asha.org/policy/RP1993-00208/

American Speech-Language-Hearing Association. (2007). *Scope of practice in speech-language pathology.* Retrieved from http://www.asha.org/policy/SP2007-00283.htm

American Speech-Language-Hearing Association. (2008a). *Guidelines for audiologists providing informational and adjustment counseling to families of infants and young children with hearing loss birth to 5 years of age* [Guidelines]. Retrieved from http://www.asha.org/policy/GL2008-00289.htm

American Speech-Language-Hearing Association. (2008b). *III. Standards for accreditation of graduate education programs in audiology and speech-language pathology.* Retrieved from http://www.asha.org/academic/accreditation/accredmanual/section3/

American Speech-Language-Hearing Association. (2010). *Code of ethics* [Ethics]. Retrieved from http://www.asha.org/policy

American Speech-Language-Hearing Association. (2012). *ASHA 2012 schools survey: SLP caseload characteristics.* Retrieved from http://www.asha.org/uploadedFiles/Schools-2012-Caseload.pdf

American Speech-Language-Hearing Association. (2014a). *Advocacy.* Retrieved from http://www.asha.org/advocacy/

American Speech-Language-Hearing Association. (2014b). *Aphasia.* Retrieved from http://www.asha.org/public/speech/disorders/aphasia.htm

American Speech-Language-Hearing Association. (2014c, May 12). *ASHA comments on the DSM-5 for the National Institutes of Health.* Retrieved from http://www.asha.org/uploadedFiles/ASHA-Comments-on-DSM-5-for-NIH.pdf

American Speech-Language-Hearing Association. (2014d). *ASHA/N-CEP evidence-based systematic reviews.* Retrieved from http://www.asha.org/members/ebp/EBSRs/

American Speech-Language Hearing Association. (2014e). *Augmentative and alternative communication (AAC).* Retrieved from http://www.asha.org/public/speech/disorders/AAC/

American Speech-Language-Hearing Association. (2014f). *Bilingual service delivery.* Retrieved from http://www.asha.org/PRPSpecificTopic.aspx?folderid=8589935225&section=Key_Issues

American Speech-Language-Hearing Association. (2014g). *Clinical topics: Autism.* Retrieved from http://www.asha.org/Practice-Portal/Clinical-Topics/Autism/

American Speech-Language-Hearing Association. (2014h). *Dysarthria.* Retrieved from http://www.asha.org/public/speech/disorders/dysarthria/

American Speech-Language-Hearing Association. (2014i). *End-of-life issues in speech-language pathology.* Retrieved from http://www.asha.org/slp/clinical/endoflife/

American Speech-Language-Hearing Association (2014j). *Evidence-based practice (EBP).* Retrieved from: http://www.asha.org/members/ebp/

American Speech-Language-Hearing Association. (2014k). *Family adjustment to aphasia.* Retrieved from http://www.asha.org/public/speech/disorders/FamilyAdjustmentAphasia/

American Speech-Language-Hearing Association. (2014l). *Feeding and swallowing disorders (dysphagia) in children.* Retrieved from http://www.asha.org/public/speech/swallowing/feeding-and-swallowing-disorders-in-children/#what_causes

American Speech-Language-Hearing Association. (2014m). *Frequently asked questions: Speech-language pathology assistants (SLPAs).* Retrieved from http://www.asha.org/associates/SLPA-FAQs.htm#e1

American Speech-Language-Hearing Association. (2014n). *Issues in ethics: Cultural and linguistic competence.* Retrieved from http://www.asha.org/Practice/ethics/Cultural-and-Linguistic-Competence/

American Speech-Language-Hearing Association. (2014o). *Language-based learning disabilities.* Retrieved from http://www.asha.org/public/speech/disorders/LBLD/

American Speech-Language-Hearing Association. (2014p). *Multicultural affairs and resources.* Retrieved from http://www.asha.org/practice/multicultural/

American Speech-Language-Hearing Association. (2014q). *Phonemic inventories across languages.* Retrieved from http://www.asha.org/practice/multicultural/Phono/

American Speech-Language-Hearing Association (2014r). *Practice issues.* Retrieved from http://www.asha.org/practice/multicultural/issues/

American Speech-Language-Hearing Association. (2014s). *Practice portal.* Retrieved from http://www.asha.org/PRPDefault.aspx?utm_source=asha&utm_medium=email&utm_campaign=pp092214

American Speech-Language-Hearing Association. (2014t). *Self-assessment for cultural competence.* Retrieved from http://www.asha.org/practice/multicultural/self/

American Speech-Language-Hearing Association. (2014u). *Stuttering.* Retrieved from http://www.asha.org/public/speech/disorders/stuttering.htm

American Speech-Language-Hearing Association. (2014v). *Swallowing disorders (dysphagia) in adults.* Retrieved from http://www.asha.org/public/speech/swallowing/Swallowing-Disorders-in-Adults/#causes

American Speech-Language-Hearing Association. (2014w). *Traumatic brain injury (TBI).* Retrieved from http://www.asha.org/public/speech/disorders/TBI/

American Speech-Language-Hearing Association Ad Hoc Committee on Service Delivery in the Schools. (1993). Definitions of communication disorders and variations. *Asha, 35*(Suppl. 10), 40–41.

American Tinnitus Association. (2014). *ATA's top 10 most frequently asked questions.* Retrieved from http://www.ata.org/for-patients/faqs

Annie E. Casey Foundation. (2014). *The changing child population of the United States.* Retrieved from http://www.aecf.org/resources/the-changing-child-population-of-the-united-states/

Arizona Behavioral Health Associates. (2015). *What Is Biofeedback?* Retrieved from http://psycho-therapy.com/bio.html

Armour, J. (2007, March 27). The audiologist as an expert witness. *The ASHA Leader.* Retrieved from http://www.asha.org/Publications/leader/2007/070327/f070327b.htm

Bates, E. (1976). *Language and context: The acquisition of pragmatics.* New York, NY: Academic Press.

Battle, D. E. (2012). *Communication disorders in multicultural and international populations.* St. Louis, MO: Mosby.

Benton, A. L. (1981). Aphasia: Historical perspectives. In M. T. Sarno (Ed.), *Acquired aphasia*. New York, NY: Academic Press.

Bernthal, J. E., Bankson, N. W., & Flipson, P. (2012). *Articulation and phonological disorders: Speech sound disorders in children* (7th ed.). Boston, MA: Pearson.

Beukelman, D. R., Yorkston, K. M., & Dowden, P. A. (2007). *Communication augmentation*. Baltimore, MD: Brookes.

Bleile, J. M., & Wallach, H. (1992). A sociolinguistic investigation of the speech of African American preschoolers. *American Journal of Speech–Language Pathology, 1*(2), 54–62.

Blissymbolics. (2014). *Omniglot: The online encyclopedia of writing systems and languages*. Retrieved from http://www.blissymbolics.org/index.php/about-blissymbolics

Bloom, C., & Cooperman, D. (1999). *Synergistic stuttering therapy: A holistic approach*. Woburn: MA: Butterworth-Heinemann.

Bloom, L., Rocissano, L., & Hood, L. (1976). Adult-child discourse: Developmental interaction between information processing and linguistic knowledge. *Cognitive Psychology, 8*, 521–552.

Bowen, C. (2013). *Dysarthria in children and young people*. Retrieved from http://speech-language-therapy.com/index.php?option=com_content&view=article&id=90:dysarthrias&catid=11:admin&Itemid=123

Boys Town National Research Hospital. (2014). *Multidisciplinary team evaluations*. Retrieved from https://www.boystownhospital.org/hearingservices/childhoodDeafness/Pages/Multidisciplinary TeamEval.aspx

Brorson, K. (2008, November 21). *SLPs perceptions of classroom-based language intervention results*. Paper presented at the 2008 American Speech-Language-Hearing Association convention, Chicago, IL.

Brown, R. (1973). *A first language: The early stages*. Cambridge, MA: Harvard University Press.

Bruner, J. (1975). The ontogenesis of speech acts. *Journal of Child Language, 2*, 1–9.

Brutton, G. J., & Vanryckeghem, M. (2006). *The behavior assessment battery for school-age children who stutter*. San Diego, CA: Plural.

Buekelman, D. R., Fager, S., Ball, L., & Dietz, A. (2007). AAC for adults with acquired neurological conditions: A review. *Augmentative and Alternative Communication, 23*(3), 230–242.

Calculator, S., & Jorgensen, C. (1994). *Including students with severe disabilities in schools*. San Diego, CA: Singular.

Calvin, W. H., & Ojemann, G. A. (1994). *Conversations with Neil's brain: The neural nature of thought & language*. Retrieved from http://williamcalvin.com/bk7/bk7.htm

Carroll, L. (1871). *Through the looking glass, and what Alice found there*. London, England: Macmillan.

Casby, M. W. (1992). An intervention approach for naming problems in children. *American Journal of Speech–Language Pathology, 1*(3), 35–42.

CBS. (2011, February 1). *Understanding stuttering* [Online video]. Retrieved from https://www .youtube.com/watch?v=VaSZbcf9tX4

Center for Parent Information and Resources. (2014a, February). *Intellectual disability* [NICHCY Disability Fact Sheet 8]. Retrieved from http://www.parentcenterhub.org/repository/intellectual/

Center for Parent Information and Resources. (2014b). *Speech and language impairments*. Retrieved from http://www.parentcenterhub.org/repository/speechlanguage

Center for Parent Information and Resources. (2014c). *Individuals with Disabilities Education Improvement Act of 2004 (IDEA)*. Retrieved from http://www.parentcenterhub.org/wp-content/uploads/repo_items/IDEA2004regulations.pdfCenters for Disease Control and Prevention. (2014). *Attention-deficit/hyperactivity disorder* (ADHD). Retrieved from http://www.cdc.gov/ncbddd/adhd/facts.html

Centers for Disease Control and Prevention. (2015, April 27). *Developmental disabilities*. Retrieved from http://www.cdc.gov/ncbddd/developmentaldisabilities/index.html

Cirrin, F. M., Schooling, T. L., Nelson, N. W., Diehl, S. F., Flynn, P. F., Staskowski, M., . . . Adam- czyk, D. F. (2010). Evidence-based systematic review: Effects of different service delivery models on communication outcomes for elementary school-age children. *Language, Speech, and Hearing Services in Schools, 41*, 233–264. doi:10.1044/ 0161-1461(2009/08-0128)

Colorado Department of Education. (2010). *Colorado K-12 speech or language impairment guidelines for assessment and eligibility, including the birth–21 rating scales.* Retrieved from http://www.cde .state.co.us/cdesped/sli_guidelines

Darley, F. L., Aronson, A. E., & Brown, J. R. (1975). *Motor speech disorders.* Philadelphia, PA: Saunders.

Deaf websites. (2014). *Auditory nerve damage.* Retrieved from http://www.deafwebsites.com/hearing-loss/auditory-nerve-damage.html

Deem, J. F., & Miller, L. (2000). *Manual of voice therapy* (2nd ed.). Austin, TX: PRO-ED.

Deep stealth. (2012, February 9). *Finding your female voice consultation,* (Pt. 7, epilogue [Online video]. Retrieved from https://www.youtube.com/watch?v=ysarXXO2GwU

Department of Statistics, University of California, Berkeley. (2014). *Glossary of statistical terms.* Retrieved from http://www.stat.berkeley.edu/~stark/SticiGui/Text/gloss.htm

Dikeman, K. J., & Kazandijan, M. S. (2004, October 19). Managing adults with tracheostomies and ventilator dependence: Current concepts. *The ASHA Leader,* 6–7, 19–20.

Duchan, J. F. (2001, May 12). *Learning leveling and leveling learning [Graduation speech].* Buffalo, NY: Department of Communicative Disorders and Sciences, University of Buffalo. Retrieved from http://www.acsu.buffalo.edu/~duchan/leveling.html

Duchan. J. F. (2003, November). *Identity based therapies.* Paper presented at the American Speech-Language-Hearing Association. Retrieved from http://www.acsu.buffalo.edu/~duchan/identity_based_therapies.html

Duchan, J. (2011). *A history of speech–language pathology: Twentieth century.* Retrieved from http://www.acsu.buffalo.edu/~duchan/history.html

Dyches, T. T., (2011). Assessing diverse students with autism spectrum disorders. *The ASHA Leader.* Retrieved from http://www.asha.org/Publications/leader/2011/110118/Assessing-Diverse-Students-With-Autism-Spectrum-Disorders

Eldridge, M. (1968). *A history of the treatment of speech disorders.* Edinburgh, Scotland: Livingstone.

Elliot, C. (2011, November 26). *Tongue cancer in young people: What to expect post operation: Speaking after surgery* [Online video]. Retrieved from https://www.youtube.com/watch?v=pju_5bmaEwo

Elliot, C (2012, October 24). *Tongue cancer in young people: What to expect after 1 year—Update October 25, 2012* [Online video]. Retrieved from https://www.youtube.com/watch?v=pKxuCS-9fXc

Engelter, S. T., Gostynski, M., Papa, S., Maya, F., Claudia, B., Vladeta, A. G., . . . Lyrer, P. A. (2006, June). Epidemiology of aphasia attributable to first ischemic stroke: Incidence, severity, fluency, etiology, and thrombosis. *Stroke, 37*(6), 1379–1384.

Ervin, M. (2001). SLI–What we know and why it matters. *The ASHA Leader.* Retrieved from http://www.asha.org/Publications/leader/2001/010626/sli.htm

Fact Monster. (2014). *Embolus.* Retrieved from http://www.factmonster.com/encyclopedia/science/embolus.html

Fairbanks, G. (1960). *Voice and articulation drillbook* (2nd ed.). New York, NY: Harper & Row.

Faroqi-Shah, Y., Frymark, T., Mullen, R., & Wang, B. (2010, July). Effect of treatment for bilingual individuals with aphasia: A systematic review of the evidence. *Journal of Neurolinguistics, 23*(4), 319–341. doi:10.1016/j.jneuroling.2010.01.002

Federal Communications Commission. (2014). *711 for telecommunications relay service.* Retrieved from http://www.fcc.gov/guides/711-telecommunications-relay-service

Felsenfeld, S., Broen, P. A., & McGue, M. (1992). A 28-year follow-up study of adults with a history of moderate phonological disorder: Linguistic and personality results. *Journal of Speech and Hearing Research, 35,* 1114–1125.

Flahive, L., & Hodson, B. (2013). Speech sound disorders: An overview of acquisition, assessment, and treatment. In N. C. Singleton & B. Shulman (Eds.), *Language development: Foundations, processes, and clinical application* (2nd ed., pp. 185–202). Sudberry, MA: Jones & Bartlett.

Fox, P. T., Ingham, R., Ingham, J. C., Hirsch, T. B., Downs, J. H., Martin, C., . . . Lancaster, J. L. (1996, July 11). A PET study of the neural systems of stuttering. *Nature, 382,* 158–162, doi:10.1038/382158a0

Fox, P. T., Inghan, R. J., Inghan, J. C., Zamarripa, F., Xiong, J.-H., & Lancaseter, J. L. (2000, October). Brain correlates of stuttering and syllable production: A PET performance-correlation analysis. *Brain, 123* (Pt. 10), 1985–2004.

Free Dictionary. (2014). *The chickens have come home to roost.* Retrieved from http://idioms .thefreedictionary.com/chickens%20come%20home%20to%20roost

Friendship Circle. (2011). *7 assistive communication apps in the iPad app store.* Retrieved from http:// www.friendshipcircle.org/blog/2011/02/07/7-assistive-communication-apps-in-the-ipad-app-store/

Fry, K. (2011, July 5). New program combines political, legislative advocacy. *The ASHA Leader.* Retrieved from http://www.asha.org/Publications/leader/2011/110705/New-Program-Combines-Political,-Legislative-Advocacy.htm

Fusaro, M. (2010). *Harvard Graduate School of Education usable knowledge: Mapping the literacy development of bilingual children.* Retrieved from http://www.gse.harvard.edu/news/uk/10/01/mapping-literacy-bilingual-children

Gallaudet University. (2014). *History of Gallaudet University.* Retrieved from http://www.gallaudet .edu/history.html

Gallaudet University Laurent Clerc National Deaf Education Center. (2008). Retrieved from http:// www.fda.gov/medicaldevices/productsandmedicalprocedures/implantsandprosthetics/cochlearimplants/ucm062843.htm

Gallaudet University Laurent Clerc National Deaf Education Center. (2014). *Effects of various types of hearing loss.* Retrieved from http://www.gallaudet.edu/clerc_center/information_and_resources/info_to_go/hearing_loss_information/effects_of_hearing_loss.html

Gillam, R. G., & Bedore, L. M. (2000). Communication across the lifespan. In R. B. Gillam, T. P. Marquardt, & F. N. Martin. (Eds.), *Communication sciences and disorders: From science to clinical practice* (pp. 25–61). San Diego, CA: Singular.

Gillam, R. B., Logan, K. J., & Pearson, N. A. (2009). *Test of childhood stuttering.* Austin, TX: PRO-ED.

Goldman, R., & Fristoe, M. (2000). *Goldman-Fristoe test of articulation* (2nd ed.). San Antonio, TX: Pearson.

Gordon, P. A., & Luper, H. L. (1992a). The early identification of beginning stuttering: I. Protocols. *American Journal of Speech-Language Pathology, 1*(3), 48–53.

Gordon, P. A., & Luper, H. L. (1992b). The early identification of beginning stuttering: II. Problems. *American Journal of Speech-Language Pathology, 1*(3), 49–55.

Grandin, T. (2009) How does visual thinking work in the mind of a person with autism? A personal account. *Philosophical Transactions of the Royal Society, 364,* paras. 2–3. Retrieved from http:// www.grandin.com/inc/visual.thinking.mind.autistic.person.html

Griffin Laboratories. (2008, May 20). *TruTone artificial speech aid for a laryngectomee* [Online video]. Retrieved from https://www.youtube.com/watch?v=AYydnhu6NbU

Gudykunst, W. B. (1998). *Bridging differences, effective intergroup communication* (3rd ed.). London, England: Sage.

Gustason, G. (1983). *Teaching and learning Signing Exact English.* Los Alamitos, CA: Modem Signs Press.

Hall, E. T. (1966). *The hidden dimension.* Garden City, NY: Doubleday.

Hanks, H. (2014). *Phonological processes.* Retrieved from http://mommyspeechtherapy.com/?p=2158

Healthline. (2014). *What is dysarthria?* Retrieved from http://www.healthline.com/symptom/speech-articulation-problems

H.E.A.R. (2014). *H.E.A.R. mission statement.* Retrieved from http://www.hearnet.com/about/about_ hearmission.shtml

Hearing Health Foundation. (2014). *Hearing loss & tinnitus statistics.* Retrieved from http://hearing-healthfoundation.org/statistics

Hinckley, J. H. (2007). *Narrative-based practice in speech-language pathology: Stories of a clinical life.* San Diego, CA: Plural.

Hodson, B. W. (2004). *Hodson assessment of phonological patterns* (3rd ed.). Austin, TX: PRO-ED.

Hodson, B. (2006). Identifying phonological patterns and projecting remediation cycles: Expediting intelligibility gains of a 7 year old Australian child. *Advances in Speech–Language Pathology, 8*(3), 257–264.

Hofstra University. (2011, May 11). *Living with aphasia: Ivan's story* [Online video]. Retrieved from https://www.youtube.com/watch?v=NTHM7-UgDr0

Hulit, L. M., & Howard, M. R. (2006). *Born to talk: An introduction to speech and language development* (4th ed.). Boston, MA: Allyn & Bacon.

International Association of Logopedics and Phoniatrics. (2014). *IALP.* from http://www.ialp.info

International Cluttering Society. (2014). *What is cluttering?* Retrieved from http://www.mnsu.edu/comdis/ica1/papers/icabrochure.pdf

Internet Stroke Center. (2014). *What is aphasia?* Retrieved from http://www.strokecenter.org/patients/caregiver-and-patient-resources/aphasia-information/

Johnston, J. (2006). *Thinking about child language: Research to practice.* Eau Claire, WI: Thinking Publications.

Khan, L., & Lewis, L. (2002). *Khan–Lewis phonological analysis* (2nd ed.). San Antonio, TX: Pearson.

Kiran, S., & Goral, M. (2012, June). One disorder, multiple languages. *The ASHA Leader* Retrieved from http://www.asha.org/Publications/leader/2012/120605/One-Disorder-Multiple-Languages.htm

Kiran, S., & Roberts, P. (2009). Semantic feature analysis treatment in Spanish–English and French–English bilingual aphasia. *Aphasiology, 24*(2), 231–261.

Klingbeil, G. M. (1939a). The historical background of the modern speech clinic: Aphasia. *Journal of Speech Disorders, 4*, 26–284.

Klingbeil, G. M. (1939b). The historical background of the modem speech clinic: Stuttering and stammering. *Journal of Speech Disorders, 4*, 115–132.

Kolb, R. (2013, June 20). *Navigating deafness in a hearing world: Rachel Kolb at TEDxStanford* [Online video]. Retrieved from https://www.youtube.com/watch?v=uKKpjvPd6Xo

Kubler-Ross, E. (1997). *On death and dying.* Riverside, NJ: Simon & Schuster.

Kuster, J. (2005a). *Other related fluency disorders: Neurogenic stuttering.* Retrieved from http://www.mnsu.edu/comdis/kuster/related.html

Kuster, J. (2005b). *The stuttering homepage.* Retrieved from http://www.mnsu.edu/comdis/kuster/stutter.html

Larson, V. L., & McKinley, N. L. (2003). *Communication solutions for older students: Assessment and intervention strategies.* Austin, TX: PRO-ED.

Lee, V., & Hoaken, P. N. S. (2007). Cognition, emotion, and neurobiological development: Mediating the relation between maltreatment and aggression. *Child Maltreatment, 12*, 281–298.

Leonard, R., Goodrich, S., McMenamin, P., & Donald, P. (1992). Differentiation of speakers with glossectomies by acoustic and perceptual measures. *American Journal of Speech–Language Pathology, 1*(4), 56–63.

Light, J., & McNaughton, D. (2010). The changing face of augmentative and alternative communication: Past, present, and future challenges. *Augmentative and Alternative Communication, 28*(4), 197–204.

Lin, F. R., Yaffe, K., Xia, J., Xue, Q.L., Harris, T. B., Purchas-Helzner, E., . . . Simonsick, E. M. (2013, February 25). Hearing loss and cognitive decline in older adults. *JAMA Internal Medicine, 173*(4), 293–299. doi:10.1001/jamainternmed.2013.1868

Luterman, D. M. (2008). *Counseling persons with communication disorders and their families* (5th ed.). Austin, TX: PRO-ED.

MacPherson, M. K., & Smith, A. (2013, February). Influences of sentence length and syntactic complexity on the speech motor control of children who stutter. *Journal of Speech, Language, and Hearing Research, 56*, 89–102. doi:10.1044/1092-4388(2012/11-0184)

Matthews, C. B. (1993). *Marketing speech–language pathology and audiology services.* San Diego, CA: Singular.

Mayo Clinic. (2014). *Hearing loss.* Retrieved from http://www.mayoclinic.org/diseases-conditions/hearing-loss/in-depth/hearing-aids/ART-20044116?pg=2

McCreery, R. W., Venediktov, R. A., Coleman, J. J., & Leech, H. M. (2012, December). An evidence-based systematic review of directional microphones and digital noise reduction earing aids in school-age children with hearing loss. *American Journal of Audiology, 21*, 295–312. doi:10.1044/1059-0889(2012/12-0014)

McFarlane, L-A. (2012, Spring). Motivational interviewing: Practical strategies for speech-language pathologists and audiologists. *Canadian Journal of Speech-Language Pathology and Audiology, 36*(1), 8–15.

Medscape. (2014). *Acute otitis media: Background.* Retrieved from http://emedicine.medscape.com/article/859316-overview#aw2aab6b2b2

Merrill Advanced Studies Center. (2014). *Top 10 things you should know . . . about children with specific language impairment.* Retrieved from http://merrill.ku.edu/top-10-things-you-should-know

Miller, L., Gillam, R. B., & Peña, E. C. (2001). *Dynamic assessment and intervention: Improving children's narrative skills.* Austin, TX: PRO-ED.

Miller, W. R., & Rollnick, S. (Eds.). (2002). *Motivational interviewing: Preparing people for change* (2nd ed.). New York, NY: Guilford Press.

Murdoch, B. (2010). The cerebellum and language: Historical perspective and review. *Cortex, 46,* 858–868. doi:10.1016/j.cortex.2009.07.018

National Aphasia Association. (2013, October 9). *Patience, listening and communicating with aphasia patients* [Online video]. Retrieved from https://www.youtube.com/watch?v=aPTTjRTmgq0

National Center for Learning Disabilities. (2014). *What is dyslexia?* Retrieved from http://www.ncld.org/types-learning-disabilities/dyslexia/what-is-dyslexia

National Center on Birth Defects and Developmental Disabilities. (2005). *Facts about intellectual disability.* Retrieved from http://www.cdc.gov/ncbddd/actearly/pdf/parents_pdfs/IntellectualDisability.pdf

National Health Service Choices. (2014). *Aphasia—Complications.* Retrieved from http://webarchive.nationalarchives.gov.uk/+/www.nhs.uk/Conditions/Aphasia/Pages/Complications.aspx

National Institute on Deafness and Other Communication Disorders. (2004, February). *Telecommunications relay services.* Retrieved from http://www.nidcd.nih.gov/health/hearing/telecomm.asp

National Institute on Deafness and Other Communication Disorders. (2010a). *Quick statistics: Voice, speech, language.* Retrieved from http://www.nidcd.nih.gov/health/statistics/vsl/Pages/stats.aspx

National Institute on Deafness and Other Communication Disorders. (2010b). *Voice, speech, and language charts and tables.* Retrieved from http://www.nidcd.nih.gov/health/statistics/vsl/Pages/charts.aspx#sli

National Institute on Deafness and Other Communication Disorders. (2014a). *Cochlear implants.* Retrieved from http://www.nidcd.nih.gov/health/hearing/coch.asp

National Institute on Deafness and Other Communication Disorders. (2014b). *Ear infections in children.* Retrieved from http://www.nidcd.nih.gov/health/hearing/pages/earinfections.aspx

National Institute on Deafness and Other Communication Disorders. (2014c). *Otosclerosis.* Retrieved from http://www.nidcd.nih.gov/health/hearing/pages/otosclerosis.aspx

National Institute on Deafness and Other Communication Disorders. (2014d). *Spasmodic dysphonia.* Retrieved from http://www.nidcd.nih.gov/health/voice/Pages/spasdysp.aspx

National Institute on Deafness and Other Communication Disorders. (2015). *Specific language impairments.* Retrieved from http://www.nidcd.nih.gov/health/voice/pages/specific-language-impairment.aspx

National Institute on Neurological Disorders and Stroke. (2015a). *NINDS muscular dystrophy information page.* Retrieved from http://www.ninds.nih.gov/disorders/md/md.htm

National Institute on Neurological Disorders and Stroke. (2015b). *NINDS myasthenia gravis information page.* Retrieved from http://www.ninds.nih.gov/disorders/myasthenia_gravis/myasthenia_gravis.htm

National Institute on Neurological Disorders and Stroke. (2015c). *NINDS Parkinson's disease information page.* Retrieved from http://www.ninds.nih.gov/disorders/parkinsons_disease/parkinsons_disease.htm

National Stroke Association. (2014a). *Aphasia.* Retrieved from http://www.stroke.org/site/PageServer?pagename=aphasia

National Stroke Association. (2014b). *Fatigue.* Retrieved from http://www.stroke.org/site/PageServer?pagename=fatigue

National Stroke Association. (2014c). *Seizures and epilepsy.* Retrieved from http://www.stroke.org/site/PageServer?pagename=seizures

National Stroke Association. (2014d). *Vision loss.* Retrieved from http://www.stroke.org/site/PageServer?pagename=vision_loss

National Stuttering Association. (2014a). *If you stutter, you're not alone!* Retrieved from http://www .westutter.org/if-you-stutter-youre-not-alone/

National Stuttering Association. (2014b). *Stuttering treatment can help . . . And early intervention is best!* Retrieved from http://www.westutter.org/who-we-help/stuttering-treatment-can-help-and-early-intervention-is-best/

National Theatre of the Deaf. (2014). *About the National Theatre of the Deaf.* Retrieved from http:// www.ntd.org/ntd_about.html

Ndung'u, R., & Kinyua, M. (2009). Cultural perspectives in language and speech disorders. *Disabilities Studies Quarterly, 29*(4). Retrieved from http://dsq-sds.org/article/view/986/1175

Nelson, H. D., Nygren, P., Walker, M., & Panoscha, R. (2006, February). Screening for speech and language delay in preschool children: Systematic evidence review for the US Preventive Services Task Force. *Pediatrics, 117*(2), 298–319.

Nippold, M. A., Ward-Lonergan, J. M., & Fanning, J. L. (2005). Persuasive writing in children, adolescents, and adults: A study of syntactic, semantic, and pragmatic development. *Language, Speech and Hearing Services in Schools, 36*, 125–138.

Nottingham Hearing Biomedical Research Unit. (2014). *Auditory examples—Sounds of tinnitus.* Retrieved from http://www.hearing.nihr.ac.uk/public/auditory-examples-sounds-of-tinnitus

NSDA/National Spasmodic Dysphonia Association. (2010, December 20). *Spasmodic dysphonia voice samples* [Online video]. Retrieved from https://www.youtube.com/watch?v=SqzfsKMaLqk

NYU Langone Medical Center. (2014). *Presbycusis.* Retrieved from http://medicine.med.nyu.edu/ conditions-we-treat/conditions/presbycusis

Olswang, L., & Bain, B. (1991). Intervention issues for toddlers with specific language impairments. *Topics in Language Disorders, 11*, 69–86.

Onslow, M. (1992). Identification of early stuttering: Issues and suggested strategies. *American Journal of Speech–Language Pathology, 1*(4), 21–27.

Owens, R. E., Jr. (2001). *Language development: An introduction* (5th ed.). Needham Heights, MA: Allyn & Bacon.

Owens, R. E., Jr. (2008). *Language development: An introduction.* Boston, MA: Pearson.

Palmer, C. V., Adams, S. W., Bourgeois, M., Durrant, J., & Rossi, M. (1999). Reductions in care-giver identified problem behaviors in patients with Alzheimer's disease post-hearing-aid fitting. *Journal of Speech, Language, and Hearing Research, 42*(2), 312–328.

Paul, R. (2007). *Language disorders from infancy through adolescence* (3rd ed.). St. Louis, MO: Mosby.

Paul, R., & Norbury, C. (2012). *Language disorders from infancy through adolescence: Listening, speaking, reading, writing, and communicating* (4th ed.). St. Louis, MO: Elsevier.

PBS. (2014). *Deaf culture.* Retrieved from http://www.pbs.org/wnet/soundandfury/culture/index.html

Peña, E., Summers, C., & Resendiz, M. (2007). Assessment and intervention of children from diverse cultural and linguistic backgrounds. In A. Kamhi, K. Apel, & J. Masterson (Eds.), *Clinical decision making in developmental language disorders* (pp. 99–118). Baltimore, MD: Brookes.

Penman, R., Cross, T., Milgram-Friedman, J., & Meares, R. (1983). Mothers' speech to prelingual infants: A pragmatic analysis. *Journal of Child Language, 10*, 17–34.

Pepper, L. (2014, January 1). *Myasthenia gravis: My symptoms* [Online video]. Retrieved from https:// www.youtube.com/watch?v=j80reMSwQs4

Physics Classroom. (2014). *Sound waves and music* [Online tutorial]. Retrieved from http://www .physicsclassroom.com/class/sound

Pichichero, M. E. (2000). Recurrent and persistent otitis media. *Pediatric Infectious Disease Journal, 19*(9), 911–916.

Plains Indian Sign Language. (2014). *Hand talk: American Indian sign language.* Retrieved from http:// pislresearch.com/index.html

Polloway, E. A., Miller, L., & Smith, T. E. C. (2012). *Language instruction for students with disabilities* (4th ed.). Denver, CO: Love.

Polloway, E. A., Patton, J. R., Serna, L., & Bailey, J. W. (2013). *Strategies for teaching learners with special needs* (10th ed.). Boston, MA: Pearson.

Post, J. G., & Leith, W. R. (1983). I'd rather tell a story than be one. *ASHA, 25*, 23–26.

Prince, M., Bryce, R., Albanese, E., Wimo, A., Ribeiro, W., & Ferri, C. P. (2013). The global prevalence of dementia: A systematic review and meta-analysis. *Alzheimer's Dementia, 9*(1), 63–75.

Psychology Today. (2014). *Communication disorders.* Retrieved from http://www.psychologytoday.com/conditions/communication-disorders

Purepedantry. (2007, September 18). *Broca's aphasia* [Online video]. Retrieved from https://www.youtube.com/watch?v=f2IiMEbMnPM

Purepedantry. (2007, September 18). *Wernicke's aphasia* [Online video]. Retrieved from https://www.youtube.com/watch?v=aVhYN7NTIKU

Registry of Interpreters for the Deaf. (2005). *Homepage.* Retrieved from http://www.rid.org/

Riley, G. D. (2009). *Stuttering severity instrument* (4th ed.). Austin, TX: PRO-ED.

Robbins, S. D. (1948). Chapter 10. In E. Froeschels (Ed.), *Twentieth century speech correction.* New York, NY: Philosophical Library.

Rogers, C. R. (1942). *Counseling and psychotherapy.* Boston, MA: Houghton Mifflin.

Rogers-Adkinson, D. L., & Stuart, S. K. (2007, April). Collaborative services: Children experiencing neglect and the side effects of prenatal alcohol exposure. *Language, Speech, and Hearing Services in Schools, 38,* 149–156. doi:10.1044/0161-1461(2007/015)

Roseberry-McKibbin, C., & Hegde, M. N. (2010). *Advanced review of speech–language pathology* (3rd ed.). Austin, TX: PRO-ED.

Ryan, C. (2011). *Language use in the United States: American community survey reports.* Retrieved from http://www.census.gov/prod/2013pubs/acs-22.pdf

Sacks, O. (1985). *The man who mistook his wife for a hat.* New York, NY: Touchstone.

Sarno, M. T. (1981). *Acquired aphasia.* San Diego, CA: Academic Press.

Scheidt, D., Kob, M., Willmes, K., & Neuschaefer-Rube, C. (2004). *Do we need voice therapy for female-to-male transgenders?* Retrieved from http://www.academia.edu/3094379/Do_We_Need_Voice_Therapy_for_Female-To-Male_Transgenders

Schuster, L. I., Ruscello, D. M., & Smith, K. D. (1992). Evoking /r/ using visual feedback. *American Journal of Speech-Language Pathology, 1*(3), 29–34.

Shallice, T. (1987). Impairments of semantic processing: Multiple dissociations. In M. Coltheart, G. Sartori, & R. Job (Eds.), *The cognitive neuropsychology of language* (pp. 111–127). Hillsdale, NJ: Erlbaum.

Shields, C. (1997). *Behind objective description: Special education and the reality of lived experience* (Unpublished doctoral thesis). University of Toronto.

Silverman, F. H. (1998). *Research design and evaluation in speech–language pathology and audiology* (4th ed.). Boston, MA: Allyn & Bacon.

Silverman, F. H., Gazzolo, M., & Peterson, Y. (1990). Impact of a T-shirt message on stutterer stereotypes: A systematic replication. *Journal of Fluency Disorders, 15,* 35–37.

Simkin, Z., & Conti-Ramsden, G. (2006). Evidence of reading difficulty in subgroups of children with specific language impairment. *Child Language Teaching and Therapy, 22*(3), 315–331.

Smith. D. D. (2006). *Introduction to special education: Making a difference* (6th ed.). Boston, MA: Allyn & Bacon.

Sommer, M., Koch, M. A., Paulus, W., Weiller, C., & Buchel, C. (2002). Disconnection of speech-relevant brain areas in persistent developmental stuttering. *Lancet, 360*(9330), 380–383.

Stockman, I. J., Boult, J., & Robinson, G. (2004, July 20). Multicultural issues in academic and clinical education: A cultural mosaic. *The ASHA Leader, 20,* 6–7.

Strand, E., Stoeckel, P., & Baas, B. (2006). Treatment of severe childhood apraxia of speech: A treatment efficacy study. *Journal of Medical Speech–Language Pathology, 14*(4), 297–307.

Sturm, J. M., & Nelson, N. W. (1997). Formal classroom lessons: New perspectives on a familiar discourse event. *Language, Speech, and Hearing Services in Schools, 18,* 259.

Stuttering Foundation. (2011, February 18). *Stuttering: For kids, by kids* [Online video]. Retrieved from https://www.youtube.com/watch?v=Po-WMo8vXRY

Stuttering Foundation. (2014a). *Differential diagnosis.* Retrieved from http://www.stutteringhelp.org/differential-diagnosis

Stuttering Foundation. (2014b). *FAQ.* Retrieved from http://www.stutteringhelp.org/faq

Stuttering Foundation. (2014c). *Why go to speech therapy?* Retrieved from http://www.stutteringhelp.org/why-go-speech-therapy

Stuttering Foundation. (2015). *Early intervention important for children who stutter.* Retrieved from http://www.stutteringhelp.org/content/early-intervention-important-children-who-stutter

Sullivan, P. M., & Knutson, J. F. (2000). Maltreatment and disabilities: A population-based epidemiological study. *Child Abuse & Neglect, 24*(10), 1257–1273.

Tannen, D. (1992). *Gender and discourse.* Toronto, Ontario, Canada: Oxford University Press.

Templin, M. C. (1957). *Certain language skills in children: Their development and interrelations* (Child Welfare Monograph Series No. 26). Minneapolis: The University of Minnesota Press.

Thomas, J. (2011, September 21). *Stroboscopy: Normal female vocal cords* [Online video]. Retrieved from https://www.youtube.com/watch?v=9Tlpkdq8a8c

Toner, M. A., & Shadden, B. B. (2012, April–June). Foreword: End-of-life care for adults: What speech–language pathologists should know. *Topics in Language Disorders, 32*(2), 107–110, doi:10.1097/TLD.0b013e3182593739

Toriello, H. V., Reardon, W., & Gorlin, R. J. (Eds.). (2004). *Hereditary hearing loss and its syndromes.* New York, NY: Oxford University Press.

Uccelli, P., & Paez, M. M. (2007). Narrative and vocabulary development of bilingual children from kindergarten to first grade: Developmental changes and associations among English and Spanish skills. *Language, Speech, and Hearing Services in Schools, 38,* 225–236.

University of Michigan Aphasia Program. (2014). *A caregiver curriculum for living with partners with aphasia.* Retrieved from http://www.michiganspeechhearing.org/docs/A%20Caregiver%20Curriculum%20for%20Living%20with%20Partners%20with%20Aphasia.pdf

U.S. Census Bureau. (2010). *Overview of race and Hispanic origin: 2010.* Retrieved from http://www.census.gov/prod/cen2010/briefs/c2010br-02.pdf

U.S. Census Bureau. (2014). *U.S. and world population clock.* Retrieved from http://www.census.gov/popclock/

U.S. Department of Education. (2006, August 14). Rules and regulations. *Federal Register, 71*(156). Retrieved from http://www.gpo.gov/fdsys/pkg/FR-2006-08-14/pdf/06-6656.pdf

U.S. Department of Labor, Bureau of Labor Statistics. (2014). *Occupational outlook handbook: Speech–language pathologists.* Retrieved from http://www.bls.gov/ooh/healthcare/speech-language-pathologists.htm

U.S. Food and Drug Administration. (2014). *Benefits and risks of cochlear implants.* Retrieved from http://www.fda.gov/medicaldevices/productsandmedicalprocedures/implantsandprosthetics/cochlearimplan,s/ucm062843.htm

Van Riper, C. (1973). *The treatment of stuttering.* Englewood Cliffs, NJ: Prentice Hall.

Van Riper, C. (1979). *A career in speech pathology.* Englewood Cliffs, NJ: Prentice Hall.

Van Riper, C., & Erickson, R. L. (1996). *Speech correction: An introduction to speech pathology and audiology* (9th ed.). Boston, MA: Allyn & Bacon.

Vickers, C. P. (2010, June). Social networks after the onset of aphasia: The impact of aphasia group attendance. *The Aphasiology Archive, 24*(6/8), 902–913. doi:10.1080/02687030903438532

Washington, M. (2014, May 18). *The thing is, I stutter: Megan Washington at TEDxSydney 2014* [Online video]. Retrieved from https://www.youtube.com/watch?v=9MegHiL93B0

Weber-Fox, C. (2005). *New research on the roots of stuttering: Language processing and speech motor control—Complex interactions in stuttering.* Retrieved from http://www.stutteringhelp.org/Default.aspx?tabid=96

Weber-Fox, C., Hampton Wray, A., & Arnold, H. (2013). Early childhood stuttering and electrophysiological indices of language processing. *Journal of Fluency Disorders, 38,* 206–221

Weiss, A. L. (2004). Why we should consider pragmatics when planning treatment for children who stutter. *Language, Speech, and Hearing Services in Schools, 35,* 34–45.

Welc, J. B. (2010). *Understanding the impact of abuse and neglect on speech and language development.* American Speech-Language-Hearing Association Convention paper. Retrieved from http://www.asha.org/events/convention/handouts/2010/1206-welc-julia/

Westby C. E. (2007, April). Child maltreatment: A global issue. *Language, Speech, and Hearing Services in Schools, 38,* 140–148. doi:10.1044/0161-1461(2007/014)

Williams, A. L. (2006). *SCIP: Sound contrasts in phonology.* Greenville, SC: Super Duper.

World Health Organization. (2001). *International classification of functioning, disability and health.* Geneva, Switzerland: Author.

World Health Organization. (2014a). *Dementia.* Retrieved from http://www.who.int/mediacentre/factsheets/fs362/en/

World Health Organization. (2014b). *Disabilities.* Retrieved from http://www.who.int/topics/disabilities/en/

Yaruss, J. S. (1998). Real-time analysis of speech fluency: Procedures and reliability training. *American Journal of Speech–Language Pathology, 7,* 25–37. doi:10.1044/1058-0360.0702.25

Yaruss, J. S., & Quesal, R. (2010). *Overall assessment of the speaker's experience of stuttering* (OASES). San Antonio, TX: Pearson.

index

A

AAC. *See* Augmentative and alternative communication (AAC)

AAE (African American English), 84

AAF (altered auditory feedback), 185–186

Abduct, 120

ABI (auditory brainstem implant), 215

Ablative surgery, 163–164

ABR (auditory brainstem response), 208

Abstract-concrete imbalance, 105, 205

Abuse and language disorders, 82–83

Academic coursework requirements for professionals, 244–246

Academic success and the importance of literacy, 68–69

Accessory behaviors, 181

Accreditation of programs, 244

Acoustic tumors, 202

Acquired dysarthria, 143–144

Acquired stuttering, 179

Adages, 58

Addition, 168

Adduct, 120

ADHD. *See* Attention-deficit/hyperactivity disorder (ADHD)

Administrators as professionals, 239, 240

Adolescent

    language development. *See* Adolescent language development

    language intervention, 91–92

    language tests for, 271–272

    in school. *See* Schools

Adolescent language development, 59–65

    characteristics, 59, 61, 65

    contrasts and trends, 62–63

    discourse, 64, 65

    figurative language and slang, 63, 65

    overview, 59–61

    pragmatics, 61, 63, 65

    semantics, 64, 65

    syntax and writing, 64, 65

Adult language disorders, 95–114

    anomic aphasia, 103, 227

    assessment, 108–110

    augmentative and alternative communication, 112–113

    bilingual clients with aphasia, 113–114

    brain damage and resulting aphasia, 98–99

    Broca's aphasia–nonfluent, 101–103

    conductive aphasia, 103–104

    global aphasia, 104

    intervention, 110–112

    Jabberwocky, 101, 102

    language characteristics of aphasia, 99–100

    left-hemisphere damage, characteristics of, 104–106

    neurology of aphasia, 96–98

    overview, 31, 95–96

    right-hemisphere deficits, 106–108

    transcortical aphasia, 104

    Wernicke's aphasia (receptive aphasia), 100–101

Adverbial conjunctives, 75

Adverbs, 75

Advocates, 237–238

AEPs (auditory evoked potentials), 212

African American English (AAE), 84

Afrikaans language, 7

Age and language use, 34

Aging and hearing loss, 200

Alphabet

    American Fingerspelling Alphabet, 219, 220

    International Phonetic Alphabet, 159, 160

    phonetic, 160

    for written communication, 6

ALS (amyotrophic lateral sclerosis), 143

ALS (assistive listening system), 218

Altered auditory feedback (AAF) device, 185–186

Alveolar ridge, 155

Alzheimer's disease, 108

American Academy of Private Practice in Speech Language Pathology and Audiology, 251–252

American Community Survey, 24

American Fingerspelling Alphabet, 219, 220

American Indian Sign Language, 287

American Psychiatric Association (APA), 78

American Sign Language (ASL)

    communication system for hearing impairments, 80

    defined, 219

    fluency of deaf children and families, 190, 207

    as intervention strategy, 287

    use at schools for the deaf, 250

prevalence of specific language impairment, 71–72

specific language impairment in kindergarten children, 79

National Institute on Neurological Disorders and Stroke, 123

National Outcomes Measurement System (NOMS), 298

National Stroke Association, 98, 104–105

National Theatre of the Deaf, 207–208

Negation forms of language, 42

Negative reactions to people with communication disorders, 21

Negative relationship, 307

Neglect and language disorders, 82–83

Neoplasms, 99, 205–206

Neurodevelopmental disorder, 79

Neurofibrillary tangles, 108

Neurogenic acquired stuttering, 179

Neurogenic stuttering, 178–179

Neurological disfluency, 179

Neuromas, 202

NIDCD. *See* National Institute on Deafness and Other Communication Disorders (NIDCD)

Noise and hearing loss, 201

NOMS (National Outcomes Measurement System), 298

Nonreversible passive sentences, 55

Nonstandardized assessments, 26

Nonverbal language
language development, 38–39
proxemics, 39

Normal distribution, 307

Normal limits, 277–279

Normal vs. abnormal disfluencies, 174–176
amount of tension present, 175
characteristics of normal speaking, 174
distribution in speech sequence, 176
duration of individual moments of disfluency, 175
frequency of occurrence, 175
speakers' awareness/attitude of disfluency, 175–176

Norm-referenced tests. *See* Standardized (norm-referenced) assessments

Norms, 87

Nottingham Hearing Biomedical Research Unit, 199

O

OAE (otoacoustic emissions test), 208

Objective attitude, 236

Objectives of intervention, 28

Objectivity of clinicians, 262

Observations

aphasia assessment, 109

for assessment, 88–89

of the client in familiar environment, 26

informal, 274–275

Occipital lobe, 97

Occlude, 129

Occupational therapist, 235

Omission, 168

Oncologist, 134

Onset of the disorders, 16

Optometrist, 235

Oral cavity
function of, 118
to produce speech, 8–9
resonance and, 121

Oral communication
defined, 5–6
hearing loss and, 220–221
purpose of, 218–219

Oral language and the bridge to written language, 66–68

Oral mechanism exam, 134

Oral peripheral exam, 134, 166

Orality, 131

Oral-to-literate shift, 48–49

Orofacial myofunctional disorder, 147

Oromo language, 7

Oropharynx, 118

Ossicles, 194, 195

Ossicular discontinuity, 198

Otitis media, 197–198

Otoacoustic emissions test (OAE), 208

Otolaryngologist, 27, 134

Otosclerosis, 198

Otoscopic examination, 209

Outer ear, 194, 197

Oval window, 194, 195, 196

P

Palatals, 157

Paradoxical vocal fold motion, 128

Paralinguistic signals, 38–39

Paraphasia, 104

Paraplegia, 141

Paraprofessionals, 233, 240–241, 258

"Parentese", 41

Parietal lobe, 97

Parkinson's disease, 123, 143

Participation model, 262–263

Part-word repetitions, 177

Passive sentences, 55–56

PECS (Picture Exchange Communication System), 92–93

Penetrating injuries of TBI, 81, 205

Percentile, 307

Lynda Miller

Lynda Miller began her professional life as a junior high school English teacher. Her students taught her that what she thought she knew about language, cognition, and learning was either wrong or in need of major rethinking. As a result, she has spent the remainder of her professional career studying how we humans learn to communicate, how we pay attention and learn, and the influence of social interactions on how we use communication in order to make our way in the world. Each time she learns of a new research finding related to communication (among other areas), she delights in fiddling with it to see how it fits into our understanding of the field of communication sciences and disorders.

Miller has had the pleasure of teaching not only in the public schools but also in universities in Colorado, Montana, Illinois, and Texas. She has also been enriched by the many professionals who have taken continuing education courses from her throughout the United States and Canada. Her most recent teaching has been for small groups interested in web-based instruction.

She has written a number of books and articles, and she has co-authored several assessment instruments designed to assess how children and adolescents learn and use language. The two most recent are the *Test of Early Communication and Emerging Language* (co-authored with Mary Blake Huer) and the *Test of Preschool Vocabulary* (co-authored with Steven C. Mathews). Currently her co-author, James E. Gilliam, and she are collecting data for the *Diagnostic Test of Pragmatic Language*.

Miller holds a B.A. in English literature, an M.A. in speech–language pathology, and a Ph.D. in language acquisition, cognitive development, and learning disabilities.

Franklin H. Silverman

Dr. Franklin H. Silverman, ASHA Fellow and pioneer in the field of augmentative and alternative communication, had been a member of the Marquette speech-language-pathology faculty for more than 30 years at the time of his death. He was the author of more than a dozen professional books and 150 articles in professional journals. He taught the Introductory Speech and Hearing Disorders course at Marquette University twice a year for more the 25 years and was the recipient of the University's annual faculty award for Teaching Excellence.

Dr. Silverman treated children and adults with speech and language disorders for more than 40 years and was certified by both ASHA and the State of Wisconsin.

His clinical advice had been sought both nationally and internationally, including by the Saudi royal family.

Dr. Silverman had more than 60 years of personal experience with speech disorders because he had stuttered since early childhood. Dr. Silverman will be greatly missed by his colleagues and friends.